Economic Crisis and Healthcare Services

Economic Crisis and Healthcare Services

Editor

Dimitris Zavras

MDPI • Basel • Beijing • Wuhan • Barcelona • Belgrade • Manchester • Tokyo • Cluj • Tianjin

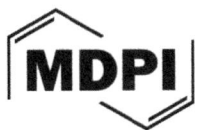

Editor
Dimitris Zavras
University of West Attica
Greece

Editorial Office
MDPI
St. Alban-Anlage 66
4052 Basel, Switzerland

This is a reprint of articles from the Special Issue published online in the open access journal *International Journal of Environmental Research and Public Health* (ISSN 1660-4601) (available at: https://www.mdpi.com/journal/ijerph/special_issues/economic_crisis_healthcare).

For citation purposes, cite each article independently as indicated on the article page online and as indicated below:

LastName, A.A.; LastName, B.B.; LastName, C.C. Article Title. *Journal Name* **Year**, *Volume Number*, Page Range.

ISBN 978-3-0365-5573-7 (Hbk)
ISBN 978-3-0365-5574-4 (PDF)

© 2022 by the authors. Articles in this book are Open Access and distributed under the Creative Commons Attribution (CC BY) license, which allows users to download, copy and build upon published articles, as long as the author and publisher are properly credited, which ensures maximum dissemination and a wider impact of our publications.

The book as a whole is distributed by MDPI under the terms and conditions of the Creative Commons license CC BY-NC-ND.

Contents

About the Editor vii

Dimitris Zavras
Access to the COVID-19 Vaccine
Reprinted from: *Int. J. Environ. Res. Public Health* **2022**, *19*, 11054, doi:10.3390/ijerph191711054 . 1

Goodluck Mselle, Peter Nsanya, Kennedy Diema Konlan, Yuri Lee, Jongsoo Ryu and Sunjoo Kang
Factors Associated with the Implementation of an Improved Community Health Fund in the Ubungo Municipality Area, Dar es Salaam Region, Tanzania
Reprinted from: *Int. J. Environ. Res. Public Health* **2022**, *19*, 5606, doi:10.3390/ijerph19095606 . . . 5

Noshaba Aziz, Jun He, Tanwne Sarker and Hongguang Sui
Exploring the Role of Health Expenditure and Maternal Mortality in South Asian Countries: An Approach towards Shaping Better Health Policy
Reprinted from: *Int. J. Environ. Res. Public Health* **2021**, *18*, 11514, doi:10.3390/ijerph182111514 . 17

Piotr Korneta and Katarzyna Rostek
The Impact of the SARS-CoV-19 Pandemic on the Global Gross Domestic Product
Reprinted from: *Int. J. Environ. Res. Public Health* **2021**, *18*, 5246, doi:10.3390/ijerph18105246 . . . 31

Muhammad Umar, Mário Nuno Mata, Adnan Abbas, José Moleiro Martins, Rui Miguel Dantas and Pedro Neves Mata
Performance Evaluation of the Chinese Healthcare System
Reprinted from: *Int. J. Environ. Res. Public Health* **2021**, *18*, 5193, doi:10.3390/ijerph18105193 . . . 43

Alberto González-García, Arrate Pinto-Carral, Jesús Sanz Villorejo and Pilar Marqués-Sánchez
Competency Model for the Middle Nurse Manager (MCGE-Logistic Level)
Reprinted from: *Int. J. Environ. Res. Public Health* **2021**, *18*, 3898, doi:10.3390/ijerph18083898 . . . 59

Yoonje Euh and Daeho Lee
How Do Pharmaceutical Companies Overcome a Corporate Productivity Crisis? Business Diversification into Medical Devices for Growth Potential
Reprinted from: *Int. J. Environ. Res. Public Health* **2021**, *18*, 1045, doi:10.3390/ijerph18031045 . . . 73

Dimitris Zavras
Studying Healthcare Affordability during an Economic Recession: The Case of Greece
Reprinted from: *Int. J. Environ. Res. Public Health* **2020**, *17*, 7790, doi:10.3390/ijerph17217790 . . . 83

Romeo-Victor Ionescu, Monica Laura Zlati and Valentin Marian Antohi
Global Challenges vs. the Need for Regional Performance Models under the Present Pandemic Crisis
Reprinted from: *Int. J. Environ. Res. Public Health* **2021**, *18*, 10254, doi:10.3390/ijerph181910254 . 105

Dimitris Zavras
Feeling Uncertainty during the Lockdown That Commenced in March 2020 in Greece
Reprinted from: *Int. J. Environ. Res. Public Health* **2021**, *18*, 5105, doi:10.3390/ijerph18105105 . . . 135

Ibrahim A. Elshaer and Alaa M. S. Azazz
Amid the COVID-19 Pandemic, Unethical Behavior in the Name of the Company: The Role of Job Insecurity, Job Embeddedness, and Turnover Intention
Reprinted from: *Int. J. Environ. Res. Public Health* **2022**, *19*, 247, doi:10.3390/ijerph19010247 . . . 145

Ibrahim A. Elshaer, Marwa Ghanem and Alaa M. S. Azazz
An Unethical Organizational Behavior for the Sake of the Family: Perceived Risk of Job Insecurity, Family Motivation and Financial Pressures
Reprinted from: *Int. J. Environ. Res. Public Health* **2022**, *19*, 6541, doi:10.3390/ijerph19116541 . . . **161**

About the Editor

Dimitris Zavras

Dimitris Zavras was born in Athens in 1968 and studied Physics at the National and Kapodistrian University of Athens.

His postgraduate studies include an M.Sc. in Applied Physics from the University of Massachusetts, an M.Sc. in Statistics from Athens University of Economics and Business, an M.Sc. in Healthcare Management from the National School of Public Health, and a Doctorate (Ph.D.) in Health Services Research and Health Economics from the University of Thessaly (Department of Economics).

He is currently an Assistant Professor at the University of West Attica and a Faculty Member of the Hellenic Open University. In the past, he has taught at the University of Peloponnese, at the Neapolis University Pafos (Cyprus), and at the Athens University of Applied Sciences.

Dimitris Zavras' research interests focus on the utilization of healthcare services, healthcare provider choice, unmet healthcare needs, and health status.

He is a member of the Hellenic Scientific Society of Health Economics and Health Policy and of the Hellenic Society of Public Health. He is also a member of the Hellenic Society for Healthcare Services Management.

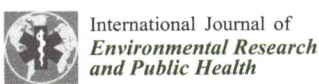

Editorial

Access to the COVID-19 Vaccine

Dimitris Zavras

Laboratory for Health Technology Assessment, Department of Public Health Policy, School of Public Health, University of West Attica, 11521 Athens, Greece; dzavras@uniwa.gr

Citation: Zavras, D. Access to the COVID-19 Vaccine. *Int. J. Environ. Res. Public Health* **2022**, *19*, 11054. https://doi.org/10.3390/ijerph191711054

Received: 31 August 2022
Accepted: 1 September 2022
Published: 3 September 2022

Publisher's Note: MDPI stays neutral with regard to jurisdictional claims in published maps and institutional affiliations.

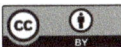

Copyright: © 2022 by the author. Licensee MDPI, Basel, Switzerland. This article is an open access article distributed under the terms and conditions of the Creative Commons Attribution (CC BY) license (https://creativecommons.org/licenses/by/4.0/).

As of 31 August 2022, 599,825,400 confirmed coronavirus disease 2019 (COVID-19) cases and 6,469,458 deaths have been reported globally [1]. The pandemic has tested humanity for more than two years. What characterizes this time period is the high death toll, the suffering [2], and the high levels of uncertainty in every aspect of the crisis. In the early phase of the pandemic, the time needed to develop and deploy vaccines was one of the sources of such uncertainty [3].

Due to the importance of COVID-19 vaccination in saving lives and in contributing to global economic recovery, this Editorial attempts to study the access to the COVID-19 vaccine.

The world's first vaccination was made available in December 2020 [4]. Reducing the spread of the disease, protecting segments of the population that are not yet vaccinated as well as those for whom vaccines have limited efficacy, and reducing severe cases that burden healthcare systems are among the benefits of vaccination against COVID-19 [5]. In addition, economic recovery will be faster in countries with higher vaccination rates [6].

However, although healthcare access is a right, there are still more than two and a half billion people around the world who are unvaccinated [4], and access to vaccines in low- and middle-income countries (LMICs) is far lower than it is in high-income countries (HICs). Consequently, rates of COVID-19 infections and deaths are higher in LMICs [7].

It is evident that access to the COVID-19 vaccine is inequitable; such global inequity is due to the concentration of vaccine development and production in high-income countries, dose-hoarding by those countries, high vaccine prices, and challenges in deploying vaccines in resource-poor settings [8]. Beyond these reasons, the existence of barriers in terms of access to healthcare may undermine the achievement of health equity [9]. According to Mooney [10], "if we are taking access to mean opportunity to use or freedom to use, it is immediately apparent that it is the potential users' perspectives on what constitutes a barrier and its height that must be used in assessing differential access", while "freedom to use describes the social possibility and the individual ability to give direction to one's will to use health services" [11].

Given that "equal access" is defined in parallel with "equal need", a question is posed: how should need be approached? The answer is that need can be considered as an expression of the risk of contracting COVID-19 [12]; people aged 60 years and over, those living in long-term care facilities, and people with underlying health conditions such as hypertension, diabetes, cardiovascular disease, etc., are considered high-risk groups for COVID-19 [13].

On the other hand, access should be approached through its dimensions and through the barriers that individuals face.

Adopting Penchansky's and Thomas's [14] framework for the dimensions of access, i.e., the five As, namely, availability, affordability, accessibility, accommodation, and acceptability, the global picture regarding the COVID-19 vaccine is as follows: (a) the availability of COVID-19 vaccines differs significantly around the world [15], and specifically, in LMICs, availability is far lower than in wealthier countries [16]; (b) in several countries, COVID-19 vaccines are provided free of charge [17], and thus, their affordability may not be an issue in monetary terms, something that is not true in some less developed nations [18];

(c) for several communities around the world, accessibility is an issue [19,20]; (d) telehealth has been adopted on a large scale for vaccination registration and for relevant medical interventions, but knowing how to further improve vaccination accommodation through telehealth while bridging the digital divide is another matter that requires immediate investigation and implementation [21]; and (e) while developing countries mainly face affordability—and accessibility-related issues regarding vaccines, developed countries face acceptability issues [22,23].

With regard to the acceptance or refusal of the COVID-19 vaccine, vaccine hesitancy is a major obstacle to high vaccination rates [24]. According to Lin et al. [25], the most common reasons for vaccination hesitation or refusal are a fear of side effects; safety; and effectiveness, while the belief that the vaccines are unnecessary; inadequate information; the unknown/short duration of vaccines; and a general anti-vaccine stance are associated with lower acceptance. In addition, vaccine acceptance on a global scale is influenced by the speed of vaccine development [26].

A fear of side effects, safety or effectiveness concerns, and beliefs related to the COVID-19 vaccine are demand-side barriers; concerns related to vaccination timing, vaccination location, and the financial cost of getting vaccinated are also demand-side barriers. Vaccine delivery and administration barriers, such as inaccessible places and people, are supply side barriers [27].

Significant predictors of COVID-19 vaccine uptake intentions are education, the existence of insurance coverage, scoring high on subjective norms, a positive attitude toward the vaccine, high perceived susceptibility to COVID-19, high perceived benefits of the vaccine, and scoring low on barriers to the vaccine [28].

Holloman [29] defined access to healthcare as the freedom from barriers to healthcare, while barriers are defined as anything that constrains, deters, delays, denies, dissuades, discourages, handicaps, or prevents the acquisition or utilization of those services that are ultimately provided by society to its members individually and collectively for the maintenance, preservation, and improvement of health.

In the case of COVID-19 vaccination, the "freedom to receive a vaccination" has been undermined to a large extent by exposure to misinformation [30]. However, we should note that a belief in misinformation may be related to prevailing generalized uncertainty. COVID-19-related uncertainty arose from various aspects of the COVID-19 crisis, i.e., health-related, economic, and social. Uncertainties related to the nature of the virus, alternative treatment options, clinical outcomes, and prevention methods [31] all concern the health dimension of the crisis. Uncertainties related to impacts on personal finances and the effectiveness and impacts of the restriction measures [32] concern the economic dimension of the crisis.

As mentioned above, barriers play a decisive role in access to healthcare, and in the actual use of services [33]. In addition, since awareness, i.e., communication and information, may be considered as the sixth dimension of access [34], providing up-to-date information would be an effective strategy against barriers such as fear or concerns related to the safety and effectiveness of the vaccine [35]. Since vaccination rates have increased in numerous communities as populations have begun to see their friends, colleagues, and neighbors get vaccinated without adverse events [36], relative information could effectively motivate individuals to get the vaccine.

COVID-19 vaccination concerns all of us, and efforts to minimize barriers to receiving it should continue. Thus, understanding such barriers and the best way to influence individuals is crucial to achieve high vaccination rates. The affordability and accessibility issues facing developing countries and the acceptability issues facing developed countries must be eliminated. "Freedom to receive a vaccination" should be translated to freedom to fight the enemy that threatens one's life, health, and well-being, and the global economy.

Conflicts of Interest: The author declares no conflict of interest.

References

1. World Health Organization. WHO Coronavirus Disease (COVID-19) Dashboard. 2022. Available online: https://covid19.who.int/ (accessed on 31 August 2022).
2. Cowden, R.G.; Davis, E.B.; Counted, V.; Chen, Y.; Rueger, S.Y.; VanderWeele, T.J.; Lemke, A.W.; Glowiak, K.J.; Worthington, E.L. Suffering, Mental Health, and Psychological Well-Being during the COVID-19 Pandemic: A Longitudinal Study of U.S. Adults with Chronic Health Conditions. *Wellbeing Space Soc.* **2021**, *2*, 100048. [CrossRef] [PubMed]
3. Altig, D.; Baker, S.; Barrero, J.M.; Bloom, N.; Bunn, P.; Chen, S.; Davis, S.J.; Leather, J.; Meyer, B.; Mihaylov, E.; et al. Economic Uncertainty before and during the COVID-19 Pandemic. *J. Public Econ.* **2020**, *191*, 104274. [CrossRef] [PubMed]
4. Mathieu, E.; Ritchie, H.; Ortiz-Ospina, E.; Roser, M.; Hasell, J.; Appel, C.; Giattino, C.; Rodés-Guirao, L. A Global Database of COVID-19 Vaccinations. *Nat. Hum. Behav.* **2021**, *5*, 947–953. [CrossRef] [PubMed]
5. Persad, G.; Emanuel, E.J. Ethical Considerations of Offering Benefits to COVID-19 Vaccine Recipients. *JAMA* **2021**, *326*, 221. [CrossRef] [PubMed]
6. Rackimuthu, S.; Narain, K.; Lal, A.; Nawaz, F.A.; Mohanan, P.; Essar, M.Y.; Charles Ashworth, H. Redressing COVID-19 Vaccine Inequity amidst Booster Doses: Charting a Bold Path for Global Health Solidarity, Together. *Glob. Health* **2022**, *18*, 23. [CrossRef]
7. Ye, Y.; Zhang, Q.; Wei, X.; Cao, Z.; Yuan, H.-Y.; Zeng, D.D. Equitable Access to COVID-19 Vaccines Makes a Life-Saving Difference to All Countries. *Nat. Hum. Behav.* **2022**, *6*, 207–216. [CrossRef]
8. Yamey, G.; Garcia, P.; Hassan, F.; Mao, W.; McDade, K.K.; Pai, M.; Saha, S.; Schellekens, P.; Taylor, A.; Udayakumar, K. It Is Not Too Late to Achieve Global COVID-19 Vaccine Equity. *BMJ* **2022**, *376*, e070650. [CrossRef]
9. Mooney, G.H. *The Health of Nations: Towards a New Political Economy*; Zed Books: London, UK; New York, NY, USA, 2012; ISBN 978-1-78032-060-1.
10. Mooney, G. Is It Not Time for Health Economists to Rethink Equity and Access? *Health Econ. Policy Law* **2009**, *4*, 209–221. [CrossRef]
11. Thiede, M. Information and Access to Health Care: Is There a Role for Trust? *Soc. Sci. Med.* **2005**, *61*, 1452–1462. [CrossRef]
12. Bolcato, M.; Rodriguez, D.; Feola, A.; Di Mizio, G.; Bonsignore, A.; Ciliberti, R.; Tettamanti, C.; Trabucco Aurilio, M.; Aprile, A. COVID-19 Pandemic and Equal Access to Vaccines. *Vaccines* **2021**, *9*, 538. [CrossRef]
13. European Centre for Disease Prevention and Control. High-Risk Groups for COVID-19. 2022. Available online: https://www.ecdc.europa.eu/en/covid-19/high-risk-groups (accessed on 7 August 2022).
14. Penchansky, R.; Thomas, J.W. The Concept of Access: Definition and Relationship to Consumer Satisfaction. *Med. Care* **1981**, *19*, 127–140. [CrossRef]
15. Hunter, D.J.; Abdool Karim, S.S.; Baden, L.R.; Farrar, J.J.; Hamel, M.B.; Longo, D.L.; Morrissey, S.; Rubin, E.J. Addressing Vaccine Inequity—COVID-19 Vaccines as a Global Public Good. *N. Engl. J. Med.* **2022**, *386*, 1176–1179. [CrossRef]
16. Clemens, J.; Aziz, A.B.; Tadesse, B.T.; Kang, S.; Marks, F.; Kim, J. Evaluation of Protection by COVID-19 Vaccines after Deployment in Low and Lower-Middle Income Countries. *eClinicalMedicine* **2022**, *43*, 101253. [CrossRef] [PubMed]
17. Chen, Z.; Zheng, W.; Wu, Q.; Chen, X.; Peng, C.; Tian, Y.; Sun, R.; Dong, J.; Wang, M.; Zhou, X.; et al. Global Diversity of Policy, Coverage, and Demand of COVID-19 Vaccines: A Descriptive Study. *BMC Med.* **2022**, *20*, 130. [CrossRef] [PubMed]
18. Reiter, R.J.; Sharma, R.; Tan, D.; Neel, R.L.; Simko, F.; Manucha, W.; Rosales-Corral, S.; Cardinali, D.P. Melatonin Use for SARS-CoV-2 Infection: Time to Diversify the Treatment Portfolio. *J. Med. Virol.* **2022**, *94*, 2928–2930. [CrossRef] [PubMed]
19. Dong, L.; Bogart, L.M.; Gandhi, P.; Aboagye, J.B.; Ryan, S.; Serwanga, R.; Ojikutu, B.O. A Qualitative Study of COVID-19 Vaccine Intentions and Mistrust in Black Americans: Recommendations for Vaccine Dissemination and Uptake. *PLoS ONE* **2022**, *17*, e0268020. [CrossRef]
20. Rosen, B.; Waitzberg, R.; Israeli, A.; Hartal, M.; Davidovitch, N. Addressing Vaccine Hesitancy and Access Barriers to Achieve Persistent Progress in Israel's COVID-19 Vaccination Program. *Isr. J. Health Policy Res.* **2021**, *10*, 43. [CrossRef]
21. Chen, X.; Wang, H. On the Rise of the New B.1.1.529 Variant: Five Dimensions of Access to a COVID-19 Vaccine. *Vaccine* **2022**, *40*, 403–405. [CrossRef]
22. Yarlagadda, H.; Patel, M.A.; Gupta, V.; Bansal, T.; Upadhyay, S.; Shaheen, N.; Jain, R. COVID-19 Vaccine Challenges in Developing and Developed Countries. *Cureus* **2022**, *14*, e23951. [CrossRef]
23. Sohil, F.; Sohail, M.U. Global Discrimination of COVID-19 Vaccine. *Hum. Vaccines Immunother.* **2022**, *18*, 2028515. [CrossRef]
24. Khairat, S.; Zou, B.; Adler-Milstein, J. Factors and Reasons Associated with Low COVID-19 Vaccine Uptake among Highly Hesitant Communities in the US. *Am. J. Infect. Control.* **2022**, *50*, 262–267. [CrossRef] [PubMed]
25. Lin, C.; Tu, P.; Beitsch, L.M. Confidence and Receptivity for COVID-19 Vaccines: A Rapid Systematic Review. *Vaccines* **2020**, *9*, 16. [CrossRef] [PubMed]
26. Danchin, M.; Buttery, J. COVID-19 Vaccine Hesitancy: A Unique Set of Challenges. *Intern. Med. J.* **2021**, *51*, 1987–1989. [CrossRef] [PubMed]
27. Tagoe, E.T.; Sheikh, N.; Morton, A.; Nonvignon, J.; Sarker, A.R.; Williams, L.; Megiddo, I. COVID-19 Vaccination in Lower-Middle Income Countries: National Stakeholder Views on Challenges, Barriers, and Potential Solutions. *Front. Public Health* **2021**, *9*, 709127. [CrossRef]
28. Guidry, J.P.D.; Laestadius, L.I.; Vraga, E.K.; Miller, C.A.; Perrin, P.B.; Burton, C.W.; Ryan, M.; Fuemmeler, B.F.; Carlyle, K.E. Willingness to Get the COVID-19 Vaccine with and without Emergency Use Authorization. *Am. J. Infect. Control.* **2021**, *49*, 137–142. [CrossRef]

29. Holloman, J.L.S., Jr. *Access to Health Care. 1983. Securing Access to Health Care: A Report on the Ethical Implications of Differences in the Availability of Health Services*; Report; U.S. Government Printing Office: Washington, DC, USA, 1983; Volume 1.
30. Dhama, K.; Sharun, K.; Tiwari, R.; Dhawan, M.; Emran, T.B.; Rabaan, A.A.; Alhumaid, S. COVID-19 Vaccine Hesitancy—Reasons and Solutions to Achieve a Successful Global Vaccination Campaign to Tackle the Ongoing Pandemic. *Hum. Vaccines Immunother.* **2021**, *17*, 3495–3499. [CrossRef]
31. Gupta, I.; Baru, R. Economics & Ethics of the COVID-19 Vaccine: How Prepared Are We? *Indian J. Med. Res.* **2020**, *152*, 153. [CrossRef]
32. Zavras, D. Studying Satisfaction with the Restriction Measures Implemented in Greece during the First COVID-19 Pandemic Wave. *World* **2021**, *2*, 379–390. [CrossRef]
33. Mooney, G.H. *Challenging Health Economics*; Oxford University Press: Oxford, UK; New York, NY, USA, 2009; ISBN 978-0-19-923597-1.
34. Saurman, E. Improving Access: Modifying Penchansky and Thomas's Theory of Access. *J. Health Serv. Res. Policy* **2016**, *21*, 36–39. [CrossRef]
35. Nawas, G.T.; Zeidan, R.S.; Edwards, C.A.; El-Desoky, R.H. Barriers to COVID-19 Vaccines and Strategies to Improve Acceptability and Uptake. *J. Pharm. Pract.* **2022**, 089719002210816. [CrossRef]
36. Nuti, S.V.; Armstrong, K. Lay Epidemiology and Vaccine Acceptance. *JAMA* **2021**, *326*, 301. [CrossRef] [PubMed]

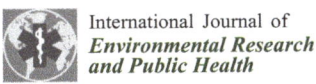

Article

Factors Associated with the Implementation of an Improved Community Health Fund in the Ubungo Municipality Area, Dar es Salaam Region, Tanzania

Goodluck Mselle [1], Peter Nsanya [1], Kennedy Diema Konlan [2,3], Yuri Lee [4], Jongsoo Ryu [5] and Sunjoo Kang [5,*]

1. Department of Health and Social Welfare, Ubungo Municipal Council, Dar es Salaam P.O. Box 55068, Tanzania; gmselle10@gmail.com (G.M.); nsanyap@gmail.com (P.N.)
2. Department of Public Health Nursing, School of Nursing and Midwifery, University of Health and Allied Sciences, Ho, Ghana; dkkonlan@uhas.edu.gh
3. Mo-Im Kim Nursing Research Institute, College of Nursing, Yonsei University, Seoul 03722, Korea
4. Department of Health and Medical Information, Myongji College, Seoul 03674, Korea; wittyyurilee@gmail.com
5. Department of Global Health, Graduate School of Public Health, Yonsei University, Seoul 03722, Korea; johnryuhira@gmail.com
* Correspondence: ksj5139@hanmail.net or ksj5139@yuhs.ac

Citation: Mselle, G.; Nsanya, P.; Konlan, K.D.; Lee, Y.; Ryu, J.; Kang, S. Factors Associated with the Implementation of an Improved Community Health Fund in the Ubungo Municipality Area, Dar es Salaam Region, Tanzania. *Int. J. Environ. Res. Public Health* **2022**, *19*, 5606. https://doi.org/10.3390/ijerph19095606

Academic Editor: Dimitris Zavras

Received: 23 March 2022
Accepted: 3 May 2022
Published: 5 May 2022

Publisher's Note: MDPI stays neutral with regard to jurisdictional claims in published maps and institutional affiliations.

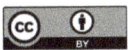

Copyright: © 2022 by the authors. Licensee MDPI, Basel, Switzerland. This article is an open access article distributed under the terms and conditions of the Creative Commons Attribution (CC BY) license (https://creativecommons.org/licenses/by/4.0/).

Abstract: Community-based health insurance schemes help households to afford healthcare services. This paper describes healthcare facilities and community factors that are associated with the Improved Community Health Fund (iCHF) scheme in the Ubungo district of Tanzania. A cross-sectional descriptive study was conducted using online questionnaires that were completed by healthcare providers and community members in public-owned healthcare facilities in the Ubungo Municipal Council district of Dar es Salaam, Tanzania, between October and November 2021. The data were analyzed using descriptive statistics and the chi-squared test of association. We found a statistically significant relationship between income level and satisfaction with the iCHF scheme. For community-related factors, income level was statistically significant in the level of involvement in iCHF implementation among local leaders. Further, income level was statistically significant in relation to community behavior/culture toward the iCHF. Occupation was statistically significant in iCHF implementation, iCHF premiums, and iCHF membership size. A statistically significant relationship was also found between income, iCHF membership size, and iCHF premiums. Moreover, people would be willing to pay the required premiums if the quality of the healthcare services under the iCHF scheme improves. Therefore, the government should allocate resources to reduce the challenges that are facing iCHF implementation, such as the preference for a user fee scheme over the iCHF, the issues that are faced by enrollment officers, and inadequate iCHF premiums and membership size.

Keywords: Improved Community Health Fund (iCHF); Ubungo municipality; healthcare providers; community health; health insurance

1. Introduction

Health finance in low-income countries (LIC) is derived from various sources, including government allocations, out-of-pocket payments, and external aid from high-income countries [1,2]. Out-of-pocket payments are direct payments that are made by citizens for the use of healthcare services. The burden of out-of-pocket payments varies depending on household size, the nature of any relevant health insurance cover, and the presence of chronic diseases in the family [3]. Out-of-pocket healthcare expenditure is large in low-income countries and poses a major barrier for community access to healthcare services. In 2018, out-of-pocket healthcare expenditure accounted for 42% of the total government healthcare budget [1], whereas social health insurance accounted for only 7% of all healthcare-related expenditure [1]. In contrast, for high-income countries, social health insurance funds accounted for 22% of their budget and only 21% was accounted for by out-of-pocket expenditure [1]. In the Universal Health 525 Coverage (UHC) report by the World Health Organization (WHO), out-of-pocket expenditure in Africa was primarily spent on medicines and medical supplies [2]. Moreover, it exceeded the 25% limit that was set by the UHC for the Sustainable Development Goal (SDG) indicator for out-of-pocket expenditure [4]. As per the Abuja Declaration, each nation must spend 15% of its total budget on healthcare, yet Tanzania only spent 8% of its budget on healthcare [4]. Tanzania also only spent USD 46 per capita on healthcare and 7.3% of the GDP on healthcare goods and services in 2014–2015, compared to 10% in Rwanda [5]. Out-of-pocket payments accounted for 26% of the total healthcare expenditure in Tanzania between 2014 and 2015. Tanzania is struggling to find the resources to create a robust healthcare budget and depends on external sources, which account for 37% of the country's total healthcare budget [6].

The Improved Community Health Fund (iCHF) is a community-based voluntary insurance program that was established in 2001 in Tanzania, which targets the populations that cannot access the National Health Insurance Fund (NHIF). In Tanzania, the NHIF primarily caters for the healthcare needs of government and private employees, who constitute only 7% of the population [7]. The NHIF covers families with up to eight children who are enrolled at dispensaries, health centers, and district hospitals for medical costs of between USD 12 and USD 65 per year. In addition, members of the NHIF benefit from outpatient care and referral systems to district or zonal hospitals. The central government, local government, and iCHF members also contribute to a matching grant [2]. The Community Health Fund (CHF) is an alternative healthcare financing measure for families who are not qualified for or cannot afford the NHIF. In 2015, the government of Tanzania set the target of enrolling 30% of the population under the CHF; however, only 16.4% were enrolled. In 2016, the government had to revise the CHF in order to increase enrollment and improve the quality of the healthcare services that were provided under the scheme. The new changes pertained to enrollment, premium amounts, collection mechanisms, and purchasing arrangements. The new version of the CHF was named the iCHF [8]. In 2018, iCHF coverage increased to 25%, with 13 million beneficiaries [7], although the number of beneficiaries was still limited according to the 2015 government projections [7]. In a study of the Mtwara region in Tanzania, healthcare facility factors, such as the absence of medicines and medical supplies, were found to cause dropouts from iCHF membership [9]. Additional challenges, such as the poor supervision of healthcare facilities by district health authorities and the mismanagement of iCHF funds, led to an insufficient enrollment of CHF members [10]. Therefore, iCHF implementation in Tanzania has faced many challenges.

To address the urgent need to examine the factors that are associated with the implementation of the iCHF, the present study of the Ubungo municipality in the Dar es Salaam region of Tanzania, where iCHF coverage is low, aimed to identify those factors. To address the factors that influence the implementation of the iCHF, specific focus needs to relate to the healthcare providers and community members who are involved in the service implementation and utilization, respectively. Therefore, this study aimed to describe the community and healthcare facility factors that influence the implementation of the iCHF in Tanzania.

2. Materials and Methods

2.1. Study Design and Setting

Using a descriptive cross-sectional design, data were collected from healthcare facilities that are registered under the iCHF. Healthcare providers who were working in a total of 21 public-owned healthcare facilities (17 dispensaries, 3 health centers, and 1 district hospital) in the Ubungo municipality were identified for the study. The Ubungo district is an urban area with a population of 1,043,549 people. The district covers a total surface area of 210 square kilometers and has 91 streets (the lowest level administrative area) and 14 wards (the mid-level administrative area) [11].

2.2. Population and Sampling

A multistage sample method was adopted for the selection of the facilities and respondents for this study. A total of 13 iCHF members were selected from each facility to participate in the study, using the simple random sample method. In using this sampling method, a sample framework of the iCHF members within each facility was first created and listed in a basket. Names were then drawn from the basket without any replacements. Those whose names were selected through this process were then contacted to respond to a questionnaire. A simple random sampling method was used to select 16 healthcare facilities out of the 21 public healthcare facilities that are under the Ubungo Municipal Council [12]. The sampling of the healthcare facilities was also performed by firstly creating a sample framework of the 21 healthcare facilities and then facilities were chosen without replacement until 16 facilities were selected. The respondents were required to provide consent prior to responding to the questionnaire. During the collection, 29 people did not return the questionnaire or did not initially provide consent to participate in the study. This represented a non-response rate of 13.9%. During data cleaning, five questionnaires were found to be completed inappropriately and hence, were also excluded from the analysis. Therefore, the effective sample size that was used for analysis was 174.

2.3. Measurements

The design and content of the online questionnaires were obtained from the existing literature on the factors that affect community-based health insurance (CBHI) [13]. The questionnaire for the healthcare providers had three parts: questions regarding the demographic characteristics of the participants, closed-ended questions regarding the healthcare facility and community-related factors (independent variables), and questions on iCHF implementation The closed-ended questions were measured using a 5-point Likert-type scale (5 = strongly agree, 4 = agree, 3 = neutral, 2 = disagree, and 1 = strongly disagree). The demographic factors that were assessed for healthcare providers were level of healthcare facility, age, sex, profession, and educational level, while those for community members were age, sex, marital status, family size, occupation, educational level, income level, and duration of iCHF enrollment. The questionnaire for the healthcare providers also elicited their rating of facility factors that influence the implementation of the iCHF on a scale of agree, neutral or disagree. Some of the healthcare facility factors that they rated included the availability of medical equipment and healthcare personnel, the effectiveness of the referral systems, and the awareness of promotion strategies. Community members were also asked to provide similar ratings on their level of satisfaction of the implementation of the iCHF, the involvement of community members in membership registration, and the influence of cultural factors on the implementation of the iCHF. Variables that were rated by both the community members and healthcare professionals included difficulty in paying iCHF premiums, membership size, and the availability of enrolment officers.

Before data collection, the questionnaire was pretested among healthcare providers and community members in the Ubungo district. The questions were uploaded via Google Forms and distributed to 20 healthcare providers at the district hospital and dispensaries and 10 community members. The questionnaire was reviewed by the Ubungo Municipal Council's Health Department Research Review Committee. The Cronbach's alpha was 0.785 for the community questionnaire and 0.707 for the healthcare provider questionnaire.

2.4. Data Analysis

The data analysis was performed using the SPSS 25.0 software after downloading the data from Google Forms into Excel spreadsheets. A descriptive analysis of the sociodemographic data was conducted using frequencies, means (M), and standard deviations (SD). A chi-squared test was performed to measure the association between sociodemographic factors and iCHF implementation. The statistical significance was set at $p < 0.05$ for a 95% confidence interval.

3. Results

3.1. Sociodemographic Characteristics

Among the participants who were healthcare providers, 75.9% worked in healthcare centers/dispensaries, 55.8% were below 39 years of age, and 70.1% were female (Table 1).

Table 1. Sociodemographic characteristics of healthcare providers.

Items	Categories	Frequency	%	Mean ± SD
Level of Healthcare Facility	District Hospital	42	24.1	
	Health Centers/Dispensaries	132	75.9	
Age	18–39	97	55.8	2.4 ± 0.7
	40–61	77	44.2	
Sex	Male	52	29.9	
	Female	122	70.1	
Profession	Doctor	77	44.3	
	Nurse and Other Workers	97	55.7	
Education Level	Certificate	34	19.7	
	Diploma	103	59.5	

Among the participants from the community, 79.4% were aged over 29 years, 52.8% were male, and 77.4% were married. The main occupations of the community members were office work (55.8%) and business (44.2%). As shown in Table 2, additional sociodemographic factors that were reported by the community members included education level, income level, and health insurance enrollment status.

Table 2. Sociodemographic characteristics of community members.

Item	Categories	Frequency	%	Mean ± SD
Age	18–28	41	20.6	2.1 ± 0.7
	29–50	158	79.4	
Sex	Male	105	52.8	
	Female	94	47.2	
Marital Status	Single	45	22.7	
	Married	153	77.4	
Family Size	1–4	118	59.3	1.5 ± 0.63
	5–8	81	40.7	
Occupation	Office Work	111	55.8	
	Business	88	44.2	
Education Level	University/College	135	67.8	
	Primary/Secondary	64	32.2	
Income Level	High	5	2.5	
	Low	194	97.5	
Enrolled Member of iCHF	1–4	174	87.4	1.1 ± 0.4
	5–8	24	12.1	

3.2. Healthcare Facility-Related Characteristics That Affect the iCHF

The findings of the present study showed that the level of the healthcare facility and the adequate availability of healthcare providers were statistically significant ($\chi^2 = 15.70$, $p < 0.00$). A total of 62.1% of the healthcare workers who were working in health centers and dispensaries agreed that there were enough workers in the healthcare facilities, as shown in Table 3. The educational level of the healthcare professionals was also statistically significant ($\chi^2 = 12.56$, $p < 0.00$) with an efficient referral system under the iCHF scheme. A total of 88.7% of the nurses and other workers agreed that the referral system was working well under the iCHF scheme. The relationship between education level and the availability of healthcare providers in a healthcare facility was statistically significant ($\chi^2 = 38.99$, $p = 0.00$). A total of 55% of the community members with university-level education agreed that there were enough healthcare providers in the healthcare facilities. The relationship between income level and iCHF awareness and promotion strategies in the community was statistically significant ($\chi^2 = 17.60$, $p < 0.00$). A total of 83% of the community members from low-income groups agreed that iCHF awareness and promotion strategies were conducted in the community. The relationship between occupation and the availability of medical supplies/equipment in a healthcare facility was statistically significant ($\chi^2 = 51.68$, $p < 0.00$), as 81.5% of the community members who were running businesses agreed that there were enough medical supplies/equipment in the healthcare facilities. Additionally, there was a statistically significant ($\chi^2 = 43.59$, $p < 0.00$) relationship between occupation and the availability of healthcare providers in a health facility. A total of 81.8% of the community members who were running businesses or were self-employed agreed that there were enough healthcare providers in the healthcare facilities. A statistically significant ($\chi^2 = 52.86$, $p < 0.00$) relationship was also identified between occupation and an efficient referral system under the iCHF scheme, as 76% of the community members who were running businesses agreed that the referral system was working well. The relationship between occupation and the awareness and promotion strategies for the iCHF in the community was also statistically significant ($\chi^2 = 37.91$, $p = 0.000$), as 47.8% of the community members who were running businesses agreed that awareness and promotion strategies for the iCHF were conducted in the community.

Table 3. Healthcare facility-related factors that affect the iCHF scheme, according to healthcare providers and community members.

	Healthcare Facility-Related Factors						
	Availability of Medical Supplies/Equipment						
Factor	Categories	Agree	Neutral	Disagree	χ^2	Cramer's V	Sig.
Education Level	Master's	51 (37.8)	40 (29.6)	44 (32.6)	44.51	0.473	0.000
	Bachelor's	14 (38.9)	5 (13.9)	17 (47.2)			
	Diploma	100 (73.0)	15 (10.9)	22 (16.1)			
	Primary/Secondary	56 (87.5)	1 (1.6)	7 (10.9)			
Income Level	High	24 (33.3)	23 (31.9)	25 (34.7)	19.45	0.313	0.000
	Low	83 (65.4)	18 (14.2)	26 (20.5)			
Occupation	Employed	35 (59.7)	37 (33.3)	39 (35.1)	51.68	0.510	0.000
	Self-employed	72 (81.8)	4 (4.5)	12 (13.6)			
	Availability of Healthcare Providers in Healthcare Facilities						
Factor	Categories	Agree	Neutral	Disagree	χ^2	Cramer's V	Sig.
Level of Healthcare Facility	District Hospital	16 (23.7)	0 (0.0)	26 (61.9)	15.70	0.300	0.000
	Health Centers/Dispensary	82 (62.1)	11 (8.3)	39 (29.5)			
Education Level	University	55 (40.7)	37 (27.4)	43 (31.9)	38.99	0.443	0.000
	Primary/Secondary	56 (87.5)	2 (3.1)	6 (9.4)			
Occupation	Employed	39 (35.1)	33 (29.7)	39 (35.1)	43.59	0.468	0.000
	Self-employed	72 (81.8)	6 (6.8)	10 (11.4)			
	Efficiency of the Referral System under the iCHF Scheme						
Factor	Categories	Agree	Neutral	Disagree	χ^2	Cramer's V	Sig.
Healthcare Professionals	Doctors	62 (80.5)	4 (5.2)	14 (13.0)	12.56	0.270	0.002
	Nurses and Other Workers	86 (88.7)	10 (10.3)	1 (1.0)			

Table 3. Cont.

	Healthcare Facility-Related Factors						
Education Level	University Primary/Secondary	59 (43.7) 57 (89.1)	45 (33.3) 3 (4.7)	31 (23) 4 (6.3)	36.99	0.431	0.000
Income Level	High Low	26 (36.1) 90 (70.9)	30 (41.7) 18 (14.2)	16 (22.2) 19 (15)	25.29	0.357	0.000
Occupation	Employed Self-employed	40 (36) 76 (51.3)	44 (39.6) 4 (21.2)	27 (24.3) 8 (9.1)	52.86	0.515	0.000
	Awareness and Promotion Strategies for the iCHF Scheme						
Factor	Categories	Agree	Neutral	Disagree	χ^2	Cramer's V	Sig.
Education Level	University Primary/Secondary	55 (40.7) 53 (82.8)	27 (20.0) 2 (3.1)	53 (39.3) 9 (14.1)	31.49	0.398	0.000
Income Level	High Low	25 (34.7) 83 (65.4)	16 (22.2) 13 (10.2)	31 (43.1) 31 (24.4)	17.60	0.297	0.000
Age	18–28 29–39 40–90	23 (56.1) 46 (44.2) 39 (72.2)	9.8 (4.0) 16 (15.4) 9 (16.7)	14 (34.1) 42 (40.4) 6 (11.1)	15.95	0.2	0.003
Occupation	Employed Self-employed	39 (35.1) 69 (47.8)	25 (22.5) 4 (4.5)	47 (42.3) 15 (17.0)	37.90	0.436	0.000
	Satisfaction with the iCHF Scheme at Healthcare Facilities						
Factor	Categories	Agree	Neutral	Disagree	χ^2	Cramer's V	Sig.
Education Level	University Bachelor's Diploma Primary/Secondary	65 (48.1) 22 (61) 125 (91.2) 56 (38.9)	23 (17) 2 (1.9) 7 (5.16) 1 (1.6)	47 (34.8) 12 (33.3) 5 (3.6) 7 (10.9)	28.80	0.38	0.000
Income Level	High Low	32 (43.8) 89 (70.1)	15 (20.8) 9 (7.1)	25 (34.7) 29 (22.8)	14.55	0.27	0.001
Occupation	Employed Self-employed	49 (44.1) 72 (5.2)	23 (20.7) 1 (1.1)	39 (35.1) 15 (23.9)	32.98	0.407	0.000
	Community-Related Factors						
	Involvement of Local Leaders in the iCHF Scheme						
Factor	Categories	Agree	Neutral	Disagree	χ^2	Cramer's V	Sig.
Education Level	University Primary/Secondary	56 (41.5) 59 (92.2)	34 (25.2) 1 (1.6)	45 (33.3) 4 (6.3)	46.02	0.481	0.000
Income Level	High Low	30 (41.7) 85 (66.9)	18 (25) 17 (13.4)	24 (33.3) 25 (19.7)	12.07	0.246	0.000
Age	18–28 29–39 40–90	27 (65.9) 48 (46.2) 40 (74.1)	3 (7.3) 22 (21.2) 10 (18.5)	11 (26.8) 34 (32.7) 4 (11.1)	17.94	0.212	0.001
Occupation	Employed Self-employed	40 (64.1) 75 (85.2)	30 (19.5) 5 (5.7)	41 (36.9) 8 (9.1)	48.72	0.495	0.000
	Community Behavior/Culture Toward the iCHF Scheme						
Factor	Categories	Agree	Neutral	Disagree	χ^2	Cramer's V	Sig.
Education Level	University Primary/Secondary	51 (37.8) 41 (64.1)	18 (13.3) 0 (0.0)	66 (48.9) 23 (35.9)	16.65	0.289	0.000
Income Level	High Low	20 (33.3) 72 (58.7)	6.5 (15.3) 7 (11.5)	41 (56.9) 48 (37.8)	16.92	0.292	0.000
Occupation	Employed Self-employed	38 (34.2) 54 (61.4)	15 (13.5) 3 (3.4)	58 (52.3) 31 (35.2)	16.35	0.288	0.000

A statistically significant ($\chi^2 = 46.02$, $p < 0.00$) relationship was found between education level and the involvement of local leaders, as shown in Table 3. A total of 59% of the community members with secondary- or primary-level education agreed that community leaders were involved in iCHF implementation. In addition, the relationship between education level and community behavior/culture toward the iCHF was statistically significant ($\chi^2 = 16.65$, $p < 0.00$), as 41% of the community members with secondary- or primary-level education agreed that members of the community seek to register with the iCHF after they have had an illness (Table 3). A statistically significant ($\chi^2 = 12.07$, $p < 0.000$) relationship was also found between income level and the involvement of local leaders in iCHF implementation. A total of 85% of the community members with low income levels agreed that local leaders participated in iCHF implementation. Moreover, the relationship between income level and community behavior/culture toward the iCHF was statistically significant ($\chi^2 = 16.92$, $p < 0.00$). A total of 72% of the community members with low income levels agreed that members of the community seek to register with the iCHF after an illness.

3.3. Institution-Related Factors That Affect the iCHF

A statistically significant ($\chi^2 = 14.01$, $p = 0.001$) relationship was identified between education level and ability to pay the iCHF premiums. A total of 50% of the community members with university-level education agreed that the iCHF premiums were affordable. The relationship between education level and iCHF membership size was also statistically significant ($\chi^2 = 14.01$, $p < 0.00$). A total of 46% ($\chi^2 = 14.01$, $p < 0.001$) of the community members with university-level education disagreed that iCHF membership should require the payment of premiums (Table 4). The relationship between income level and iCHF membership size was statistically significant ($\chi^2 = 21.818$, $p = 0.000$) as well. A total of 75% of the community members with low income levels disagreed regarding iCHF membership size. Finally, the relationship between income level and ability to pay the iCHF premiums was statistically significant ($\chi^2 = 18.68$, $p = 0.00$). A total of 68% of the community members with low income levels agreed that the iCHF premiums were affordable. A statistically significant ($\chi^2 = 19.08$, $p < 0.001$) relationship was found between occupation and ability to pay the iCHF premiums. A total of 61.4% of the community members who were running businesses agreed that the iCHF premiums were affordable. The relationship between occupation and iCHF membership size was statistically significant ($\chi^2 = 21.289$, $p < 0.00$) as well. A total of 65.9% of the community members who were running businesses disagreed that iCHF membership was acceptable.

Table 4. Institution-related factors that affect the iCHF, according to healthcare providers and community members.

	Institutional-Related Factors						
		Ability to Pay the iCHF Premiums					
Factor	Categories	Agree	Neutral	Disagree	χ^2	Cramer V	Sig.
Education Level	University	50 (37.0)	39 (28.9)	46 (34.1)	14.01	0.265	0.001
	Primary/Secondary	40 (62.5)	6 (9.4)	18 (28.1)			
Income Level	High	22 (30.6)	28 (38.9)	22 (30.6)	18.67	0.306	0.000
	Low	68 (53.5)	17 (28.7)	42 (33.1)			
Occupation	Employed	36 (32.4)	35 (35.1)	40 (36.0)	19.08	0.310	0.000
	Self-employed	54 (61.4)	10 (11.4)	24 (27.3)			

Table 4. Cont.

		Institutional-Related Factors					
		iCHF Membership Size					
Factor	Categories	Agree	Neutral	Disagree	χ^2	Cramer V	Sig.
Education Level	University	50 (37.0)	31 (23.0)	54 (40.0)	20.329	0.320	0.000
	Primary/Secondary	19 (29.7)	1 (1.6)	44 (68.8)			
Income Level	High	27 (37.5)	22 (30.6)	23 (31.9)	21.818	0.331	0.000
	Low	42 (33.1)	10 (7.9)	75 (59.1)			
Occupation	Employed	44 (39.6)	27 (24.3)	40 (36.0)	21.289	0.327	0.000
	Self-employed	25 (28.4)	5 (5.7)	58 (65.9)			
		Availability of Enrollment Officers for the iCHF Scheme					
Factor	Categories	Agree	Neutral	Disagree	χ^2	Cramer V	Sig.
Education Level	University	56 (41.5)	34 (25.2)	45 (33.3)	46.026	0.481	0.000
	Primary/Secondary	59 (92.2)	1 (1.6)	4 (6.3)			
Income Level	High	21 (29.2)	24 (33.3)	27 (37.5)	25.439	0.358	0.000
	Low	21 (92.2)	15 (11.9)	29 (23.0)			
Occupation	Employed	82 (65.1)	37 (33.6)	44 (40.0)	67.748	0.585	0.000
	Self-employed	74 (45.8)	2 (2.3)	12 (13.6)			

4. Discussion

The present study identified the factors that influenced the implementation of the Improved Community Health Fund project in the Ubungo municipality of Dar es Salaam, Tanzania. The results of this study confirmed the availability of sufficient healthcare providers at various levels of healthcare facilities, thereby demonstrating the increased healthcare service provision under the iCHF scheme. The role of healthcare providers was found to be essential for the quality of the services that were provided. Therefore, it is pertinent that government interventions are aimed at improving healthcare service provision in communities by enhancing the quantity and quality of healthcare workers. This would also help to increase the confidence of community members in adopting insurance schemes, such as the iCHF. To ensure this occurs, the government should invest more financial resources into improvements in healthcare service provision, which would automatically increase the coverage and enrollment of iCHF members. Our findings regarding the importance of the availability of qualified healthcare providers were consistent with studies that were conducted in the Iramba and Liwale districts of Tanzania, where the development of healthcare providers influenced the excellent performance of the iCHF scheme [14].

Additionally, the necessary medical equipment/supplies were considered to be essential for healthcare and iCHF provision, as members would receive better healthcare services under the scheme. This finding was consistent with a study that was conducted in Ethiopia, where the presence of medical equipment led to an increase in the enrollment of iCHF members [15]. With the increasing quantity and quality of equipment and personnel within healthcare facilities, community confidence in orthodox medicine is likely to improve, along with an increase in enrollment in health insurance schemes. This is particularly true for resource-strapped African countries, in which the use of traditional alternative medicine and treatment has been a barrier to service acquisition. Most alternative medical practices in poor countries lack scientific rigor and are conducted in unsanitary and unsafe environments. This study demonstrated that other factors that affect the implementation of the iCHF included insufficient supplies and a lack of trained professionals. The iCHF would perform better if healthcare facilities had sufficient medical supplies/equipment and healthcare providers. In Ethiopia, the community perceived a poor quality of healthcare under the community-based health insurance scheme due to the unavailability of medicines/medical supplies, long wait times, and inadequate healthcare providers [13]. In Tanzania, poor healthcare outcomes under the iCHF were caused by a lack of healthcare providers, long wait times, and a lack of medications [16,17].

This study indicated that the referral systems under the iCHF were functioning well in the healthcare facilities that were included in the research. This could be due to the proximity of the hospitals in the municipality, the availability of ambulances, and the presence of several referral hospitals and a national hospital in the area. This finding contrasted with many studies that were conducted in other parts of Tanzania, where the referral systems under the iCHF have been reported to be not working well. This could be caused by the absence of referral or zonal hospitals in those areas and the limited number of ambulances, especially in rural areas [18,19]. Healthcare referral systems are essential for improving community perceptions of the benefits that are associated with insurance facilities in low-resource settings.

Community awareness and promotion strategies contributed to the implementation of the iCHF at the community level by increasing iCHF enrollment [20]. This finding was consistent with studies that were conducted in three Dodoma districts in Tanzania, which showed higher levels of community awareness [21,22]. However, the factors that influence enrollment in community-based health insurance schemes are numerous and interact in complex ways to influence individual decisions. In a study that was conducted in northwest Ethiopia, community awareness programs about saving and credit decisions contributed significantly to the implementation of the community health insurance scheme [21]. In another study in southern Ethiopia, community leaders played a crucial role in enrolling and implementing community-based health insurance [13]. A study in Tanzania indicated that most of the information on iCHF implementation was obtained from local leaders [21]. Another study in Dodoma, Tanzania, indicated that the implementation of the iCHF scheme improved after the involvement of community leaders. District authorities ensured that all local leaders were registered with the iCHF scheme and were informed as to its importance for the local community [23]. Therefore, in addition to an increased awareness of the health insurance scheme, other factors and barriers that influence enrollment need to be further investigated in future studies.

The income and education levels of the community members were important factors that influenced the adoption of iCHF, as the participants with high income and education levels perceived the healthcare services under the iCHF scheme to be of good quality, regardless of the iCHF premiums or iCHF membership size. The results of studies in northwest [24,25] and southwest Ethiopia [26] were consistent with the current findings that the iCHF premiums were acceptable to the community if the scheme could ensure quality healthcare services. However, a study in Rwanda opposed this finding because it was found that a change in the premiums could cause low enrollment rates, especially in rural areas [27]. In addition, high premium costs could contribute to differences in healthcare provision between urban and rural areas due to varying income levels. The results from a previous study in Tanzania were consistent with the current findings that the low levels of iCHF membership in three districts were caused by poor healthcare services and low enrollment. However, in another study, the iCHF premiums were influenced by the user fee and people who were not members of the CHF scheme preferred it because the quality of the healthcare services was good [27].

Strengths and Limitations

The present study was successful in identifying factors that affect the implementation of the iCHF at both the community member and healthcare provider levels, unlike many of the other studies, which have focused on the factors that affect community health while ignoring the role of healthcare providers. However, a key limitation of this study was the inability to determine the causal relationship between the factors that impact iCHF adoption due to the cross-sectional nature of the study. The factors that were associated with the implementation of the iCHF were multiple dimensional and the level of impact of each variable could only be ascertained through longitudinal studies or those that implement experimental designs. Due to this, we could not determine the level of impact of each factor on the implementation of the iCHF in Tanzania. Therefore, it is important that experimental research designs are employed to test the contribution and efficacy of each influencing factor in terms of an individual's choice to use the iCHF. However, regardless of these limitations, we highlighted the factors that are associated with the implementation of the iCHF in Tanzania.

5. Conclusions

This study demonstrated that multiple dimensional factors influence the implementation of the iCHF in Tanzania. These factors range from individual to community factors, which interact dynamically to influence the implementation of the iCHF. For healthcare providers, the factors that affect the implementation of the iCHF scheme that were identified in the present study included the level of the healthcare facility, the education level of the healthcare providers, and the referral system in the hospital. For community members, the factors included education level, age, and income level. All health, community, and institutional factors were affected at both the healthcare facility and community levels. It is important that future research uses experimental designs or longitudinal follow-up approaches to identify the level of influence of each factor on the implementation of the iCHF. To have an effective iCHF, stakeholders must focus on mitigating these factors while efforts are made to improve the education and awareness of the tenants of the fund. The education of community members about the iCHF must focus on those in the lower socioeconomic groups, which have limited formal education. Healthcare institutions must also be empowered to implement effective referral systems that can ensure prompt care for patients.

Author Contributions: This work was carried out in collaboration with all authors. G.M. conceptualized the study, developed the initial research question, conducted the literature review, and developed the study design in discussion with S.K. and Y.L. Data collection and data curation were supported by P.N. and K.D.K. G.M. wrote the original draft of this manuscript and all of the relevant data in the tables were collected under the supervision of S.K., Y.L. and J.R. All authors have read and agreed to the published version of the manuscript.

Funding: This research received no external funding.

Institutional Review Board Statement: Permission was granted by Ubungo Municipal Council's Health and Social Welfare Department on 4 October 2021.

Informed Consent Statement: Informed consent was obtained from all subjects who were involved in the study. A researcher explained the aims and objectives of the study to the healthcare providers and community members before the questionnaire was distributed. A consent form was signed by all participants, which informed them of their voluntary participation, right to withdraw from the study at any time, and right to freedom of choice, expression, anonymity, and confidentiality during the study.

Data Availability Statement: The data are available upon reasonable request from the corresponding author.

Acknowledgments: We gratefully acknowledged the efforts of Myung-Ken Lee, former director, Whiejong M. Han, director of the Global Health Policy and Finance Program at the Graduate School of Public Health, Yonsei University, and the entire staff for their support of this study, as well as the scholarship support of the KOICA.

Conflicts of Interest: The authors declare no conflict of interest.

Disclosure: This article is a condensed form of the first author's master's degree thesis for the Graduate School of Public Health, Yonsei University, Seoul, South Korea.

References

1. Vrijburg, K.; Hernández-Peña, P. *Global Spending on Health: Weathering the Storm 2020*; World Health Organization Working Paper; World Health Organization: Geneva, Switzerland, 2020; ISBN 9789240017788.
2. Borghi, J.; Makawia, S.; Kuwawenaruwa, A. The administrative costs of community-based health insurance: A case study of the community health fund in Tanzania. *Health Policy Plan.* **2015**, *30*, 19–27. [CrossRef] [PubMed]
3. Attia-Konan, A.R.; Oga, A.S.S.; Touré, A.; Kouadio, K.L. Distribution of out of pocket health expenditures in a sub-Saharan Africa country: Evidence from the national survey of household standard of living, Côte d'Ivoire. *BMC Res. Notes* **2019**, *12*, 25. [CrossRef] [PubMed]
4. World Health Organization (WHO). Primary Health Care on the Road to Universal Health Coverage: 2019 Monitoring Report: Executive Summary. Available online: https://www.who.int/docs/default-source/documents/2019-uhc-report-executive-summary (accessed on 21 October 2021).
5. Eastern Africa National Networks of AIDS Service Organizations. Status of Health Financing in East Africa. Available online: https://eannaso.org (accessed on 4 February 2022).
6. Wang, H.; Juma, M.A.; Rosemberg, N.; Ulisubisya, M.M. Progressive pathway to universal health coverage in Tanzania: A call for preferential resource allocation targeting the poor. *Health Syst. Reform.* **2018**, *4*, 279–283. [CrossRef] [PubMed]
7. Ministry of Health, Community Development, Gender, Elderly and Children (MOHCDGEC). *Mid Term Review of the Health Sector Strategic Plan IV 2015–2020 Technical Report Health Financing*; Ministry of Health, Community Development, Gender, Elderly and Children, United Republic of Tanzania: Dodoma, Tanzania, 2019; Available online: http://old.tzdpg.or.tz/fileadmin/documents/dpg_internal/dpg_working_groups_clusters/cluster_2/health/JAHSR_2019/MTR_HSSP_IV_Health_Finance_Thematic_Report_2019.09101.pdf (accessed on 4 February 2022).
8. Asantemungu, R.; Maluka, S. An assessment of the implementation of the re-structured community health fund in Gairo District in Tanzania. *Tanzan. J. Dev. Stud.* **2020**, *18*, 27–41.
9. Ndomba, T. Uptake of community health fund: Why is Mtwara District lagging behind? *J. Glob. Health Sci.* **2019**, *1*, e50. [CrossRef]
10. Mpambije, C.J. Decentralisation of health systems and the fate of community health Fund in Tanzania: Critical review of high and low performing districts. *Sci. J. Public Health* **2017**, *5*, 136. [CrossRef]
11. Ubungo Municipal Council (UMC) Profile. Municipal Director, Dar-es-Salaam, Tanzania: Ubungo Municipal Council Kibamba Area, Morogoro Road Postal Address: P. O. Box 55068 Dar es Salaam. 2016. Available online: https://www.ubungomc.go.tz (accessed on 4 February 2022).
12. UMC. *Regional Joint Meeting Presentation*; Ubungo Municipal Council: Dar es Salaam, Tanzania, 2021.
13. Abdilwohab, M.G.; Abebo, Z.H.; Godana, W.; Ajema, D.; Yihune, M.; Hassen, H. Factors affecting enrollment status of households for community based health insurance in a resource-limited peripheral area in Southern Ethiopia. Mixed method. *PLoS ONE* **2021**, *16*, e0245952. [CrossRef] [PubMed]
14. Joseph, C.; Maluka, S.O. Do management and leadership practices in the context of decentralisation influence performance of community health fund? Evidence from Iramba and Iringa districts in Tanzania. *Int. J. Health Policy Manag.* **2017**, *6*, 257. [CrossRef] [PubMed]
15. Shigute, Z.; Mebratie, A.D.; Sparrow, R.; Alemu, G.; Bedi, A.S. The effect of Ethiopia's community-based health insurance scheme on revenues and quality of care. *Int. J. Environ. Res. Public Health* **2020**, *17*, 8558. [CrossRef] [PubMed]
16. Kamuzora, P.; Gilson, L. Factors influencing implementation of the Community Health Fund in Tanzania. *Health Policy Plan.* **2007**, *22*, 95–102. [CrossRef] [PubMed]
17. Marwa, B.; Njau, B.; Kessy, J.; Mushi, D. Feasibility of introducing compulsory community health fund in low resource countries: Views from the communities in Liwale district of Tanzania. *BMC Health Serv. Res.* **2013**, *13*, 298. [CrossRef] [PubMed]
18. Kivelege, G. *Community Health Fund and Quality Health Services in Morogoro District, Tanzania*; Sokoine University of Agriculture: Morogoro, Tanzania, 2015.
19. Kigume, R.; Maluka, S. The failure of community-based health insurance schemes in Tanzania: Opening the black box of the implementation process. *BMC Health Serv. Res.* **2021**, *21*, 646. [CrossRef] [PubMed]
20. Atafu, A.; Kwon, S. Adverse selection and supply-side factors in the enrollment in community-based health insurance in Northwest Ethiopia: A mixed methodology. *Int. J. Health Plan. Manag.* **2018**, *33*, 902–914. [CrossRef] [PubMed]
21. Kapologwe, N.A.; Kagaruki, G.B.; Kalolo, A.; Ally, M.; Shao, A.; Meshack, M.; Stoermer, M.; Briet, A. Barriers and facilitators to enrollment and re-enrollment into the community health funds/Tiba Kwa Kadi (CHF/TIKA) in Tanzania: A cross-sectional inquiry on the effects of socio-demographic factors and social marketing strategies. *BMC Health Serv. Res.* **2017**, *17*, 308. [CrossRef] [PubMed]
22. Modest, A.R.; Ngowi, A.F.; Katalambula, L. Enrollment Status and Determinants of Improved Community Health Fund Among Households in Dodoma Tanzania. *Int. J. Innov. Sci. Res. Technol.* **2021**, *6*, 807–815.
23. Ajuaye, A.; Verbrugge, B.; Van Ongevalle, J.; Develtere, P. Understanding the limitations of "quasi-mandatory" approaches to enrolment in community-based health insurance: Empirical evidence from Tanzania. *Int. J. Health Plan. Manag.* **2019**, *34*, 1304–1318. [CrossRef] [PubMed]
24. Mirach, T.H.; Demissie, G.D.; Biks, G.A. Determinants of community-based health insurance implementation in west Gojjam zone, Northwest Ethiopia: A community based cross sectional study design. *BMC Health Serv. Res.* **2019**, *19*, 544. [CrossRef] [PubMed]

25. Eseta, W.A.; Lemma, T.D.; Geta, E.T. Magnitude and Determinants of Dropout from Community-Based Health Insurance Among Households in Manna District, Jimma Zone, Southwest Ethiopia. *Clin. Outcomes Res.* **2020**, *12*, 747–760. [CrossRef] [PubMed]
26. Mukangendo, M.; Nzayirambaho, M.; Hitimana, R.; Yamuragiye, A. Factors Contributing to Low Adherence to Community-Based Health Insurance in Rural Nyanza District, Southern Rwanda. *J. Environ. Public Health* **2018**, *2018*, 2624591. [CrossRef] [PubMed]
27. Renggli, S.; Mayumana, I.; Mshana, C.; Mboya, D.; Kessy, F.; Tediosi, F.; Pfeiffer, C.; Aerts, A.; Lengeler, C. Looking at the bigger picture: How the wider health financing context affects the implementation of the Tanzanian Community Health Funds. *Health Policy Plan.* **2019**, *34*, 12–23. [CrossRef]

Article

Exploring the Role of Health Expenditure and Maternal Mortality in South Asian Countries: An Approach towards Shaping Better Health Policy

Noshaba Aziz [1], Jun He [1,*], Tanwne Sarker [2] and Hongguang Sui [3]

1. College of Economics and Management, Nanjing Agricultural University, Nanjing 210095, China; noshabaaziz@yahoo.com
2. School of Economics and Finance, Xi'an Jiaotong University, Xi'an 710049, China; sarker@stu.xjtu.edu.cn
3. School of Economics, Shandong University, Jinan 250100, China; hongguang.sui@sdu.edu.cn
* Correspondence: hejun@njau.edu.cn

Abstract: Accomplishing unremitting favorable health outcomes, especially reducing maternal mortality, remains a challenge for South Asian countries. This study explores the relationship between health expenditure and maternal mortality by using data set consisting of 18 years from 2000 to 2017. Fully modified ordinary least squares (FMOLS) and dynamic ordinary least squares (DOLS) models were employed for the empirical analysis. The outcomes revealed that a 1% rise in health expenditure increased the maternal mortality rate by 1.95% in the case of FMOLS estimator and 0.16% in the case of DOLS estimator. This reflects that the prevailing health care system is not adequate for reducing maternal mortality. Moreover, the meager system and the priorities established by an elitist system in which the powerless and poor are not considered may also lead to worsen the situation. In addition, the study also added population, economic growth, sanitation, and clean fuel technology in the empirical model. The findings revealed that population growth has a significant long-term effect on maternal mortality—an increase of 40% in the case of FMOLS and 10% in the case of DOLS—and infers that an increase in population growth has also dampened efforts towards reducing maternal mortality in the South Asian panel. Further, the results in the case of economic growth, sanitation, and clean fuel technologies showed significant long-term negative effects on maternal mortality by 94%, 7.2%, and 11%, respectively, in the case of the FMOLS estimator, and 18%, 1.9%, and 5%, respectively, in the case of the DOLS estimator. The findings imply that GDP and access to sanitation and clean fuel technologies are more nuanced in declining maternal mortality. In conclusion, the verdict shows that policymakers should formulate policies considering the fundamental South Asian aspects warranted to reduce maternal mortality.

Keywords: health expenditure; maternal mortality; sanitation; clean technologies; South Asian countries

1. Introduction

Human capital is an imperative factor for attaining the desired economic growth and development of any country [1]. Under the concept of the neoclassical growth model, human capital, particularly good human health, markedly influences a country's per capita income in the long run [2]. The health status of any given country depends upon maternal and infant mortality rates, which play a crucial role in evaluating the country's population health, quality of care, socioeconomic status, and poverty [3]. Moreover, maternal health is likely to bring economic benefits for the whole family and society. But recently, mothers' poor health, especially maternal deaths, have remained an unavoidable phenomenon that occurs at relatively high rates in many developing countries despite a steep reduction in maternal mortality worldwide since 1990 [4–6]. The maternal mortality ratio numerically shows the maternal deaths during a given time period per 100,000 live births during the same time period. It illustrates the maternal death risks relative to the number of live births and basically captures the death risk in a single pregnancy or a single live birth. According to the World Health Organization (WHO), around 810 women die during pregnancy every year, and about 94% of them belong to developing countries [7].

Globally, the maternal mortality ratio has declined from 342 to 311 (by nearly 38%) from 2000 to 2017 [7]. However, South Asian countries and sub-Saharan African countries face disproportionately higher maternal mortality ratios than other regions of the world, making up around 85% of all maternal-related deaths. The third Sustainable Development Goal (SDG 3) of reducing the deaths to 70 per 100,000 live births and ensuring that all human beings, at all ages, achieve healthy lives by 2030, has intensified their struggles to promote the health sector [8]. In this regard, a good health care system is focused, and has been is shown that the health care system comprises various sectors, of which the most important is health financing [3]. Evidence has confirmed that financing in the health sector considerably supports the economy [9]. This implies that spending in the health care system improves peoples' health and generates employment opportunities, increases social and political stability, and ultimately leads to the growth and development of the whole economy [10–12].

Despite significant investments in the health sector, expenditure on health in governments' financial plans in developing regions, including South Asian countries, is still under-represented due to resource scarcity [13]. Even if South Asian countries develop and progress at the same pace, the global SDG target of decreasing maternal deaths to 70 per 100,000 live births by 2030 is hard to accomplish. Over the past few decades, keeping in view the importance of the health of the people and its role in the national economy, scholars and researchers have devoted their attention to evaluating the link between health expenditure and health outcomes. In this vein, many studies have been conducted before (see, for example, [14–21]). Some studies showed that health expenditure leads to better health outcomes [22], while others found no such relationship [23,24]. The link between health expenditure with health outcomes is uncertain, as health expenditure and health care patterns alter considerably; therefore, the debate over health care expenditure and health outcomes remains questionable [25], which warrants more investigation. Moreover, the rise in health expenditure in developing countries has demonstrated that maternal mortality rates are still higher, which has prompted authors to identify the core cause of maternal mortality, so health expenditure is appropriately directed and utilized.

Based on the above discussion, the current study was designed to explore the following research question: "Does health expenditure contribute to decreased maternal mortality in South Asian countries?" Exploring this question will enable policymakers to prepare strategies accordingly to accomplish the sustainable development goal of reducing maternal mortality, as health expenditure is regarded as the clearest policy variable [26]. Investigating health care outcomes in South Asian countries is remarkably important, not only due to the relationship of health with economic growth but also poor health leads to disparity between actual income and real opportunities, as it decreases the degree to which a given income level can be transformed into the ability to live a life of an acceptable quality [27]. Perkins, Radelet, Lindauer, and Block [28], and Booth and Cammack [29] also pointed out that the health sector is among the most pervasive markets that may lead to failure because of the problems of principal agents, negative externalities, collective actions, and information failures, which require government interventions. Moreover, most preceding studies ignored other macro-level factors of maternal mortality, such as population growth, economic growth, sanitation, and access to clean fuel technologies. Thus, the current study may help to unpack the association of health expenditure with maternal mortality by incorporating these factors for the South Asian region.

As discussed above, many previous studies have explored the relationships between health outcomes (mortality) by using different datasets and have used different research methods and found diverse findings, particularly for the maternal mortality ratio [24,30–34]. However, a recent study pointed out that an investigation of this kind must account for "unobserved heterogeneity" [34]. Even so, many studies have ignored the heterogeneity and even cross-sectional dependency within the panel data. Therefore, to fix the cross-sectional dependency and heterogeneity issues in the panel data and add a contribution to the health economics literature, the present study applied fully modified ordinary least squares (FMOLS) and dynamic ordinary least squares (DOLS). The recent study of Aziz et al. [35] also used this phenomenon to assess the determinants of undernourishment in a South Asian panel. As per the authors' knowledge, this is the first study attempting to scrutinize the long-run effects of health expenditure on maternal mortality in a South Asian panel via this empirical approach.

2. Literature Review

This section is an attempt to review the previous efforts of scholars and researchers on the subject matter of the current study. This section concisely reviews the studies available in the literature.

According to previous studies, the health expenditure level in a nation is one of the key measures for determining the health investment level; hence, it is acknowledged as an imperative input factor, like diet and exercising, for enhancing health. An extensive body of literature has scrutinized the association between health expenditure and health outcomes across countries. Despite these efforts, the pivotal link between health expenditure and health outcomes is still not clear. It is generally presumed that increasing health expenditure will inevitably improve health outcomes. In this regard, Aldogan, Austill, and Kocakülâh [36] observed prominent health outcomes such as infant, under-five, and maternal mortality rates due to government spending in the MENA region from 1990 to 2010, by using pooled ordinary least regression, random effects, and Hausman–Taylor instrumental variable models. Betrán et al. [30] argued that with the exception of developed countries, variability of national maternal mortality estimates is large even within sub-regions. In another study, Anyanwu and Erhijakpor [9] used data from 47 African countries between 1999 and 2004, and statistically revealed that health expenditure significantly and negatively influenced the infant and under-five mortality rates. In developing countries, Bokhari, Gai, and Gottret [37], using the instrumental variable approach, implied that economic growth and government expenditure on health are important factors for boosting public health. Nketiah-Amponsah [38] studied 46 sub-Saharan African countries over the period 2000–2015 and unveiled that a 1% increase in health expenditure per capita reduced under-five mortality by 0.5% and maternal mortality by 0.35%, while improving life expectancy by 0.06%. Likewise, Arthur and Oaikhenan [39] also indicated that health expenditure meaningfully boosted the expectancy of life and lessened maternal mortality and under-five mortality.

On the other side, several other studies found no causal association between expenditure on health and health outcomes [24,40]. Ashiabi, Nketiah-Amponsah, and Senadza [41], in another study, investigated the impact of both public and private health expenditure on maternal and child health for 40 sub-Saharan African countries for the years 2000–2010. The study used a fixed effect model and indicated that there was no significant effect of health expenditure on maternal mortality. Bradley, Elkins, Herrin, and Elbel [42] used a pooled cross-sectional analysis of OECD countries from the year 1995 to 2005. The main outcomes were life expectancy at birth, infant mortality, low birth weight, maternal mortality and potential years of lost life. The findings revealed that health service expenditure adjusted for GDP and two health outcomes were significantly associated, while in the case of social services expenditure adjusted for GDP; only three of five indicators were found to be significant. Several other studies have also shown contrary findings in low- and high-income countries. For example, Self and Grabowski [43] revealed that health expenditure significantly influenced health only in low- to middle-income countries. The countries belongs to different income groups have differences in health expenditures as well which corresponds to different health outcomes. Likewise, Rana, Alam, and Gow [34] indicated that the association of health expenditure with health outcomes was resilient only for countries with a low income. Lower-income countries are more susceptible to poor health due to negative shocks to health expenditure. Gupta, Verhoeven, and Tiongson [44], by using demographic health surveys from 44 countries, established that the poor experience worse health than the non-poor, and their empirical findings stated that public spending alone is not enough to improve health status. Gupta [45] argued that public spending enhances health and education in developing and emerging economies. Ullah et al. [46] findings confirm that public healthcare spending significantly impacts health outcomes in Pakistan both in the short-run and long-run. Using a fixed effect model, Nixon and Ulmann [19], in a panel of 15 European Union members over the period 1980–1995, showed that health care expenditure and infant mortality rates were strongly associated, while the results for life expectancy were found to be marginally associated. The findings indicated that factors such as lifestyle, diet, and the environment also influence health outcomes, as these factors vary significantly between low-income and high countries. Therefore, the relationship between health expenditure and health outcomes at different income levels was found to be inconclusive. In another study of Nigeria, Yaqub, Ojapinwa, and Yussuff [47] stated that public expenditure was significant for enhancing health unless corruption in the country was controlled. By using both ordinary least squares and two-stage least squares, the study proposed that lowering infant mortality and under-five mortality rate and raising the life expectancy in Nigeria would only be possible if corruption in the country reduced considerably.

Based on the literature review mentioned above, it is apparent that the results on heath expenditure and health outcome are inconclusive and there has been variance in the use of specific econometric methods. To explore the phenomenon empirically by using advanced econometric techniques, the current study utilized the data of South Asian countries. Finally, by using a more robust empirical strategy, the current study offers new empirical evidence concerning health expenditures and it impact on maternal mortality in the South Asian panel.

3. Materials and Methods

3.1. Data Sources

Based on the availability, the data set of eight South Asian countries including Pakistan, Bangladesh, Bhutan, Nepal, Sri Lanka, India, Maldives and Afghanistan was collected. The maternal mortality ratio (MMR) was used as an outcome variable; this numerically shows the women died during pregnancy or pregnancy-related causes or within 42 days of pregnancy termination per 100,000 live births, while the predictor variables included total health expenditure (HE), population (POP), economic growth (LNGDP), basic sanitation (BS), and access to clean technologies (CT). Health expenditure was measured in current USD. Economic growth (LNGDP) was measured in constant 2010 USD and was used in natural logarithmic form for empirical analysis. The variable population (POP) was measured as the annual percentage growth in the population. The other variables, basic sanitation (BS) and clean technologies (CT), measured the proportion of the population using at least basic sanitation services and clean fuel technologies for cooking.

The data for the desired variables used in the current study were sourced from the World Bank Development Indicators databank from 2000 to 2017. Furthermore, the quarterly data were used for applying the quadratic match sum method. Many previous studies have used this method [48]. This method is appropriate for altering low-frequency data into high-frequency data, as it allows adjustments for seasonal deviation by dropping end-to-end data deviation. The trends of maternal mortality and health expenditure in South Asian countries are portrayed below. The Figure 1 below reveals that though maternal mortality has slightly declined in all regions, the most apparent decline is seen for Afghanistan compared with other regions, and the least were seen in Sri Lanka and Maldives.

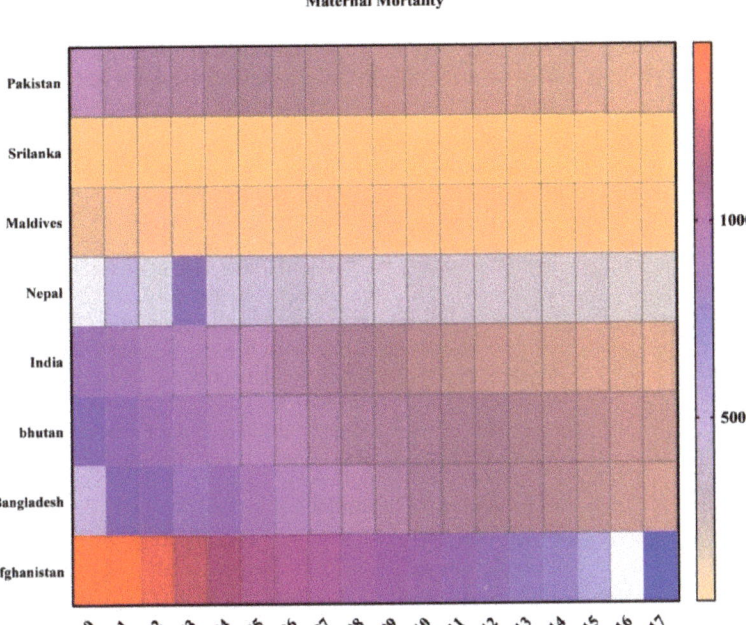

Figure 1. Trends of Maternal Mortality in the South Asian Panel.

3.2. Model Specification

It is a crucial and well recognized fact that a better understanding of various aspects in the economy leads to the formulation of effective economic policy, including the nexus among maternal mortality, health expenditure, economic growth, population, basic sanitation, and clean technologies. As the present study intended to explicate the long-run relationship of health expenditure effects on maternal mortality in South Asian regions while controlling for population, economic growth, basic sanitation, and access to clean technologies, the subsequent model was designed to analyze the relationship empirically:

$$MMR_{i,t} = \alpha_0 + \beta_1 MMR_{i,t-1} + \beta_2 HE_{i,t} + \beta_3 LNGDP_{i,t} + \beta_4 POP_{i,t} + \beta_5 BS_{i,t} + \beta_6 CT_{i,t} + \mu_{i,t} \tag{1}$$

where MMR, HE, LNGDP, POP, BS, and CT signify the maternal mortality ratio, health expenditure, economic growth, population, basic sanitation, and clean fuel technology, respectively. In this model, the maternal mortality ratio represents the dependent variable; βk (k = 1, 2, 3, 4, 5) are the coefficients of the lag of maternal mortality ratio, health expenditure, economic growth, population, basic sanitation, and clean fuel technology; and $\mu_{i,t}$ shows the error term. Our models remained confined to these variables to avoid over fitting the model and to allow our core variables of interest to show the association.

Determination of the long-run relationships among the study variables was undertaken via the following essential steps. Firstly, panel unit root tests were used to examine the stationarity properties of the variables. Testing stationarity is vital for both time and panel data because non-stationary data lead to spurious results [49]. Thus, Im, Pesaran, and Shin's test [50] for unit roots was applied to test the stationarity [51–53]. However, it has been argued that such unit root tests for panel data may not be accurate due to the probability of cross-sectional dependency. Therefore, second-order generation tests such as cross-sectional IPS (CIPS) were also used, along with a cross-dependency test (CD), as these tests can be executed under the notion of cross-sectional dependency as well as heterogeneity [54], which was unnoticed by Im, Pesaran, and Shin [50]. Many earlier studies have used this method [55,56].

Once the stationarity had been checked, the next step was to test the variables' cointegration. Cointegration expresses the association among the studied variables in the long run. The cointegration test of [57] for panel data involves two stages. In the first stage, it monitors short-run parameters and individual deterministic trends to control the heterogeneity. On the basis of the estimated residuals, statistics of different tests can be derived, i.e., pooled (within-dimension) data to test the common process, and grouped (between-dimensions) data to test individual processes. The four statistics included in a within-dimensions approach were panel v, panel ρ, panel PP, and panel ADF. In contrast, the three statistics included in the between dimensions approach were group O, group PP, and group ADF. The cointegration test only indicated the long-run associations among the variables and did not indicate the direction of the variables used in the study.

To indicate the direction, the study primarily used fixed effect and random effect models [58], but as the panel data suffered from cross-sectional dependency, FMOLS and DOLS were used, as in Kao and Chiang [59]. FMOLS and DOLS are appropriate for panel data. FMOLS is a non-parametric technique that deals with serial correlation, while DOLS is a parametric method that deals with endogeneity.

4. Results and Discussion

4.1. Descriptive Statistics

The variables used in the current study and their descriptive statistics are presented in Table 1. The findings reveal that maternal mortality's maximum and minimum values are around 1450 and 36, respectively, for the sample countries. The sampled countries' health expenditure had a mean value of about 105, with a standard deviation of 184, a maximum of 946, and a minimum value of 8.36. The mean value of economic growth was USD 24.18; the mean value for population was nearly 1.83 and its standard deviation was about 1.067. Clean fuel technologies and basic sanitation had a mean value of 32.16 and 53.63, with a standard deviation of 20.24 and 23.83, respectively.

Table 1. Descriptive Statistics.

	Maternal Mortality	Health Expenditure	Economic Growth	Population	Clean Fuel Technologies	Basic Sanitation
Mean	312.4028	105.0910	24.18627	1.834289	32.16650	53.63868
Median	236.5000	40.11737	24.24980	1.562703	26.56000	48.65390
Maximum	1450.000	946.8112	28.60913	4.668361	94.56000	99.37300
Minimum	36.00000	8.362380	20.31048	−0.266960	7.240000	15.12425
Std. Dev.	302.9920	184.0360	2.209372	1.067289	20.24544	23.83500
Skewness	1.957352	2.931312	0.159694	0.850876	1.503814	0.484218
Kurtosis	6.467059	10.90132	2.181728	3.393813	4.979517	2.010786
Jarque–Bera	164.0724	580.8078	4.629465	18.30628	77.24570	11.49848
Probability	0.000000	0.000000	0.098793	0.000106	0.000000	0.003185

Source: Authors' estimations.

4.2. Unit Root Tests

Before performing the regression analysis, the variables' stationarity was required to be checked. First, the variables' stationarity properties were checked using the conventional unit root tests of Im, Pesaran, and Shin [50]. In Table 2, the findings of the unit root test with individual intercepts and individual intercepts with trend terms are illustrated. The findings reveal that basic sanitation and clean technologies have a unit root problem at the level but become stationary at first difference. The study then proceeded to inspect the cointegration among variables.

Table 2. Results of the stationarity analysis.

Variable	Im, Pesaran, and Shin			
	I (0)		I (1)	
	Intercept	Intercept with Trend	Intercept	Intercept with Trend
Maternal Mortality	−3.44394 ***	1.28452	−3.37734 ***	−6.50037 ***
Health Expenditure	6.53287	−1.45462 *	−5.33655 ***	−5.31860 ***
Economic Growth	1.32175	−20.9478 ***	−33.4276 ***	−30.2320 ***
Population	−3.65753 ***	−7.00708 ***	−9.68864 ***	−12.4179 ***
Basic Sanitation	5.17881	1.69497	−4.75597 ***	−17.7165 ***
Clean Technologies	3.39259	1.21140	−4.34171 ***	−9.37003 ***

Note: ***, * show significance at the 1% and 10% levels, respectively.

Before checking cointegration, the present study used the cross-sectional dependency. It has been argued that orthodox unit root tests do not offer robust outcomes in data series with cross-sectional dependence. Therefore, according to the cross-section dependency test results, it was apparent that there was cross-sectional dependence, as the results were found to be significant for all variables at the 1% significance level (see Table 3). For panel data with cross-sectional dependence, it is recommended to use a cross-sectional unit root test IPS (CIPS), rather than the conventional Im, Pesaran, and Shin unit root test. Therefore, the current study used the CIPS results, which assumed cross-section dependency within the panel data and revealed that all variables became stationary at first difference.

Table 3. Cross-sectional dependence and CIPS unit root test results.

Variables	CD Test	p-Value	CIPS Test	
			Level	First Difference
Maternal Mortality	22.01677	0.000	−2.606 ***	−4.253 ***
Health Expenditure	21.45441	0.000	−0.909	−3.654 ***
Economic Growth	16.55560	0.000	−2.653 ***	−4.603 ***
Population	5.181234	0.000	−3.334 ***	−1.659 ***
Basic Sanitation	22.39049	0.000	−0.451	−2.028 *
Clean Technologies	21.89715	0.000	−0.269	−3.935 ***

Note: ***, * signifies significance at the 1% and 10% levels, respectively.

4.3. Panel Cointegration Test

Once the stationarity features of all variables had been proven, panel data cointegration was valid to apply. To check the cointegration, the study used the panel cointegration test of Pedroni [57]. The results in Table 4 revealed that four tests out of seven were significant at the 1% level. Based on these test results, it is apparent that variables are co-integrated in the long run.

Table 4. Results of Pedroni co-integration (Engle-Granger based) in the South Asian panel.

MMR = f (HE+ LNGDP + POP + BS+ CT)		
Estimates	Stats.	Prob.
Panel v-statistics	−0.4468	0.673
Panel rho-statistics	2.04059	0.979
Panel PP-statistics	−11.393	0.000
Panel ADF-statistics	−6.6653	0.000
Alternative hypothesis: individual AR coefficient		
Group rho-statistic	2.97338	0.999
Group PP-statistic	−14.826	0.000
Group ADF-statistic	−3.5834	0.002

Note: The panel cointegration null hypothesis is no cointegration.

4.4. Panel Estimation Results

4.4.1. Fixed Effect and Random Effect Results

As a preliminary analysis, the conventional panel data models, i.e., fixed and random effects were applied. The results of the fixed effect model showed that health expenditure, economic growth, and population positively influenced maternal mortality in South Asian countries by 43%, 58%, and 71%, respectively, while in the case of random effects, the coefficients were similar: 42%, 44%, and 72%, respectively. The findings for health expenditure are unexpected and reveal that an increase in health expenditure increased maternal mortality in the South Asian panel. In contrast, access to sanitation and clean fuel technologies were proven to reduce maternal mortality. The random effect model also reported the same findings, with similar coefficients in the sample countries. Hausman's [60] test was also executed, and indicated that the fixed effect model was more appropriate for the current study (see Table 5). However, as the panel data suffered from cross-sectional dependency and heterogeneity, as the countries are diverse and are not identical in their demographic aspects, health infrastructure, medical technology, and the prevalence of diseases, relying on fixed effects may give biased results. Therefore, the study proceeded towards using fully modified ordinary least squares and dynamic ordinary least squares. These methods are beneficial for overcoming heteroscedasticity and autocorrelation in the panel data [61,62]

Table 5. Panel regression results.

	Fixed Effect				Random Effect			
Variables	Coefficient	Std. Error	T-Stat	p-Value	Coefficient	Std. Error	T-Stat	p-Value
Health Expenditure	0.4347	0.1183	3.67	0.000	0.4284	0.1190	3.6	0.000
Economic Growth	58.853	13.533	4.35	0.000	44.911	12.554	3.58	0.000
Population	71.887	12.736	5.64	0.000	72.051	12.923	5.58	0.000
Basic Sanitation	−4.415	1.0606	−4.16	0.000	−4.258	1.0396	−4.1	0.000
Clean Fuel Technologies	−8.577	1.4936	−5.74	0.000	−8.273	1.4802	−5.59	0.000
Constant	−775.0	320.65	−2.42	0.017	−456.6	308.21	−1.48	0.138
R^2	0.2783				R^2	0.3399		
Prob > F	0.0000				Prob > chi-sq	0.0000		
Hausman test Prob > chi2	0.0000							

Source: Estimations by the authors.

4.4.2. FMOLS and DOLS Results

Table 6 reports the estimation results of FMOLS and DOLS and indicates that though the magnitude of the coefficients is diverse, the signs are almost similar. There is a consensus that increased health expenditure crucially reduces maternal mortality. However, in South Asian countries, the outcomes are quite surprising, showing that a 1% rise in health expenditure led to an upsurge of the mortality rate by 1.95% for FMOLS and 0.16% for the DOLS estimator. The results in the case of economic growth were, as expected, significant and vigorous, and negatively affected maternal mortality. The outcomes show that an increase in GDP by 1% negatively influenced maternal mortality by 94% in FMOLS. The results in the case of population were expected and revealed that a 1% increase in population growth increased maternal mortality by 40% in the case of FMOLS and 10% in the case of DOLS. In the context of basic sanitation and clean fuel technologies, the results were found to be negatively significant: 7% and 11% in the case of FMOLS and 1.9% and 5.6% in the case of the DOLS estimator.

Table 6. FMOLS and DOLS long-run results.

Variables	FMOLS			DOLS		
	Coefficient	Std. Error	T-Stat	Coefficient	Std. Error	T-Stat
Health Expenditure	1.9592 ***	0.1910	10.255	0.1675 **	0.0803	2.0813
Economic Growth	−94.264 ***	26.727	−3.526	−18.22	13.392	−1.360
Population	40.640 ***	7.3916	5.4981	10.61 **	4.9330	2.1513
Basic Sanitation	−7.2306 **	3.2193	−2.245	−1.960 **	0.8554	−2.291
Clean Fuel Technologies	−11.581 ***	1.4931	−7.756	−5.691 ***	1.0351	−5.498

Note: ***, ** indicates significance at the 1% and 5% levels, respectively.

4.5. Discussion

This study contributes to the rising debate regarding maternal mortality and health expenditure. The data from eight South Asian countries over 2000–2017 is used for the FMOLS and DOLS estimation techniques. The study findings revealed that there is rise in the maternal mortality ratio in developing countries and it is less likely to obtain better health facilities. The results further imply that majority of females in developing countries belong to resource-poor settings, and even when the females reach a health center, they face innumerable hurdles such as inappropriate and inadequate care, and also other factors such as failures in the delivery of health services, a shortage of equipment or personnel, and—worst of all—faulty management. Despite increasing health expenditure in the sampled region, the unsatisfactory and meager quality of management and substandard health care services may dampen efforts to reduce maternal mortality. The result further suggests that though funds allocated for health care have increased in South Asian countries, the funds might be poorly distributed and mismanaged. Previous studies also found that a large share of the health budget is spent on pharmaceuticals, which reduces the share for other health programs [63]. Various other studies have shown contradictory findings regarding healthcare expenditure and health outcomes. For instance, Rana et al. [34], and Anand and Ravallion [64] revealed a positive link between health expenditure and the health sector's performance. Nketiah-Amponsah [38] showed that an increase in expenditure on health of 1% resulted in reducing maternal mortality by 0.35% and under-five mortality by 0.5%, and improved life expectancy by 0.06%.

Regarding infant mortality, the study revealed that total expenditure on health significantly reduced infant mortality in South Asian countries [65]. In contrast, Filmer, Pritchett, and Musgrove [24,40] found no association between these variables. Likewise, Zakir and Wunnava [66], and Nolte and Mckee [67] also found no association between health expenditure and health outcomes. Moreover, the health expenditure effects in the sampled region can additionally be attributed to the fact that there are culturally significant beliefs regarding prenatal care services. Most of the women in South Asian countries perceive prenatal care to be worse for their offspring in the womb. Thus, on the basis of empirical estimations, it was concluded that health and betterment in maternal health are not associated with increased health expenditure. Still, the value, cost, reliability, and acceptability of health facilities also matter.

Similarly, the positive coefficient of population growth revealed the expected finding that an increase in population also leads to increased maternal mortality. South Asia comprises a considerable proportion of the global population and includes some of the peak child and maternal mortality rates internationally. The reason could be that when households have more family members, they may be less likely to provide adequate nutrition and healthcare services [68,69]. Such an alarming growth rate could lead to absolute scarcity of food, shelter, clothing, and, more importantly, health services. The exploitation of resources becomes worse due to population pressure and creates many social problems. Due to the large population size, most health services are required to be shared, and a large portion of the health expenditure is spent on curative medicines, which mostly reach the people of urban areas. Moreover, the majority of the population in developing countries belongs to resource-poor settings and face hurdles in obtaining government of health care services due to the great mass of inhabitants, so maternal death prevention entails fundamental changes not only through increased health expenditure but also proper resource allocation and delivery of health services. People from resource-poor settings will have to be fought for to achieve equity and social justice [70–73].

Setting health expenditure and population growth aside, the significance of economic growth, access to sanitation, and clean fuel technologies in decreasing mortality rate cannot be disregarded. This suggests that maternal mortality can be reduced with an increase in income. Moreover, dietary preferences and lifestyle can also be enhanced with an increased share of income [74,75]. Many prior studies have stated a similar verdict and revealed that economic growth increases the average income, which intensifies accessibility and consumption of goods and services, and eventually improves peoples' health [76,77]. Increased income can help women seek experienced health experts and recognize the perils of not receiving satisfactory healthcare during pregnancy. The study of Pritchett and Summers [78] also showed that per capita GDP positively and significantly influenced health. Usually, in developing countries, people face financial constraints and cannot afford health expenses, so they prefer to spend on food commodities. Therefore, in this case, government spending can improve the health of poor people. Health is an essential human right, so economic growth can lessen maternal mortality in South Asian regions. Bloom, Canning, Kotschy, Prettner, and Schünemann [79] also showed that income positively affects health and improves life expectancy. The findings also showed that individual income plays a vital role in improving people's health in South Asian countries.

Further, several studies have shown a link between sanitation and improved health outcomes [80,81]. Many former researchers have considered access to water and sanitation for dropping the morbidity of diarrhea, and infants and under-five mortality [82–84]. The existing studies proposed that well-executed interventions in socioeconomic conditions, particularly in areas where primary settings are meager, can reduce maternal mortality. The results correspond well with those for sub-Saharan Africa found by Pickbourn and Ndikummana [85], where mortality rates and diarrhea morbidity were greater than in other regions. The individuals whose water and hygienic sanitation improved are among the lowest in the world. Thus, the findingsindicatethat investments in socioeconomic determinants such as sanitation and clean technologies are also likely to improve the maternal health status of the South Asian region.

5. Conclusions and Policy Recommendations

The mother's health is crucial for a child's cognitive growth and time spent caring for children. Given the rising maternal mortality rates in South Asian countries, reducing maternal mortality remains a noteworthy challenge for human development in South Asian countries. The current study unpacked the myth of increased health expenditure and reduced maternal mortality in South Asian countries by utilizing panel data from 2000–2017. The current study applied heterogeneous panel estimation techniques to examine the overlooked time-invariant heterogeneity and cross-dependency across countries.

The outcomes revealed that increased health expenditure and population growth were associated with an increased maternal mortality ratio. Health expenditure is a vital matter that can govern policy decisions at the national and international levels. Nevertheless, as indicated above, merely increasing health expenditure is insufficient; access, price, and consistency may influence the extent to which they are used, as well as, most importantly, their accessibility by deprived women. Thus, it is essential to go beyond simply expanding. Though increasing governments' health care spending is essential for reducing mortality and enhancing health outcomes, the results for the sample countries indicate that governments should support the accountability and transparency of the amounts allocated for maternal health care services. In the nonexistence of transparent financial support, the possibility of achieving the SDG in South Asian countries will be difficult. This evidence should support officials in the health sector in countries with rising rates of maternal mortality to lower the mortality rate, either directly by increasing access to better health amenities for underprivileged women or indirectly by increasing the financial capability of officials to allow sufficient funds to the maternal health sector in general and programs for the prevention of mortality in particular [86]. The government should allocate a larger portion of the health budget for maternal health. Health services should accompany a suitable allocation of funds for women's health at the community level. Women from resource-poor settings who are in utmost need of health advice and at the highest peril of death have limited health facilities. They can better avail these facilities if such services accessible adjacent to their home town, preferably in their neighborhoods. What is required is the placement of a number of health workers at the community level who are armed with proper training for maternal health care. This is possibly one of the best methods for taking advantage of resources. Additionally, our outcomes also focus on the significance of economic growth, and access to sanitation and clean fuel technologies in lowering maternal mortality. The results indicate that the governments of South Asian countries should improve the infrastructure and increase access to water and sanitation to end preventable deaths of mothers. The prevention of maternal deaths requires extensive socioeconomic modifications beyond the boundaries of the health care system alone, and these aspects can make childbirth and pregnancy safer naturally.

The findings of this study area new addition to the literature concerning health expenditure and maternal mortality in similar nations of South Asia. The findings show that each region has its challenges for health, and how sensibly expenditure on health is directed is the crux of the matter. Another area of action is improving the quality of health care facilities and competent people. This encompasses more than guaranteeing equipment availability; it also requires making the health services more publicly liable. The prevailing healthcare system adds to the rising maternal mortality due to meager and incompetent arrangements or meager administrative competencies. It also reflects the priorities established by an elitist system in which the powerless and poor do not count.

This study has also certain notable limitations. For example, the analysis only added a few control variables and ignored other potential confounding variables, such as the literacy rate, the physician to population ratio, and many other aspects of health. The reason for this was the high rate of missing data for these variables, which resulted in the exclusion of these variables from the model. Moreover, it is also likely that not all of the indicators of the World Bank databank are recounted each year. Thus the World Bank data might not remain consistent with the annually reported data of the Ministry of Health of each country. Further, the World Development data only give the data at the national level and, in this case, may not be helpful for showing the situation at the individual and community levels. Moreover, the present study utilized data from an South Asian panel, so the outcome may not be generalized to other developing countries. Regardless of these limitations, it is expected that the current study will provide impactful and meaningful results for policy makers to devise strategies, keeping in view the fundamental South Asian aspects warranted to reduce maternal mortality.

Author Contributions: Conceptualization, writing and methods, N.A.; supervision and funding acquisition, J.H.; review and editing, T.S.; review and analysis, H.S. All authors have read and agreed to the published version of the manuscript.

Funding: This research was funded by National Natural Science Foundation of China, grant number 713111025 and Postdoctoral Science Foundation of China, grant number 2021M691610.

Institutional Review Board Statement: Not applicable.

Informed Consent Statement: Not applicable.

Data Availability Statement: The data will be available on request.

Conflicts of Interest: The authors declare no conflict of interest.

References

1. Kiross, G.T.; Chojenta, C.; Barker, D.; Loxton, D. The effects of health expenditure on infant mortality in sub-Saharan Africa: Evidence from panel data analysis. *Health Econ. Rev.* **2020**, *10*, 5. [CrossRef] [PubMed]
2. Romer, D. *Advanced Macroeconomics*, 5th ed.; McGraw-Hill Education: New York, NY, USA, 2018.
3. Owusu, P.A.; Sarkodie, S.A.; Pedersen, P.A. Relationship between mortality and health care expenditure: Sustainable assessment of health care system. *PLoS ONE* **2021**, *16*, e0247413. [CrossRef] [PubMed]
4. How Maternal Mortality Has Been Reduced in South Asia. Available online: https://www.weforum.org/agenda/2015/01/how-maternal-mortality-has-been-reduced-in-south-asia/ (accessed on 15 January 2015).
5. Alkema, L.; Chou, D.; Hogan, D.; Zhang, S.; Moller, A.B.; Gemmill, A.; Fat, D.M.; Boerma, T.; Temmerman, M.; Mathers, C.; et al. Global, regional, and national levels and trends in maternal mortality between 1990 and 2015, with scenario-based projections to 2030: A systematic analysis by the UN Maternal Mortality Estimation Inter-Agency Group. *Lancet* **2016**, *387*, 462–474. [CrossRef]
6. Hill, K.; Johnson, P.; Singh, K.; Amuzu-Pharin, A.; Kharki, Y. Using census data to measure maternal mortality: A review of recent experience. Demographic. *Demogr. Res.* **2018**, *39*, 337–364. [CrossRef] [PubMed]
7. WHO. *Maternal Mortality*; WHO: Geneva, Switzerland, 2019.
8. Le Blanc, D. Towards Integration at Last? The Sustainable Development Goals as a Network of Targets. *Sustain. Dev.* **2015**, *23*, 176–187. [CrossRef]
9. Anyanwu, J.C.; Andrew, E.O.E. Health expenditures and health outcomes in Africa. *Afr. Dev. Rev.* **2009**, *21*, 400–433. [CrossRef]
10. WHO. *New Perspectives on Global Health Spending for Universal Health Coverage*; WHO: Geneva, Switzerland, 2017.
11. Si, R.; Lu, Q.; Aziz, N. Impact of COVID-19 on peoples' willingness to consume wild animals: Empirical insights from China. *One Health* **2021**, *12*, 100240. [CrossRef]
12. Si, R.; Yao, Y.; Zhang, X.; Lu, Q.; Aziz, N. Investigating the Links Between Vaccination Against COVID-19 and Public Attitudes Toward Protective Countermeasures: Implications for Public Health. *Front. Public Health* **2021**, *9*, 1040. [CrossRef]
13. WHO. *World Health Statistics*; WHO: Geneva, Switzerland, 2010.
14. Babazono, A.; Hillman, A. A comparison of international health outcomes and health care spending. *Int. J. Technol. Assess. Health Care* **1994**, *10*, 376–381. [CrossRef] [PubMed]
15. Berger, M.C.; Messer, J. Public financing of health expenditures, insurance, and health outcomes. *Appl. Econ.* **2002**, *34*, 2105–2113. [CrossRef]
16. Crémieux, P.Y.; Meilleur, M.C.; Ouellette, P.; Petit, P.; Zelder, M.; Potvin, K.C. Public and private pharmaceutical spending as determinants of health outcomes in Canada. *Health Econ.* **2005**, *14*, 107–116. [CrossRef] [PubMed]
17. Hitiris, T.; Posnett, J. The determinants and effects of health expenditure in developed countries. *J. Health Econ.* **1992**, *11*, 173–181. [CrossRef]
18. Zeynep, O. Determinants of health outcomes in industrialised countries: A pooled, cross-country, time-series analysis. *OECD Econ. Stud.* **2000**, *30*, 53–77.
19. Nixon, J.; Ulmann, P. The relationship between health care expenditure and health outcomes. Evidence and caveats for a causal link. *Eur. J. Health Econ.* **2006**, *7*, 7–18. [CrossRef]
20. Bhutta, Z.A.; Gupta, I.; De'silva, H.; Manandhar, D.; Awasthi, S.; Hossain, M.; Salam, M.A.; Lanka, S. Education and debate Maternal and child health: Is South Asia ready for change? Situational analysis. *BMJ Br. Med. J.* **2004**, *328*, 816–819. [CrossRef] [PubMed]
21. Nair, V.; Jayasinghe, S.; Behranwala, A.; Unger, J.; Ana, J. Health in South Asia. *Br. Med. J.* **2004**, *328*, 1497. [CrossRef] [PubMed]
22. Baldacci, E.; Clements, B.J.; Gupta, S.; Cui, Q. Social Spending, Human Capital, and Growth in Developing Countries. *World Dev.* **2008**, *36*, 1317–1341. [CrossRef]
23. Aid, the Incentive Regime, and Poverty Reduction. Available online: https://papers.ssrn.com/sol3/papers.cfm?abstract_id=597236 (accessed on 20 April 2016).
24. Filmer, D.; Pritchett, L. The impact of public spending on health: Does money matter? *Soc. Sci. Med.* **1999**, *49*, 1309–1323. [CrossRef]
25. Novignon, J.; Olakojo, S.A.; Nonvignon, J. The effects of public and private health care expenditure on health status in sub-Saharan Africa: New evidence from panel data analysis. *Health Econ. Rev.* **2012**, *2*, 22. [CrossRef]
26. Ssozi, J.; Amlani, S. The Effectiveness of Health Expenditure on the Proximate and Ultimate Goals of Healthcare in Sub-Saharan Africa. *World Dev.* **2015**, *76*, 165–179. [CrossRef]
27. Sen, A. Development as Freedom. In *The Globalization and Development Reader: Perspectives on Development and Global Change*; Oxford University Press: Oxford, UK, 1999.
28. Perkins, D.; Radelet, S.; Lindauer, D.; Block, S. *Economics of Development*; W.W. Norton & Company: New York, NY, USA, 2013.
29. Booth, D.; Cammack, D. *Governance for Development in Africa*; Zed Books: New York, NY, USA, 2013.
30. Betrán, A.P.; Wojdyla, D.; Posner, S.F.; Gülmezoglu, A.M. National estimates for maternal mortality: An analysis based on the WHO systematic review of maternal mortality and morbidity. *BMC Public Health* **2005**, *5*, 1–12. [CrossRef] [PubMed]
31. Chirowa, F.; Atwood, S.; Van der Putten, M. Gender inequality, health expenditure and maternal mortality in sub-Saharan Africa: A secondary data analysis. *Afr. J. Prim. Health Care Fam. Med.* **2013**, *5*, 471. [CrossRef]
32. Akca, N.; Sonmez, S.; Yilmaz, A. Determinants of health expenditure in OECD countries: A decision tree model. *Pak. J. Med. Sci.* **2017**, *33*, 1490–1494. [CrossRef] [PubMed]

33. Bhalotra, S. Spending to save? State health expenditure and infant mortality in India. *Health Econ.* **2007**, *16*, 911–928. [CrossRef] [PubMed]
34. Rana, R.H.; Alam, K.; Gow, J. Health Expenditure, Child and Maternal Mortality Nexus: A Comparative Global Analysis. *BMC Int. Health Hum. Rights* **2018**, *18*, 29. [CrossRef] [PubMed]
35. Aziz, N.; He, J.; Raza, A.; Sui, H.; Yue, W. Elucidating the Macroeconomic Determinants of Undernourishment in South Asian Countries: Building the Framework for Action. *Front. Public Health* **2021**, *9*, 696789. [CrossRef] [PubMed]
36. Aldogan, M.; Austill, A.D.; Kocakülâh, M.C. The excellence of activity-based costing in cost calculation: Case study of a private hospital in Turkey. *J. Health Care Financ.* **2014**, *41*, 1–27.
37. Bokhari, F.; Gai, Y.; Gottret, P. Government health expenditures and health outcomes. *Health Econ.* **2007**, *16*, 257–273. [CrossRef]
38. Nketiah-Amponsah, E. The Impact of Health Expenditures on Health Outcomes in Sub-Saharan Africa. *J. Dev. Soc.* **2019**, *35*, 134–152. [CrossRef]
39. Arthur, E.; Oaikhenan, H.E. The effects of health expenditure on health outcomes in Sub-Saharan Africa (SSA). *Afr. Dev. Rev.* **2017**, *29*, 524–525. [CrossRef]
40. Musgrove, P. Public and private roles in health: Theory and financing patterns. In *HNP Discussion Paper Series*; The World Bank: Washington, DC, USA, 1996.
41. Ashiabi, N.; Nketiah-Amponsah, E.; Senadza, B. The Effect of Health Expenditure on Selected Maternal and Child Health Outcomes in Sub Saharan Africa. *Int. J. Soc. Econ.* **2016**, *43*, 1386–1399.
42. Bradley, E.H.; Elkins, B.R.; Herrin, J.; Elbel, B. Health and social services expenditures: Associations with health outcomes. *BMJ Qual. Saf.* **2011**, *20*, 826–831. [CrossRef] [PubMed]
43. Self, S.; Grabowski, R. How effective is public health expenditure in improving overall health? A cross-country analysis. *Appl. Econ.* **2003**, *35*, 835–845. [CrossRef]
44. Gupta, M.; Verhoeven, M.; Tiongson, M. Public spending on health care and poor. *Health Econ.* **2003**, *12*, 685–696. [CrossRef] [PubMed]
45. Gupta, S.; Verhoeven, M.; Tiongson, E.R. The effectiveness of government spending on education and health care in developing and transition economies. *Eur. J. Polit. Econ.* **2002**, *18*, 717–737. [CrossRef]
46. Ullah, I.; Ullah, A.; Ali, S.; Poulova, P.; Akbar, A.; Shah, M.H.; Rehman, A.; Zeeshan, M.; Afridi, F. Public Health Expenditures and Health Outcomes in Pakistan: Evidence from Quantile Autoregressive Distributed Lag Model. *Risk Manag. Healthc. Policy* **2021**, *14*, 3893. [CrossRef]
47. Yaqub, J.; Ojapinwa, T.; Yussuff, R. Public health expenditure and health outcome in Nigeria: The impact of governance. *Eur. Sci. J.* **2012**, *8*, 198–201.
48. Aziz, N.; Sharif, A.; Raza, A.; Rong, K. Revisiting the role of forestry, agriculture, and renewable energy in testing environment Kuznets curve in Pakistan: Evidence from Quantile ARDL approach. *Environ. Sci. Pollut. Res.* **2020**, *27*, 10115–10128. [CrossRef]
49. Granger, C.W.J.; Newbold, P. Spurious regressions in econometrics. *J. Econ.* **1974**, *2*, 111–120. [CrossRef]
50. Im, K.S.; Pesaran, M.H.; Shin, Y. Testing for Unit Roots in Heterogeneous Panels. *J. Econ.* **2003**, *115*, 53–74. [CrossRef]
51. Khan, Z.A.; Koondhar, M.A.; Aziz, N.; Ali, U.; Tianjun, L. Revisiting the effects of relevant factors on Pakistan's agricultural products export. *Agric. Econ.* **2020**, *66*, 527–541.
52. Ahmed, M.; Aziz, N.; Tan, Z.; Yang, S.; Raza, K.; Kong, R. Green growth of cereal food production under the constraints of agricultural carbon emissions: A new insights from ARDL and VECM models. *Sustain. Energy Technol. Assess.* **2021**, *47*, 101452.
53. Si, R.; Aziz, N.; Raza, A. Short and long-run causal effects of agriculture, forestry, and other land use on greenhouse gas emissions: Evidence from China using VECM approach. *Environ. Sci. Pollut. Res.* **2021**, 1–12. [CrossRef]
54. Pesaran, M.H. A simple panel unit root test in the presence of cross-section dependence. *J. Appl. Econom.* **2007**, *22*, 265–312. [CrossRef]
55. Aziz, N.; Sharif, A.; Raza, A.; Jermsittiparsert, K. The role of natural resources, globalization, and renewable energy in testing the EKC hypothesis in MINT countries: New evidence from Method of Moments Quantile Regression approach. *Environ. Sci. Pollut. Res.* **2020**, *28*, 13454–13468. [CrossRef]
56. Aziz, N.; Mihardjo, L.W.W.; Sharif, A.; Jermsittiparsert, K. The role of tourism and renewable energy in testing the environmental Kuznets curve in the BRICS countries: Fresh evidence from methods of moments quantile regression. *Environ. Sci. Pollut. Res.* **2020**, *27*, 39427–39441. [CrossRef]
57. Pedroni, P. Panel cointegration: Asymptotic and finite sample properties of pooled time series tests with an application to the PPP hypothesis. *Econ. Theory* **2004**, *20*, 597–625. [CrossRef]
58. Raza, A.; Sui, H.; Jermsittiparsert, K.; Zukiewicz-Sobczak, W.; Sobczak, P. Trade liberalization and environmental performance index: Mediation role of climate change performance and greenfield investment. *Sustainability* **2021**, *13*, 9734. [CrossRef]
59. Kao, C.; Chiang, M.H. On the estimation and inference of a cointegrated regression in panel data. In *Advances in Econometrics*; Baltagi, B.H., Fomby, T.B., Eds.; Emarald: Bradford, UK, 2000; pp. 179–222.
60. Hausman, J.A. Specification Tests in Econometrics. *Econometrica* **1978**, *46*, 1251–1271. [CrossRef]
61. Haseeb, A.; Xia, E.; Baloch, M.A.; Abbas, K. Financial development, globalization, and CO_2 emission in the presence of EKC: Evidence from BRICS countries. *Environ. Sci. Pollut. Res.* **2018**, *25*, 31283–31296. [CrossRef]
62. Dogan, B.; Madaleno, M.; Tiwari, A.K.; Hammoudeh, S. Impacts of export quality on environmental degradation: Does income matter? *Environ. Sci. Pollut. Res.* **2020**, *27*, 13735–13772. [CrossRef] [PubMed]

63. Fokunang, C.N.; Ndikum, V.; Tabi, O.Y.; Jiofack, R.B.; Ngameni, B.; Guedje, N.M.; Tembe-Fokunang, E.A.; Tomkins, P.; Barkwan, S.; Kechia, F.; et al. Traditional medicine: Past, present and future research and development prospects and integration in the National Health System of Cameroon. *Afr. J. Tradit. Complement. Altern. Med.* **2011**, *8*, 284–295. [CrossRef] [PubMed]
64. Anand, S.; Ravallion, M. Human Development in Poor Countries: On the Role of Private Incomes and Public Services. *J. Econ. Perspect.* **1993**, *7*, 133–150. [CrossRef]
65. Rahman, M.; Khanam, R.; Rahman, M. Health care expenditure and health outcome nexus: New evidence from the SAARC-ASEAN region. *Glob. Health* **2018**, *14*, 113. [CrossRef] [PubMed]
66. Zakir, M.; Wunnava, P. Factors affecting infant mortality rates: Evidence from cross-sectional data. *Appl. Econ. Lett.* **1999**, *6*, 271–273. [CrossRef]
67. Nolte, E.; McKee, M. *Does Health Care Save Lives? Avoidable Mortality Revisited*; The Nuffield Trust: London, UK, 2004.
68. Bhandari, A. Women's status and global food security: An overview. *Sociol. Compass* **2017**, *11*, e12479. [CrossRef]
69. Fatema, K.; Lariscy, J.T. Mass Media Exposure and Maternal Healthcare Utilization in South Asia. *SSM Popul. Health* **2020**, *11*, 100614. [CrossRef] [PubMed]
70. Aziz, N.; Ren, Y.; Rong, K.; Zhou, J. Women's empowerment in agriculture and household food insecurity: Evidence from Azad Jammu & Kashmir (AJK), Pakistan. *Land Use Policy* **2021**, *102*, 105249.
71. Aziz, N.; Nisar, Q.A.; Koondhar, M.A.; Meo, M.S.; Rong, K. Analyzing the women's empowerment and food security nexus in rural areas of Azad Jammu & Kashmir, Pakistan: By giving consideration to sense of land entitlement and infrastructural facilities. *Land Use Policy* **2020**, *94*, 104529.
72. Wei, W.; Sarker, T.; Zukiewicz-Sobczak, W.; Roy, R.; Alam, G.M.; Rabbany, M.; Hossain, M.S.; Aziz, N. The Influence of Women's Empowerment on Poverty Reduction in the Rural Areas of Bangladesh: Focus on Health, Education and Living Standard. *Int. J. Environ. Res. Public Health* **2021**, *18*, 6909. [CrossRef]
73. Si, R.; Lu, Q.; Aziz, N. Does the stability of farmland rental contract & conservation tillage adoption improve family welfare? Empirical insights from Zhangye, China. *Land Use Policy* **2021**, *107*, 105486.
74. Joshi, P.K.; Parappurathu, S.; Kumar, P. Dynamics of food consumption and nutrient insecurity in India. *Proc. Indian Natl. Sci. Acad.* **2016**, *82*, 1587–1599.
75. Kumar, A.K.S. Why are levels of child malnutrition not improving? *Econ. Polit. Wkly.* **2007**, *42*, 1337–1345.
76. Bhutta, Z. *Pakistan National Nutrition Survey 2011*; UNICEF Pakistan: Islamabad, Pakistan, 2012; pp. 1–84.
77. Headey, D.; Ecker, O. Rethinking the measurement of food security: From first principles to best practice. *Food Secur.* **2013**, *5*, 327–343. [CrossRef]
78. Pritchett, L.; Summers, L. Wealthier is Healthier. *J. Hum. Resour.* **1996**, *31*, 841–868. [CrossRef]
79. Bloom, D.E.; Canning, D.; Kotschy, R.; Prettner, K.; Schünemann, J.J. *Health and Economic Growth: Reconciling the Micro and Macro Evidence (No. w26003)*; National Bureau of Economic Research: Cambridge, MA, USA, 2019.
80. Botting, M.J.; Porbeni, E.O.; Joffres, M.R.; Johnston, B.C.; Black, R.E.; Mills, E.J. Water and sanitation infrastructure for health: The impact of foreign aid. *Glob. Health* **2010**, *6*, 12. [CrossRef]
81. Wayland, J. *A Drop in the Bucket? The Effectiveness of Foreign Aid in the Water, Sanitation, and Hygiene (WASH) Sector*; American University: Washington, DC, USA, 2013.
82. Esrey, S.A.; Habicht, J.P.; Latham, M.C.; Sisler, D.G.; Casella, G. Drinking water source, diarrheal morbidity, and child growth in villages with both traditional and improved water supplies in rural Lesotho, southern Africa. *Am. J. Public Health* **1988**, *78*, 1451–1455. [CrossRef]
83. Fewtrell, L.; Kaufmann, R.B.; Kay, D.; Enanoria, W.; Haller, L.; Colford, J.M. Water, sanitation, and hygiene interventions to reduce diarrhoea in less developed countries: A systematic review and meta-analysis. *Lancet Infect. Dis.* **2005**, *5*, 42–52. [CrossRef]
84. Fink, G.; Günther, I.; Hill, K. The effect of water and sanitation on child health: Evidence from the demographic and health surveys 1986–2007. *Int. J. Epidemiol.* **2011**, *40*, 1196–1204. [CrossRef]
85. Pickbourn, L.; Ndikumana, L. Does Health Aid Reduce Infant and Child Mortality from Diarrhoea in Sub-Saharan Africa? *J. Dev Stud.* **2019**, *55*, 2212–2231. [CrossRef]
86. Irfan, M. Poverty in South Asia. *Pak. Dev. Rev.* **2000**, *39*, 1141–1151. [CrossRef]

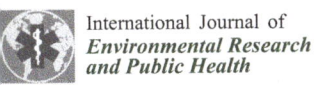

Article

The Impact of the SARS-CoV-19 Pandemic on the Global Gross Domestic Product

Piotr Korneta * and Katarzyna Rostek

Faculty of Management, Warsaw University of Technology, 02-524 Warszawa, Poland; katarzyna.rostek@pw.edu.pl
* Correspondence: piotr.korneta@pw.edu.pl

Abstract: The rapid, unexpected, and large-scale expansion of the SARS-CoV-19 pandemic has led to a global health and economy crisis. However, although the crisis itself is a worldwide phenomenon, there have been considerable differences between respective countries in terms of SARS-CoV-19 morbidities and fatalities as well as the GDP impact. The object of this paper was to study the influence of the SARS-CoV-19 pandemic on global gross domestic product. We analyzed data relating to 176 countries in the 11-month period from February 2020 to December 2020. We employed SARS-CoV-19 morbidity and fatality rates reported by different countries as proxies for the development of the pandemic. The analysis employed in our study was based on moving median and quartiles, Kendall tau-b coefficients, and multi-segment piecewise-linear approximation with Theil–Sen trend lines. In the study, we empirically confirmed and measured the negative impact of the SARS-CoV-19 pandemic on the respective national economies. The relationship between the pandemic and the economy is not uniform and depends on the extent of the pandemic's development. The more intense the pandemic, the more adaptive the economies of specific countries become.

Keywords: SARS-CoV-19; pandemic; crisis management; GDP; gross domestic product; multi-segment Theil–Sen

Citation: Korneta, P.; Rostek, K. The Impact of the SARS-CoV-19 Pandemic on the Global Gross Domestic Product. *Int. J. Environ. Res. Public Health* **2021**, *18*, 5246. https://doi.org/10.3390/ijerph18105246

Academic Editors: Dimitris Zavras and Paul B. Tchounwou

Received: 29 March 2021
Accepted: 8 May 2021
Published: 14 May 2021

Publisher's Note: MDPI stays neutral with regard to jurisdictional claims in published maps and institutional affiliations.

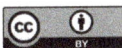

Copyright: © 2021 by the authors. Licensee MDPI, Basel, Switzerland. This article is an open access article distributed under the terms and conditions of the Creative Commons Attribution (CC BY) license (https://creativecommons.org/licenses/by/4.0/).

1. Introduction

The SARS-CoV-19 pandemic has rapidly spread around the world and has posed significant threats to public health, as well as social and economic standing of many countries. The unexpected onset of the global health crisis caused many scholars to change their research domains towards pandemic-related areas. A significant number of studies have already been conducted in terms of the medical aspects of the coronavirus-2019, including the understanding of coronavirus-2019 pathogenic mechanism [1], its transmission routes [2], and different patterns of symptom development [3–6]. Several researchers have already identified obesity; ageing; and comorbidities such as cardiovascular diseases, cancers, and diabetes as risk factors in SARS-CoV-19 patients [7–10]. The SARS-CoV-19 fatality rate is estimated at around 4% of infected patients but varies between respective countries from 0 to 20% [11,12]. Such a large range of fatality discrepancies might result from different demographic, economic, and political variables specific to different countries [12]. Finally, it is noteworthy that thanks to the extensive work performed by scientists and pharmaceutical companies, the vaccination process is already underway around the world [13].

As research in the healthcare perspective is starting to yield significant effects, it is now time to focus our attention on the economy and the significant consequences the pandemic has had in this context. A number of scholars have already studied the impact of the global health crisis on financial markets whose sharp fluctuations during the pandemic have led to confusion and uncertainty among investors [14–16]. Results reported by other researchers indicate that the SARS-CoV-19 pandemic has changed consumer behaviors [17]. The first papers on the impact of the SARS-CoV-19 pandemic on the condition of the healthcare industry have also already appeared. It has been claimed that the pandemic has had both positive and negative effects on respective branches of the healthcare industry, but the latter are nonetheless predominant [18]. The negative impact of the pandemic on the economies of various countries has already been acknowledged in both local [19–21] and global terms [22–24]. The first gross domestic product (GDP) forecasts have also been already provided [25]. It is believed that the decline of global economy stems from two primary factors [23]. The first relates to the various forms of isolation imposed by the governments, such as social distancing, shutdowns of events and corporate offices, and lockdowns. The second is the uncertainty about how bad the situation can get. According to information provided by the International Monetary Fund (IMF), the global gross domestic product is estimated to have declined by around -3.5%. We should note, however, that the data provided by IMF indicate significant discrepancies between economic effects observed in respective countries [26]. Such differences may result from two major factors. Firstly, the degree to which the economies of specific countries have been affected by the pandemic. This can be measured relative to SARS-CoV-19 morbidity and fatality rates. The second factor relates to the various restrictions introduced in particular countries [27,28], availability of public aid [29,30], and interconnections developed between the economies of various countries during the pandemic [31,32].

Since 2020 is already over and real data reflecting changes in the global GDP are now available, scientists can commence studies in this area. The objective of our paper was to consider the impact of the SARS-CoV-19 pandemic on national economies. We selected SARS-CoV-19 morbidity and fatality rates as viable proxies of pandemic development in specific countries, while GDP fluctuations served as a measure of the economy's condition. In order to achieve the objective of the paper, we formulated the following two hypotheses:

H1: *There is a negative correlation between the SARS-CoV-19 pandemic development and GDP growth.*

H2: *The relationship between the pandemic and GDP fluctuations is not a linear one.*

The first of the formulated hypotheses is based on the postulates of other scholars [22–24] who reported on the negative effects of the pandemic on the global economy. The second results from the assumption that the actions taken by governments might affect the severity of the impact that the pandemic has had on the economies of respective countries [27–32]. To our best knowledge, this study is the first to explore correlations between SARS-CoV-19 morbidity and fatality rates on the one hand, and the economies of specific countries on the other. Notably, the objective of this paper was not to analyze the sources of morbidity and fatality rates discrepancies between respective countries, but rather to study how such differences affect their economies.

The paper analyzed data relating to 176 countries from six different continents in a 11-month period from February 2020 to December 2020. Because of significant data dispersion, we had to use robust statistical methods in our analysis. We employed moving medians and quartiles to determine the form of the relationship between the degree of pandemic development and the change of gross domestic product in specific countries, in their respective ranges. We employed the Kendall tau-b to determine the significance of correlations. Next, we calculated multi-segment Theil–Sen linear approximations to fit the obtained relations.

The rest of the paper is structured in the following way: In Section 2, research methods and their different components such as the database and sample of observations, variables, and design of the study are provided. Section 3 presents results derived from empirical data. Section 4 provides the discussion and indicates limitations of our study. Finally, we provide conclusions and implications.

2. Materials and Methods

2.1. Database and Sample of Observations

The data used in this study were obtained from two well recognized sources: the open access database "Our World in Data" [33] and the "International Monetary Fund" [26]. From the latter, information on the change of gross domestic product in 2020 as of 7 March 2021 as compared to 2019 by different countries was obtained. The "Our World in Data" database compiles official information relating to the SARS-CoV-19 pandemic, including the number of reported new SARS-CoV-19 cases and deaths and PCR testing around the world [33]. From this database, accessed on March 7, 2021, we obtained 59,787 daily observations relating to 176 countries in a 11-month period from February 2020 to December 2020. Since this database provided no information regarding other countries, we were not in a position to analyze all the countries worldwide. We aggregated the obtained daily observations into 176 yearly observations. As a result, the studied figures comprised 82.5 million and 1.8 million diagnosed SARS-CoV-19 cases and reported deaths, respectively, and related the same to the world population of 7.6 billion. Table 1 presents the breakdown of observation samples used in the study, divided by continent, with the numbers of SARS-COV-19 new cases and deaths reported and the respective number of countries considered.

Table 1. Description of the study sample by continent.

Continent	New Cases	Deaths	Population	Number of Countries
Africa	2,753,352	65,360	1,333,308,499	53
Asia	19,659,852	334,364	4,518,306,798	41
Europe	23,796,060	545,361	748,015,042	42
North America	23,013,002	512,367	575,845,728	20
Australia and Oceania	31,440	945	41,417,217	8
South America	13,194,159	362,651	430,457,607	12
Total	82,447,865	1,821,048	7,647,350,891	176

2.2. Variables

The variables used in this study, their acronyms, number of observations, and descriptions of calculations are presented in Table 2. The first two of the studied variables are SARS-CoV-19 case rate (CCR) and SARS-CoV-19 fatality rate (CFR). We calculated these variables for each country. Since the populations of respective countries differ, we divided newly diagnosed SARS-CoV-19 cases and deaths per 1000 residents. A similar approach has already been used by other scholars [34]. We employed CCR and CFR variables to measure the pandemic. The last of the variables selected for the study was the change in gross domestic product relative increase (GDP). This ratio indicates the market value of all goods and services produced in a specific period. Hence, the change in GDP relative increase is a good proxy of the change in the world's economy.

Table 2. Variables used in the study.

Acronym	Variable	Description
CCR	SARS-CoV-19 cases rate	New SARS-CoV-19 cases reported in a country per 1000 of the population of the country
CFR	SARS-CoV-19 fatality rate	New SARS-CoV-19 deaths reported in a country per 1000 of the population of the country
GDP	Gross domestic product	The difference of gross domestic product in 2020 and 2019, divided by gross domestic product in 2019, calculated for each country

2.3. Design and Data Analysis

Once the variables had been selected, we analyzed descriptive statistics. In the next step of the study, we plotted the relationships between respective variables on graphs.

Visualization of the contemplated relationships was achieved by employing the moving median and first and third quartiles in order to determine different correlations between the considered variables in different ranges [35]. We calculated the median values for both variables in a moving window containing data from 50 observations. The division of our relations into segments helped us to identify ranges of pandemic intensity with different effects on the GDP. In practice, it is important to identify what pandemic intensity has a dominant effect on the change of global gross domestic product. The approach of dividing infected individuals according to the 80/20 rule has been suggested to explain transmission events during the SARS epidemic [36]. After identifying the relation between variables in different ranges, we calculated the Kendall tau-b [37–39] coefficients. Kendall tau-b rank correlation coefficient is widely used as a distribution-free measure of the strength and direction of association that exists between two variables. In order to analyze data using Kendall tau-b, one should measure two variables on an ordinal or continuous scale (interval or ratio variables), and data should follow a monotonic relationship. We calculated Kendall tau-b rank correlation coefficient in intervals where monotonic relationship was indicated by the moving median and quartiles. Our variables thus satisfy the requirements of Kendall tau-b, which can be used to determine the strength and direction of the association [40–43]. The values of Kendall's rank correlation coefficient around 0.1 are typically obtained in the analysis of meteorological data, where they vary between 0.012 and 0.159 [44]. Decision about the statistical significance was made using empirical significance level (p-value) compared to $\alpha = 5\%$. We used one-tailed Mann–Kendall test [41,42].

Next, we applied the multi-segment linear regression with the Theil–Sen robust lines to characterize different relations between our independent and dependent variables in different ranges [45]. This regression model was selected because it is resistant to the effects of outliers and non-normality in residuals. The multi-segment model is the most suitable choice if more than one regression relation is necessary to characterize different relations that may occur in different regimes of explanatory variables. The nonparametric estimate of the slope of the line, identified as the Theil–Sen (or Kendall–Theil or Sen) slope in the literature, is calculated as the median of all possible pairwise slopes between points [45–49]. The line intercept was calculated by using the median slope and the median of the independent and dependent variables [47,49]. The multi-segment Theil–Sen regression technique was comprehensively described by Granato [50] and has been used by other researchers [50,51]. Furthermore, the Theil–Sen estimator is considerably more accurate than non-robust simple linear regression, especially for heteroskedastic and skewed data. It should also be noted that the Theil–Sen estimator provides better results than the non-robust least squares method, even for normally distributed data [47]. Finally, we obtained multi-segment piecewise-linear approximation to the studied relationships between considered variables. The Theil–Sen procedure has already been used in other studies in the fields of economy [51] and health [52,53].

3. Results

Presented in Table 3 are the descriptive statistics of the variables used in this study, calculated for each country in the relevant period. On average, 15.749 (CCR) per 1000 persons were infected with SARS-CoV-19 in 2020, and 76.819 was the maximum. Great differences in mortality between respective countries are revealed in the min, median, and max values of the SARS-CoV-19 fatality rate (CFR). The highest mortality of 1.739 deaths per 1000 people was reported in San Marino, closely followed by Belgium, where the fatality rate in the studied period reached 1.685 per 1000. The (arithmetic) mean of the GDP fluctuation was -5.694 (%) and was negative in 153 countries, with only 23 states reporting positive values.

Table 3. Descriptive statistics.

Variable	Mean	SD	Median	Min	Max	Skewness	Kurtosis
CCR	15.749	18.874	7.263	0.003	76.819	1.239	0.659
CFR	0.295	0.392	0.083	0	1.739	1.42	1.181
GDP	−5.694	7.181	−5.1	−66.7	26.2	−3.271	30.415

Table 4 presents the results of statistical tests for the relationships between CCR, CFR, and GDP in two identified ranges for each variable. We showed the Kendall tau-b values with their p-values (one side). In the selected ranges, we performed linear approximation of the studied relationships using the Theil–Sen procedure. The obtained values of Theil–Sen slopes (m) and intercepts (b) are given in Table 4. This two-segment piecewise-linear approximation well describes the considered relationships in the two identified ranges.

Table 4. Results of statistical tests using the Kendall tau-b of relations between CCR, CFR, and the change in GDP relative increase (GDP) with Theil–Sen slopes (m) and intercepts (b) of trend lines approximating these relations.

Variable	Range	Kendall Tau-B	p	Theil–Sen m Slope	Theil–Sen b Intercept
		Gross Domestic Product (GDP)			
CCR	<7	−0.1274	0.0383	−0.4851	−2.7409
CCR	>7	−0.0339	0.3231	−0.008	−6.2276
		Gross Domestic Product (GDP)			
CFR	<0.2	−0.1401	0.0161	−12.9928	−3.2868
CFR	>0.2	−0.1421	0.0456	−1.3475	−5.8339

The scatterplot in Figure 1 was fitted with the multi-segment Theil–Sen regression model. The number of segments, coefficient of regression lines, and the convergence points were calculated and adjusted according to the procedure described by Granato [50]. The two-line model, without discontinuity plotted on the scatterplot, was a good fit. One can notice that this relationship differs considerably for the CCR variable up to 7 and above. It can thus be well represented by two straight lines, i.e., by two-segment approximation. The Kendall tau-b for the first of approximated lines (CCR < 7) amounts to −0.1274, which confirms the negative trend. The low p-value, below 0.05, confirms that these results are statistically significant. The slope of the approximated line is −0.4851. Such a high value of the approximated slope indicates that the GDP is very sensitive to any changes of the CCR variable in the studied range. The relationship between GDP and CCR in the second of the identified ranges (CCR > 7) was statistically insignificant as the p-value was above 0.3. These results are endorsed by the Theil–Sen trend line, which was flat (the slope was 0.008), indicating that there was no relationships between CCR and GDP in the second range, i.e., for CCR above 7.

Figure 2 shows the relation between SARS-CoV-19 fatality rate (CFR) and GDP. As can be seen, the contemplated relationship can be divided into two different ranges and approximated with two straight trend lines. The first range comprised CFR observations below 0.2. Here, the Theil–Sen trend line (m = −12.9928) was sharp and fast declining. The relationship between CFR and GDP was negative. The Kendall tau-b coefficient was −0.1401. This confirmed that this relationship was negative and statistically significant (p-values below 0.05). The relation between CFR and GDP for GDP> 0.2 was well fitted by the Theil–Sen straight line with the slope of m = - 1.3475 and the intercept b = −5.8339. This result was endorsed by the Kendall tau-b, which was −0.1421. The results are statistically significant with p = 0.0456.

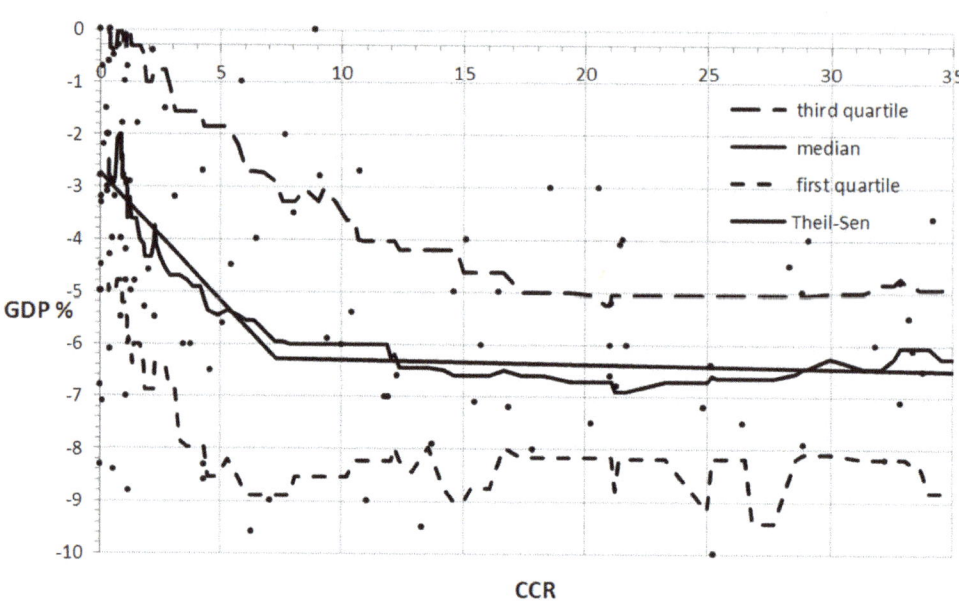

Figure 1. The relation between CCR and GDP with the moving median, first and third quartiles, and two-segment linear Theil–Sen approximation.

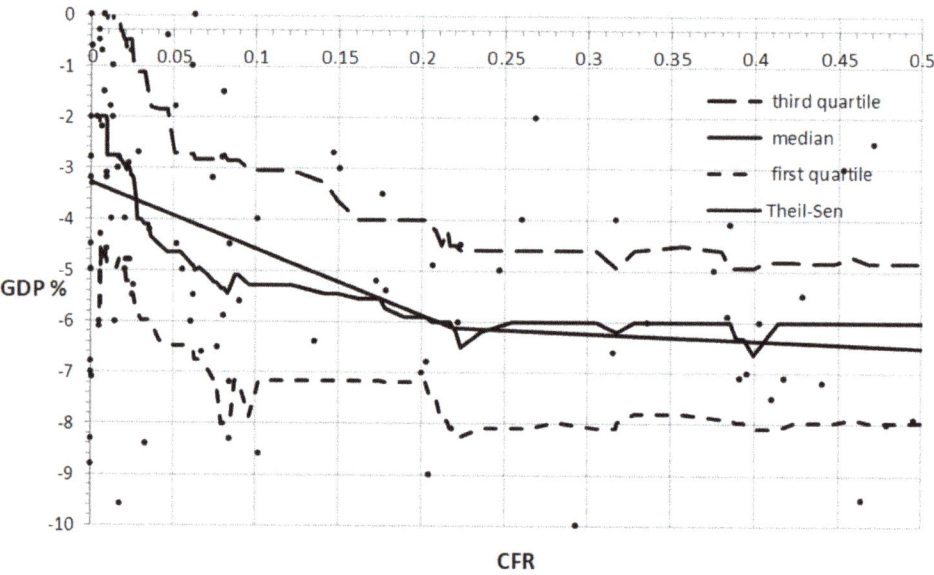

Figure 2. The relation between CCR and GDP with the moving median, first and third quartiles, and two-segment linear Theil–Sen approximation.

4. Discussion

As already discussed and confirmed in the literature, the global health crisis caused by coronavirus-2019 has negatively affected the world economy. This negative impact has already been discussed at the levels of both local economies [19–21] and globally [22–24]. Several researchers have provided the very first approximations of the global economic costs of the SARS-CoV-19 pandemic, which might total at around USD 2.7 trillion [54]. Other scholars note that the negative impact of SARS-CoV-19 on the economies has not only caused GDPs to decline but has also increased the importing and exporting costs. At the same time, it must be added that this negative impact varies greatly between respective economy sectors, with tourism and domestic services losing the most, and natural resources and agriculture being only negligibly affected. Reports also confirm considerable differences between individual countries [55]. König and Winkler provided the initial empirical evidence on the relationship between the SARS-CoV-19 pandemic and the economic crisis. Their research was based on data from the first three quarters of 2020 relating to 42 countries, using simple ordinary least squares and panel fixed effects regressions. They explained the link between the pandemic and the GDP by highlighting two major factors. The first results from restrictive measures imposed by the governments of different countries. Their results indicate that governmental restrictions lowered the GDP growth in the same quarter, with noticeable improvement in GDP dynamics in the following one. The second link between the pandemic and GDP is the health risk that leads to voluntary social distancing, which, again, lowers the GDP. They measured the health risk on the basis of fatality rates and provided initial empirical evidence suggesting that high fatality rates contribute significantly to the negative growth rates [56]. In comparison with the study by König and Winkler, our research was based on a considerably larger sample (176 versus 42 countries), related to a longer period (full year instead of three quarters), and employed a different econometric approach and databases. Our results are aligned to postulates of other scholars and empirically confirm the negative impact of the SARS-CoV-19 pandemic on the global economy. In our calculations, Kendall tau-B coefficients confirmed the negative correlation between SARS-CoV-19 fatality rates and changes in the GDP relative increase. The very low p-value (below 0.05) indicates that the obtained results are robust. We also identified a negative relationship between SARS-CoV-19 infections rate (CCR variable) and the decrease of gross domestic product. This relationship, however, was only significant for CCR values below 7, i.e., up to 7 infections per 1000 people in 2020. Therefore, the first of the formulated hypotheses, stating that *there is a negative correlation between the SARS-CoV-19 pandemic and GDP growth*, has been corroborated.

The onset of the SARS-CoV-19 pandemic and efforts aimed at limiting its further development were approached differently by decision makers in various countries. The tools most frequently employed against the pandemic included isolation, quarantine, and lockdown. In general, the more rapidly the pandemic developed in a country, the more severe restrictions were introduced by the policymakers [27,28]. SARS-CoV-19 tests have also been widely used in an effort to halt the pandemic development. Several researchers have claimed that the expansion of the pandemic can be limited by increasing the testing rate [57]. However, high costs and financial restraints caused the countries employ different testing strategies [34,58,59]. The third tool employed to reduce the negative impact of the SARS-CoV-19 pandemic on the economy entailed government programs supporting the companies and citizens during periods of isolation and lockdowns [29,30]. Finally, several scholars have also noted the development of interactions between different countries during the pandemic [31,32]. Assuming that all the aforementioned actions might affect the expansion of the pandemic, we formulated the second hypothesis, namely, that *the correlation between the pandemic and GDP fluctuations is not a linear one*. We estimated that the relationship between SARS-CoV-19 fatality rates and changes in the gross domestic product relative increase can be well fitted with two straight lines, with slopes of -12.9928 and -1.3475 and in the ranges below 0.2 deaths per 1000 (or up to 200 per 1 million) of the population and above the same, respectively. This shows that the GDP falls by 0.013 percentage points with each death per 1 million people. Once the threshold of 0.2 deaths per 1000 people is exceeded, however, the gross domestic product becomes less sensitive to new SARS-CoV-19 deaths and falls by only 0.0013 percentage points with each new death per 1 million people. The relationship between gross domestic product and SARS-CoV-19 morbidity is similar, with the threshold of 7 new infections per 1000 people. Since the slope of the approximated line was −0.4851, each new infected person per 1000 residents reduced the GDP by 0.4581. Once the threshold of seven new infections is exceeded, the contemplated relationship becomes statistically insignificant (very high p-value Kendall tau-B). Hence, the GDP change is considerably more sensitive to new SARS-CoV-19 deaths than to infections. The two distinctly identified ranges in the relationship between GDP and SARS-CoV-19 morbidity and fatality rates indicate that there is a threshold over which countries manage to adapt to the pandemic. Due to this observation, our second hypothesis must be accepted. The world economic crisis triggered by the SARS-CoV-19 pandemic is a complex and multifaceted issue and differs from other economic slowdowns in recent decades. This is because, additionally to the burden on the healthcare systems, the pandemic has directly resulted in the premature deaths of employees, large-scale workplace absenteeism, productivity reduction, negative supply shocks, manufacturing activity slowdown, global supply chain disruptions, and decimation of the tourism industry [60]. Given the complexity of this crisis, a fraction of researchers employed a high-level, comprehensive approach in their studies, while most of the others focused only on selected economy issues. Al-Thaqeb et al. claim economic policy uncertainty plays a key role in understanding the current crisis. They indicate that high uncertainty in terms of economic policy is associated with adverse effects on households, corporations, and governments, which tend to delay financial decisions due to the same reasons. This leads to lower consumption, lower loan issuance, fewer investments, and higher unemployment. They also note that the effects of political and regulatory uncertainty extend even to the commodity and crypto-currency markets. [61]. Song and Zhou also acknowledge the fact that uncertainty plays a key role in the current economic crisis. They draw attention to high periods prior to SARS-CoV-2, resulting primarily from Chinese economy problems and slow recent growth; synchronized global economy slowdown; de-globalization; and unfavorable macroeconomic settings, including deflation [62]. Stiifanić et al. studied the impact of the SARS-CoV-19 pandemic on crude oil prices and selected stock indexes: DJI, S&P 500, and NASDAQ. They employed new SARS-CoV-19 infections as the independent variable. In terms of crude oil prices, they identified uncertainty and supply shock increase in the global stocks of crude oil, which led to price slumping. They also demonstrated the existence of a link between stock market prices and the pandemic, indicating, however, that the movement of stock indexes does not reflect the real situation in the economy but is mainly based on expectations and monetary and fiscal incentives. [63]. Finally, other researchers studied the impact of the SARS-CoV-19 pandemic on selected industries, namely, travel, hospitality, sports, events, entertainment, education, and finance. Their approximations were negative for each of the studied industries [64]. In our study, we focused on the question of how the SARS-CoV-19 pandemic has affected the economies of 176 selected countries as a whole. Therefore, unlike other authors, we did not study specific industries or selected economy ratios. Instead, we considered the change in gross domestic product relative increase throughout the pandemic period in the studied countries, which we considered to provide a good proxy for the condition of economy as a whole. Our sample of countries and studied period were considerably larger than those reported in previous studies. As a result of the above and due to the robust statistical results, our findings provide global evidence on how the SARS-CoV-19 pandemic has affected the economies of respective countries.

The presented study has several limitations. Firstly, the sample for this study comprised observations relating to 176 countries. Hence, not all countries could be considered in this study. Secondly, we calculated the change in the GDP for each country on the basis of the initial calculations of 2020 GDP provided by the International Monetary Fund as of 7 March 2021. These variables might require minor adjustments. The aforementioned two limitations might change the values of coefficients calculated in the study, but not our overall results. This is because our results were robust with low p-values (below 0.05). The final limitation of this study results from the analyzed period. Since we studied observations relating to only a single year, i.e., 2020, we are not in a position to conclude on the long-term impact of the SARS-CoV-19 pandemic on the economies of the analyzed countries.

In this study, we identified the economies of the countries with regards to the SARS-CoV-19 pandemic. We did not study the underlying reasons, which we consider to be rather multifaceted in nature. Hence, further research into adaptation mechanism in the context of the pandemic could prove interesting from the scientific point of view. In this paper, we analyzed and identified global trends related to the pandemic and GDP fluctuations. To this end, we ignored local differences, timing, and intensity of the pandemic. Although such an analysis was not required for our study, we consider it to be a good indication for further research. The final indication for the continuation of our research is to study the long-term impact of coronavirus-2019 on the global economy.

5. Conclusions

The global health and economy crisis caused by coronavirus-2019 is unprecedented, both in terms of its global dimension and the depth of its impact on the economy, society, political and legal conditions, and even the environment. The severity of the aforementioned phenomena and various related factors continues to increase, while the pandemic's prolonged duration poses a very real risk of a global catastrophe. As a result, many researchers and state policymakers have shifted the domains of their professional interests towards the pandemic and its surrounding issues.

In this paper, we studied data relating to 176 countries in the pandemic period and in the previous year. The objective of this paper was to study the impact of SARS-CoV-19 pandemic on national economies. Given the fact that at the time of writing this article real data pertaining to GDP values worldwide have just been officially provided, our study is the first or one of the first to analyze the impact of SARS-CoV-19 on the economies of countries in the first year of the pandemic. We selected the SARS-CoV-19 morbidity and fatality rates as proxies for the pandemic's development and GDP fluctuations in 2020 and 2019 as representative of the state of economy. Firstly, we identified the negative and statistically significant correlations between the SARS-CoV-19 morbidity and fatality rates and GDP changes. Next, we determined that the studied relationships were not linear, with the economies growing increasingly immune to the pandemic. The more severe the development of the pandemic, the more adaptive to its negative effects the economies eventually became. This finding is especially interesting as it shows that the global economy can quickly adjust to fast-changing severe and negative conditions. Hence, our results also demonstrate how the economies of the respective countries have been developing immunity to the negative effects of coronavirus-2019. This has been due to both governmental action and agility of companies.

Our results might have practical implications for policymakers. We identified and econometrically measured the direct connection between the spread of the SARS-CoV-19 pandemic, measured with new infections and fatality rates, and the change in gross domestic product relative increase. Therefore, our results empirically confirm the intuitive approach of many policymakers, who were the first to assume that the spread of the virus should be contained and next the economic issues should follow.

Finally, it should be noted that our paper shows the possibility of applying the multi-segment Theil–Sen model to disciplines such as healthcare and economics.

Author Contributions: Conceptualization, P.K. and K.R.; methodology, P.K.; validation, P.K. and K.R.; formal analysis, P.K. and K.R.; data curation, P.K. and K.R.; writing—original draft preparation, P.K. and K.R.; writing—review and editing, P.K. and K.R.; visualization, P.K. All authors have read and agreed to the published version of the manuscript.

Funding: This research was funded/by IDUB against COVID-19 project granted by Warsaw University of Technology under the program Excellence Initiative: Research University (IDUB).

Institutional Review Board Statement: Not applicable.

Informed Consent Statement: Not applicable.

Data Availability Statement: The data used in this study were from the open access databases "Our World in Data" and "International Monetary Fund" and can be found there. Further information on data and materials used are available from the corresponding author on reasonable request.

Conflicts of Interest: The authors declare no conflict of interest.

References

1. Lopachev, A.V.; Kazanskaya, R.B.; Khutorova, A.V.; Fedorova, T.N. An Overview of the Pathogenic Mechanisms Involved in Severe Cases of COVID-19 Infection, and the Proposal of Salicyl Carnosine as a Potential Drug for its Treatment. *Eur. J. Pharmacol.* **2020**, *886*, 173457. [CrossRef] [PubMed]
2. Jia, J.S.; Lu, X.; Yuan, Y.; Xu, G.; Jia, J.; Christakis, N.A. Population Flow Drives Spatiotemporal Distribution of COVID-19 in China. *Nature* **2020**, *582*, 389–394. [CrossRef] [PubMed]
3. Huang, C.; Wang, Y.; Li, X. Clinical features of patients infected with 2019 novel coronavirus in Wuhan, China. *Lancet* **2020**, *395*, 497–506. [CrossRef]
4. Chen, N.; Zhou, M.; Dong, X. Epidemiological and clinical characteristics of 99 cases of 2019 novel coronavirus pneumonia in Wuhan, China: A descriptive study. *Lancet* **2020**, *395*, 507–513. [CrossRef]
5. Wang, D.; Hu, B.; Hu, C. Clinical characteristics of 138 hospitalized patients with 2019 novel coronavirus-infected pneumonia in Wuhan, China. *JAMA* **2020**, *323*, 1061–1069. [CrossRef]
6. Wu, Z.; McGoogan, J.M. Characteristics of and important lessons from the coronavirus disease 2019 (COVID-19) outbreak in China. Summary of a report of 72314 cases from the Chinese center for disease control and prevention. *JAMA* **2020**, *323*, 1239–1242. [CrossRef]
7. Kang, S.J.; Jung, S.I. Age-Related Morbidity and Mortality among Patients with COVID-19. *Infect. Chemother.* **2020**, *52*, 154–164. [CrossRef]
8. Li, H.; Wang, S.; Zhong, F.; Bao, W.; Yipeng, L.; Lei, L.; Hongyan, W.; Yungang, H. Age-Dependent Risks of Incidence and Mortality of COVID-19 in Hubei Province and Other Parts of China. *Front. Med.* **2020**, *7*, 190.
9. Qiurong, R.; Yang, K.; Wang, W.; Jiang, L.; Song, J. Clinical predictors of mortality due to COVID-19 based on an analysis of data of 150 patients from Wuhan, China. *Intensive Care Med.* **2020**, *46*, 846–848.
10. Pettit, N.N.; Erica, L.; MacKenzie, J.; Ridgway, P.; Pursell, K.; Ash, D.; Patel, B.; Pho, M.T. Obesity is Associated with Increased Risk for Mortality Among Hospitalized Patients with COVID-19. *Obesity* **2020**, *28*, 1806–1810. [CrossRef]
11. Rajgor, D.D.; Lee, M.H.; Archuleta, S.; Bagdasarian, N.; Quek, S.C. The many estimates of the COVID-19 case fatality rate. *Lancet Infect. Dis.* **2020**, *20*, 776–777. [CrossRef]
12. Sorci, G.; Faivre, B.; Morand, S. Explaining among-country variation in COVID-19 case fatality rate. *Sci. Rep.* **2020**, *10*, 1–11. [CrossRef]
13. Hodgson, S.H.; Mansatta, K.; Mallett, G.; Harris, V.; Emary, K.R.W.; Pollard, A.J. What Defines an Efficacious COVID-19 Vaccine? A Review of the Challenges Assessing the Clinical Efficacy of Vaccines against SARS-CoV-2. *Lancet Infect. Dis.* **2020**, *23*, 9–10. [CrossRef]
14. Adekoya, O.B.; Oliyide, J.A. How COVID-19 drives connectedness among commodity and financial markets: Evidence from TVP-VAR and causality-in-quantiles techniques. *Resour. Policy* **2021**, *70*, 101898. [CrossRef]
15. Zhang, D.; Hu, M.; Ji, Q. Financial markets under the global pandemic of COVID-19. *Financ. Res. Lett.* **2020**, *36*, 101528. [CrossRef] [PubMed]
16. Youssef, M.; Mokni, K.; Ajmi, A.N. Dynamic connectedness between stock markets in the presence of the COVID-19 pandemic: Does economic policy uncertainty matter? *Financ. Innov.* **2021**, *7*, 1–27. [CrossRef]
17. Yuan, X.; Li, C.; Zhao, K.; Xu, X. The Changing Patterns of Consumers' Behavior in China: A Comparison during and after the COVID-19 Pandemic. *Int. J. Environ. Res. Public Health* **2021**, *18*, 2447. [CrossRef]
18. Korneta, P.; Kludacz-Alessandri, M.; Walczak, R. The Impact of COVID-19 on the Performance of Primary Health Care Service Providers in a Capitation Payment System: A Case Study from Poland. *Int. J. Environ. Res. Public Health* **2021**, *18*, 1407. [CrossRef]
19. Naumann, E.; Möhring, K.; Reifenscheid, M.; Wenz, A.; Rettig, T.; Lehrer, R.; Blom, A.G. COVID-19 policies in Germany and their social, political, and psychological consequences. *Eur. Policy Anal.* **2020**, *6*, 191–202. [CrossRef]
20. Nath, H. Covid-19: Macroeconomic Impacts and Policy Issues in India. *Space Cult. India* **2020**, *8*, 1–13. [CrossRef]
21. Arndt, C.; Davies, R.; Gabriel, S.; Harris, L.; Makrelov, K.; Robinson, S.; Anderson, L. Covid-19 lockdowns, income distribution, and food security: An analysis for South Africa. *Glob. Food Secur.* **2020**, *26*, 100410. [CrossRef] [PubMed]
22. Bagchi, B.; Chatterjee, S.; Ghosh, R.; Dandapat, D. Impact of COVID-19 on global economy. In *Coronavirus Outbreak and the Great Lockdown*; Springer: Singapore, 2020; pp. 15–26.
23. Ozili, P.; Arun, T. Spillover of COVID-19: Impact on the Global Economy. *SSRN Electron. J.* **2020**. [CrossRef]
24. Reinhart, C.; Reinhart, V. The pandemic depression: The global economy will never be the same. *Foreign Aff.* **2020**, *99*, 84.
25. Jena, P.R.; Majhi, R.; Kalli, R.; Managi, S.; Majhi, B. Impact of COVID-19 on GDP of major economies: Application of the artificial neural network forecaster. *Econ. Anal. Policy* **2021**, *69*, 324–339. [CrossRef]
26. International Monetary Fund. Available online: https://www.imf.org/external/datamapper/NGDP_RPCH@WEO/OEMDC/ADVEC/WEOWORLD (accessed on 7 March 2021).

27. Goolsbee, A.; Syverson, C. Fear, lockdown, and diversion: Comparing drivers of pandemic economic decline 2020. *J. Public Econ.* **2021**, *193*, 104311. [CrossRef] [PubMed]
28. Selby, K.; Durand, M.A.; Gouveia, A.; Bosisio, F.; Barazzetti, G.; Hostettler, M.; von Plessen, C. Citizen Responses to Government Restrictions in Switzerland During the COVID-19 Pandemic: Cross-Sectional Survey. *JMIR Form. Res.* **2020**, *4*, e20871. [CrossRef] [PubMed]
29. Bennedsen, M.; Larsen, B.; Schmutte, I.; Scur, D. *Preserving Job Matches during the COVID-19 Pandemic: Firm-Level Evidence on the Role of Government Aid*; GLO Discussion Paper; EconStor: Berlin, Germany, 2020; p. 588.
30. Gordon, T.; Dadayan, L.; Rueben, K. State and local government finances in the COVID-19 era. *Natl. Tax J.* **2020**, *73*, 733–757. [CrossRef]
31. Hyun, J.; Kim, D.; Shin, S.R. The Role of Global Connectedness and Market Power in Crises: Firm-Level Evidence from the COVID-19 Pandemic. Available online: https://www.researchgate.net/publication/343794415_The_Role_of_Global_Connectedness_and_Market_Power_in_Crises_Firm-level_Evidence_from_the_COVID-19_Pandemic (accessed on 2 April 2021).
32. Verbeke, A.; Yuan, W.A. Few Implications of the COVID-19 Pandemic for International Business Strategy Research. *J. Manag. Stud.* **2020**, *58*, 597–601. [CrossRef]
33. Hasell, J.; Mathieu, E.; Beltekian, D.A. Cross-country database of SARS-COV-19 testing. *Sci. Data* **2020**, *7*, 345. [CrossRef] [PubMed]
34. Shams, S.A.; Haleem, A.; Javaid, M. Analyzing SARS-COV-19 pandemic for unequal distribution of tests, identified cases, deaths, and fatality rates in the top 18 countries. *Diabetes Metab. Syndr. Clin. Res. Rev.* **2020**, *14*, 953–961. [CrossRef]
35. Arce, G.R. *Nonlinear Signal Processing: A Statistical Approach*; Wiley: Hoboken, NJ, USA, 2005.
36. Galvani, A.P. Dimensions of superspreading. *Nature* **2005**, *438*, 293–295. [CrossRef] [PubMed]
37. Wilson, T. A Proportional-Reduction-in-Error Interpretation for Kendall's Tau-B. *Soc. Forces* **1969**, *47*, 340–342. [CrossRef]
38. Korneta, P. Determinants of sales profitability for Polish agricultural distributors. *Int. J. Manag. Econ.* **2019**, *55*, 40–51.
39. Best, D.; Roberts, D. Algorithm AS 89: The Upper Tail Probabilities of Spearman's Rho. *J. R. Stat. Soc. Ser. C (Appl. Stat.)* **1975**, *24*, 377–379. [CrossRef]
40. Signorino, C.S.; Ritter, M.J. Tau-b or Not Tau-b: Measuring the Similarity of Foreign Policy Positions. *Int. Stud. Q.* **1999**, *43*, 115–144. [CrossRef]
41. Fredricks, G.A.; Nelsen, R.B. On the relationship between Spearman's rho and Kendall's tau for pairs of continuous random variables. *J. Stat. Plan. Inference* **2007**, *137*, 2143–2150. [CrossRef]
42. Bonett, D.G.; Wright, T.A. Sample size requirements for Pearson, Kendall, and Spearman correlations. *Psychometrika* **2000**, *65*, 23–28. [CrossRef]
43. Corder, G.W.; Foreman, D.I. *Nonparametric Statistics: A Step-by-Step Approach*; Wiley: Hoboken, NJ, USA, 2014.
44. Kocsis, T.; Anda, A. Parametric or non-parametric: Analysis of rainfall time series at a Hungarian meteorological station. *Q. J. Hung. Meteorol. Serv.* **2018**, *122*, 203–216. [CrossRef]
45. Sen, P.K. Estimates of the Regression Coefficient Based on Kendall's Tau. *J. Am. Stat. Assoc.* **1968**, *63*, 1379–1389. [CrossRef]
46. Theil, H. *A Rank-Invariant Method of Linear and Polynomial Regression Analysis. I, II, III*; Akademie van Wetenschappen: Amsterdam, The Netherlands, 1950.
47. El-Shaarawi, A.H.; Piegorsch, W. *Encyclopedia of Environmetrics*; Wiley: Hoboken, NJ, USA, 2001.
48. Gilbert, R.O. *Statistical Methods for Environmental Pollution Monitoring*; Wiley: Hoboken, NJ, USA, 1987.
49. Wilcox, R. A note on the Theil–Sen regression estimator when the regressor is random and the error term is heteroscedastic. *Biom. J.* **1998**, *40*, 261–268. [CrossRef]
50. Granato, G.E. Kendall-Theil Robust Line (KTRLine—Version 1.0)—A Visual Basic Program for Calculating and Graphing Robust Nonparametric Estimates of Linear-Regression Coefficients between Two Continuous Variables: Techniques and Methods of the U.S. Geological Survey, 2006, book 4, chap. A7. Available online: https://pubs.usgs.gov/tm/2006/tm4a7/ (accessed on 29 March 2021).
51. Korneta, P. Growth, profitability and liquidity of Polish road transportation companies. In *Proceedings of the 20th International Scientific Conference Business Logistics in Modern Management*; Strossmayer, J., Ed.; University of Osijek: Osijek, Croatia, 2020; pp. 75–88.
52. Worden, L.; Wannier, R.; Hoff, N.A.; Musene, K.; Selo, B.; Mossoko, M.; Okitolonda-Wemakoy, E.; Tamfum, J.J.M.; Rutherford, G.W.; Lietman, T.M.; et al. Projections of epidemic transmission and estimation of vaccination impact during an ongoing Ebola virus disease outbreak in Northeastern Democratic Republic of Congo. *PLoS Negl. Trop. Dis.* **2019**, *13*, e0007512. [CrossRef]
53. Barth, D.; Mayosi, B.M.; Badri, M.; Whitelaw, A.; Engel, M.E. Invasive and non-invasive group A β-haemolytic streptococcal infections in patients attending public sector facilities in South Africa: 2003–2015. *South. Afr. J. Infect. Dis.* **2018**, *33*, 12–17.
54. Orlik, T.; Rush, J.; Cousin, M.; Hong, J. Coronavirus Could Cost the Global Economy $2.7 Trillion. Here's How. *Bloomberg Economics*. NiGEM, OECD. 2020. Available online: https://www.bloomberg.com/graphics/2020-coronavirus-pandemic-global-economic-risk (accessed on 2 April 2021).
55. Maliszewska, M.; Mattoo, A.; Van Der Mensbrugghe, D. The potential impact of COVID-19 on GDP and trade: A preliminary assessment. *World Bank Policy Res. Work. Pap.* **2020**, 9211. Available online: https://papers.ssrn.com/sol3/papers.cfm?abstract_id=3573211 (accessed on 2 April 2021).
56. König, M.; Winkler, A. COVID-19: Lockdowns, Fatality Rates and GDP Growth. Evidence for the First Three Quarters of 2020. *Intereconomics* **2021**, *56*, 32–39. [CrossRef] [PubMed]

57. Peto, J. Covid-19 mass testing facilities could end the epidemic rapidly. *Br. Med. J.* **2020**, *368*, 1163. [CrossRef]
58. Finch, W.H.; Finch, M.E.H. Poverty and Covid-19: Rates of Incidence and Deaths in the United States during the First 10 Weeks of the Pandemic. *Front. Sociol.* **2020**, *5*, 47. [CrossRef]
59. Liang, L.L.; Tseng, C.H.H.; Ho, H.J.; Wu, C.Y. Covid-19 mortality is negatively associated with test number and government effectiveness. *Sci. Rep.* **2020**, *10*, 12567. [CrossRef]
60. Pak, A.; Adegboye, O.A.; Adekunle, A.I.; Rahman, K.M.; McBryde, E.S.; Eisen, D.P. Economic Consequences of the COVID-19 Outbreak: The Need for Epidemic Preparedness. *Front. Public Health* **2020**, *8*, 241.
61. Al-Thaqeb, S.A.; Algharabali, B.G.; Alabdulghafour, K.T. The pandemic and economic policy uncertainty. *Int. J. Financ. Econ.* **2020**, 1–11. [CrossRef]
62. Song, L.; Zhou, Y. The COVID-19 Pandemic and Its Impact on the Global Economy: What Does It Take to Turn Crisis into Opportunity? *China World Econ.* **2020**, *28*, 1–25. [CrossRef]
63. Štifanić, D.; Musulin, J.; Miočević, A.; Šegota, S.B.; Šubić, R.; Car, Z. Impact of COVID-19 on Forecasting Stock Prices: An Integration of Stationary Wavelet Transform and Bidirectional Long Short-Term Memory. *Complexity* **2020**, 1–12. [CrossRef] [PubMed]
64. Gorain, B.; Choudhury, H.; Molugulu, N.; Athawale, R.B.; Kesharwani, P. Fighting Strategies Against the Novel Coronavirus Pandemic: Impact on Global Economy. *Front. Public Health* **2020**, *8*, 606129. [CrossRef] [PubMed]

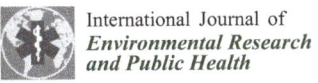

Article

Performance Evaluation of the Chinese Healthcare System

Muhammad Umar [1,*], Mário Nuno Mata [2,*], Adnan Abbas [3], José Moleiro Martins [2,4], Rui Miguel Dantas [2] and Pedro Neves Mata [5]

1. School of Economics and Management, East China Jiaotong University, Nanchang 330013, China
2. ISCAL-Instituto Superior de Contabilidade e Administração de Lisboa, Instituto Politécnico de Lisboa, Avenida Miguel Bombarda 20, 1069-035 Lisboa, Portugal; zdmmartins@gmail.com (J.M.M.); rmdantas@iscal.ipl.pt (R.M.D.)
3. School of Economics and Management, Harbin University of Science and Technology, Harbin 150080, China; adnan.abbas001@yahoo.com
4. Instituto Universitário de Lisboa (ISCTEIUL), Business Research Unit (BRU-IUL), 1649-026 Lisboa, Portugal
5. ISTA-School of Technologies and Architecture, Instituto Universitário de Lisboa (ISCTE-IUL), Avenida das Forças Armadas, 1649-026 Lisboa, Portugal; pedronmata@gmail.com
* Correspondence: umare_umare@yahoo.com (M.U.); mnmata@iscal.ipl.pt (M.N.M.)

Abstract: This study aims to evaluate the performance of the Chinese healthcare system. It uses sustainable development goal (SDG) 3, set by the United Nations to ensure healthy lives and promote well-being for all at all ages as a benchmark. It uses data of 17 variables ranging from the year 2000 to 2017 and uses a multistage methodology to evaluate the performance. In the first stage, it uses difference in mean test to know whether or not the indicators show an improvement in the second decade of the 21st century compared to the first decade. In the second phase, simple linear regression has been used to know the rate of change of performance of every indicator over the sample period. The third step compares the performance of the healthcare sector with the sustainable goals set by the UN and the fourth phase attempts to forecast performance for the next five years i.e., 2018 to 2022. As per the results, the Chinese healthcare sector has performed very well on many fronts except alcohol consumption in males, road accidents and the incidence of non-communicable diseases. Alcohol consumption by males is touching dangerous levels. Therefore, the policies should focus on educating males to lower their alcohol consumption to stay fit and healthy.

Keywords: Chinese healthcare system; sustainable development goals (SDGs); performance; evaluation

Citation: Umar, M.; Mata, M.N.; Abbas, A.; Martins, J.M.; Dantas, R.M.; Mata, P.N. Performance Evaluation of the Chinese Healthcare System. *Int. J. Environ. Res. Public Health* **2021**, *18*, 5193. https://doi.org/10.3390/ijerph18105193

Academic Editor: Dimitris Zavras

Received: 12 April 2021
Accepted: 10 May 2021
Published: 13 May 2021

Publisher's Note: MDPI stays neutral with regard to jurisdictional claims in published maps and institutional affiliations.

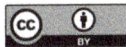

Copyright: © 2021 by the authors. Licensee MDPI, Basel, Switzerland. This article is an open access article distributed under the terms and conditions of the Creative Commons Attribution (CC BY) license (https://creativecommons.org/licenses/by/4.0/).

1. Introduction

The current pandemic has highlighted the importance of healthcare in a society. China was the first country that was hit hard by COVID-19. So, this study aims to evaluate the performance of the Chinese healthcare sector. As performance is always measured by the comparison of data with a benchmark, this study uses health-related sustainable development goals (SDG) set by the United Nations as a reference point. All UN member states unanimously adopted "The 2030 Agenda for Sustainable Development" in 2015. At the heart of this agenda are 17 SDGs that are to be achieved by 2030 [1]. The third goal amongst 17 goals is related to primary healthcare. This goal aims at achieving "healthy lives and promote well-being for all at all ages". According to studies, there exists a connection between health-related indicators, health outcomes, environment and metabolic risks [2,3].

This new agenda replaces the Millennium development goals (MDG) framework, which expired in 2015 [1]. The SDGs were developed through a highly consultative and iterative process, including many meetings with area experts, civil society, and governments. The operation of developing the SDGs' goals, targets, and indicators has not been without criticism. The common goal of scientific meetings and news media was to create more and more SDGs and to achieve the best results [4–9]. Health takes a central position in the SDGs, e.g., improvement in maternal mortality rate, neonatal death rate, incidence of malaria, tuberculosis, non-communicable diseases, rural health, equal access to treatment, reduction in non-communicable diseases, etc. The SDGs play an essential role in promoting public health through a proper approach to public policies across different sectors [3]. For example, for better education of girls, sound mental health is a pre-requisite. Burning coal harms the health of the general public. So, we may say that the ultimate objective of all the goals is to achieve better health and wellbeing for all people at all ages. Research on healthcare shows that a robust primary healthcare system forms a solid foundation to provide accessible and reasonable primary healthcare to the residents [10,11].

There are a number of studies that have evaluated the performance of global-, regional- and country-level healthcare systems. A comprehensive study conducted by using data from 173 countries concluded that the average efficiency of national health systems was 78.9% [12]. African countries had the lowest efficiency of 67% and countries in the west Pacific had the highest efficiency of 86%. Furthermore, the efficiency of national health systems depends on national economic status, the incidence of HIV/AIDS, governance and health insurance mechanisms. The study concluded that a 1% increase in social security expense as a percentage of total health expenditure results in a 1.9% increase in national health systems efficiency. Another study on 30 European countries concluded that both developed and developing countries lie on an efficient frontier and many of them are inefficient [13].

Another study conducted on 14 high-performing low- and middle-income countries (LMIC) found that most of these countries maintained or improved their performance in scope of service, quality, and access to health insurance [14]. Another study on seven high-income countries concluded that these countries face similar challenges regarding healthcare system performance but all have different policies to cope with these issues. There are some country-specific studies as well. A study on the Australian healthcare system concluded that healthcare services in Australia are among the best in the world [15]. The study highlighted resource allocation and performance in patient outcome improvements as two main challenges faced by the healthcare system. Lebanon is one of the countries that has opened its borders for Syrian refugees. The influx of the refugees has put pressure on the Lebanese healthcare system. A study conducted on the Lebanese healthcare system inferred that the healthcare system performed reasonably well despite being stressed by the influx of refugees [16].

There are some studies that have analyzed the healthcare sector of China. An editorial of The Lancet states that China has made great progress in providing equal access to healthcare and health insurance but the challenges of better quality, control of non-communicable disease and efficiency in healthcare services remains a challenge [17]. Another communication from the BMJ states that China has improved its primary healthcare, health insurance coverage and medicine policies; however, the challenges of better-quality primary healthcare, cost of medical care and inefficient use of resources remain [18]. A study conducted on healthcare system reform of Hubei province concluded that the reforms resulted in better healthcare services for Hubei province [19]. However, despite being the largest country on the planet as per population records, the comprehensive studies regarding the Chinese primary healthcare system are rare. Therefore, the current study bridges the above-mentioned gap by evaluating the performance of the Chinese healthcare system. It not only analyzes the performance of the healthcare system in the post-reforms era but entails the pre-reform period as well.

The question is, why it is important to study China's healthcare system? There are a number of reasons. First, China is the largest country by population. It is home to 1.4 billion people. Its huge population makes it an important country to study. Second, China has achieved marvelous progress in terms of economic development in the recent past. This led to many challenges for environmental and health-related development [20,21]. Third, in 2009, China's healthcare reforms objective shifted to achieve "Health for all" by expanding the underlying healthcare system [22]. The focus was to provide the best health and medical services to its citizens, which are affordable, safe, and useful. Using this National strategy, China started investing in this area and achieved excellent results from the primary healthcare system [23–29]. To strengthen these efforts, China is currently working with the World Health Organization (WHO) framework to garner quick results [30]. This system will help to organize health needs and engagement.

Fourth, China is still a developing country with nearly 30 million people living below poverty [31]. So, China faces many challenges in achieving health-related SDGs. A study called Global Burden Disease [32] showed that China ranked 88th among the 195 countries and territories evaluated on health-related SDG index. A total number of health-related SDG indicators are 41 in this study [32]. China achieved 62 in health-related SDG, a little higher than the global median index of 59.4, but it is lower than the top three countries; the top countries achieved scores of 83 in this area. Fifth, China faces many health challenges as many middle-income countries, including the highest portion of hepatitis disease. A third of 240 million people are fighting with chronic hepatitis [33] and it is mainly due to the lack of an adequate and comprehensive hepatitis disease control program. Another of the biggest health-related issues in China is smoking; 300 million smokers are living in China, which is a third of the world total, with limited measures in place to control this problem. Other important challenges regarding basic healthcare include alcohol consumption by males, road traffic accidents and the incidence of non-communicable diseases. So, there still exists many significant health-related problems in reducing social and health disparities in the context of economic growth [34].

Sixth, the Chinese government has a strong commitment to achieving health-related SDG targets. To achieve the above-mentioned goals, the State Council of China issued the Healthy China 2030 Planning Outline in 2016 [35]. The purpose of this study is multifold: to compare the performance of China with its own past, comparison of performance with the SDGs, forecasting the performance on the basis of the past and suggestions to remedy the weak areas. Many health-related SDGs have already been achieved by the China but some of them still need a lot of work to be complete.

This study uses data of 17 primary healthcare-related variables which include data regarding maternal mortality, neonatal mortality, the incidence of lethal and non-communicable diseases, abuse of drugs and alcohol, road-side accidents, and spending on healthcare. It uses a multistage methodology to evaluate the performance of the Chinese healthcare sector with its own past and the SDGs. In the first step, the study compares the performance of the Chinese basic healthcare facilities in the second decade of the 21st century with the first decade by using the difference in mean test. The second stage runs regression with goals as dependent variables and years as independent to calculate the average rate of change in performance over the sample period. The third step compares the performance of Chinese healthcare with the SDGs and the final step forecasts the expected performance ranging from 2017 to 2022. The study proposes policy suggestions to improve basic healthcare and the well-being of people in China.

The rest of this study is as follows: Section 2 explains the data and methodology used to evaluate and forecast the performance of the Chinese healthcare sector. Section 3 presents the empirical results and Section 4 concludes by providing policy suggestions for improvement.

2. Materials and Methods

2.1. Data

The data was obtained from the Health Nutrition and Population Statistics database of the World Bank, and it ranges from the year 2000 to 2017. The dataset consists of 17 variables, with each variable having 18 observations. The ultimate source of data for different variables extracted from the World Bank repository and used in this study is the WHO, UNICEF, UNFPA and United Nations Population Division and the UN. The World Bank repository is a consolidated and reliable source of data, so it has been accessed for data collection. Another reason for collecting data from the World Bank is its relative neutrality. Therefore, this study uses a very rich and reliable dataset spanning over almost two decades.

2.2. Study Variables

Table 1 mentions the abbreviations and description of variables used in this study. The maternal mortality rate is estimated by the World Bank and the data is provided by the national statistics. National estimates define the maternal mortality rate as the ratio of women who die from pregnancy-related causes during pregnancy or within 42 days of pregnancy termination per 100,000 live births. The World Bank estimates this variable by using a regression model based on maternal deaths among non-AIDS deaths in women aged 15 to 49, birth attendants, fertility, and GDP. Neonatal deaths in numbers provide information about the number of deaths of newborns before reaching 28 days in a particular year, and the neonatal mortality rate is the number of neonates dying before reaching 28 days per 1000 live births in a specific year.

Table 1. Variable abbreviations and names.

Variable	Names
MMR_EST	Maternal mortality rate, as per the World Bank estimates
MMR_NEST	Maternal mortality rate, national estimates
NN_MR	Neonatal mortality rate
NND_NUMB	Neonatal deaths in numbers
MR_U5	Mortality rate of children under the age of five years
MR_U5_FML	Mortality rate of females under the age of five years
MR_U5_ML	Mortality rate of males under the age of five years
INC_MLRA	Incidence of malaria
INC_TBC	Incidence of tuberculosis
COD_NCD	Non-communicable diseases as cause of death
ALC_PC	Alcohol consumption per capita in liters
ALC_PC_FML	Alcohol consumption by females per capita in liters
ALC_PC_ML	Alcohol consumption by males per capita in liters
MOR_RA	Mortality as a result of road accidents
CHE_GDP	Chinese health expenditure as a percentage of GDP
CHE_PC	Chinese health expenditure per capita
CHE_PC_PPP	Chinese health expenditure per capita on the basis of GDP purchasing power parity

The study also uses the data regarding the mortality rate of children who die before reaching their sixth birthday. The mortality rate under the age of five is measured as the probability per 1000 that a child will die before reaching the age of five. This study also uses the mortality rate of female and male children under the age of five. The incidence of malaria describes the number of new cases per 1000 of the population at risk in a year, and the impact of tuberculosis is estimated as several new and relapse tuberculosis cases arising in a given year, expressed as the rate per 100,000 population. Estimates include all forms of TB. Non-communicable diseases as a cause of death represent the percentage of deaths caused by cancer, diabetes mellitus, cardiovascular diseases, digestive diseases, skin diseases, musculoskeletal diseases, and congenital anomalies to the people of all ages.

The study also uses data regarding alcohol consumption. It is measured as the liters of pure alcohol consumed per capita (15 years or older) in a calendar year adjusted for tourist consumption. The data for female and male consumption have also been used for detailed analysis. Mortality as a result of road accidents is measured as the deaths caused by traffic injury per 100,000 of population. This variable informs us about road safety. Finally, the study also uses data regarding healthcare expenditure, which provides an idea about the overall healthcare of the people. Healthcare expenditure includes healthcare goods and services consumed during each year, and it does not include capital expenditure on a building, machinery, IT, or vaccines for emergencies or outbreaks. Health expenditure per capita includes current healthcare expenditure per capita in US dollars on a theoretical basis, and health expenditure per capita purchasing power basis is the current health expenditure per capita in terms of purchasing power parity (PPP).

2.3. Statistical Analysis

This study uses a multiple-step approach for the analysis. In the first step, all the variables were divided into two segments. The first portion ranges from the year 2000 to 2009, and the other section covers 2010 to 2017. So, half of the data depicts the Chinese performance regarding health-related sustainable goals in the first decade of the 21st century, and the other half shows the performance of the Chinese healthcare sector in the second decade of the 21st century. The difference in the mean test for paired observations was run to know whether or not the performance has significantly improved over the period. As the number of observations for each variable was less than 30, the rejection or acceptance of the null hypothesis of no difference in performance was decided on the basis of *t* distribution.

Simple linear regression (SLR) was used in the second step to find the rate of change of performance regarding different targets over the years. The mathematical expression for our regression model is given below.

$$Y_i = \alpha_0 + \beta_i X_i + \varepsilon$$

where Y represents the dependent variable, and subscript i represents the ith variable. α_0 shows y intercept; X shows time, which ranges from year 2000 to 2017, and ε represents the error term.

In the third step, we used two different mechanisms for forecasting. In the first mechanism, we forecasted the values for all the variables using the beta coefficient β measured by the above model and by replacing X with year 2018 to 2022. In the second mechanism, we used extrapolation to forecast out of the sample the performance of the Chinese healthcare sector. We compared the results of both methods and drew forecasts mostly based on extrapolation to incorporate nonlinearities in the forecasts.

3. Results and Discussion

Table 2 provides descriptive statistics for all the variables used in this study. As per the national estimates, the average maternal mortality rate over the sample period is 35 per 100,000 live births, far below the global target of 70 set under sustainable goals (SDG). The mean neonatal mortality rate is 11 per 1000 live births. This number is also below the global target of 12 per 1000, which is to be achieved by 2030. The under-five mortality rate of 19.84 is far below the target of 27 per 1000 live births. The statistics reveal that the incidence of TB and malaria is negligibly small with only 0.007 patients of malaria per 1000 of the population and 83.28 patients of TB per 100,000 of the population. Although malaria and TB have been curtailed, the government must keep up with its strategies to combat these diseases so that they may not emerge again.

As per the statistics, non-communicable diseases are the cause of 85.95% of deaths. As far as alcohol consumption is concerned, on average, people in China drink 7.075 L of pure alcohol each in a year. The average consumption of pure alcohol for females per capita is just 2.525 L, but this number for males is 11.45 L per capita. The alcohol consumption by males is on the rise and expected to surpass the binge drinking level of 12.98 L per capita soon. The statistics regarding alcohol consumption are based on the drinking levels defined by the National Institute on Alcohol Abuse and Alcoholism of the United States [Appendix A]. As per the statistics, the road accident mortality rate is declining and the average number of deaths per 100,000 of the population is 20.60. The average current healthcare expenditure as a percentage of GDP is 4.39%. The average health expenditure per capita is $188.77 in nominal terms and $385.33 per capita in purchasing power parity terms. Table 3 provides the pairwise correlation matrix.

Table 4 provides the results for the difference in the means test for the performance of the Chinese healthcare sector in the first decade of the 21st century and the second decade. As per the World Bank estimates, the average maternal mortality rate over the first decade was 48.40 per 100,000 live births, but the average maternal mortality rate over the second decade is only 29.25 per 100,000 live births. It shows a significant decline in maternal mortality rate over the sample period. National estimates regarding maternal mortality rate provide an even better picture. The maternal mortality rate is 50% lesser in the second decade compared to the first. The average neonatal mortality rate was 14.87 per 1000 live births in the first decade, and it dropped to 6.37 in the second decade, which shows a significant improvement over the period.

Table 2. Descriptive statistics.

	Mean	Median	STDV	Minimum	Maximum	Skewness	Kurtosis
MMR_EST	39.889	39.000	11.198	25.000	58.000	0.181	1.619
MMR_NEST	35.136	33.050	12.933	18.000	53.000	0.172	1.468
NN_MR	11.094	9.700	5.374	4.700	21.400	0.561	2.023
NND_NUMB	184,179	164,952	85,038	78,087	347,408	0.516	2.030
MR_U5	19.844	17.750	8.679	9.300	36.800	0.574	2.097
MR_U5_FML	19.356	17.615	8.600	8.700	34.700	0.396	1.789
MR_U5_ML	21.867	20.085	9.499	9.900	38.700	0.372	1.781
INC_MLRA	0.007	0.010	0.005	0.000	0.010	−0.707	1.500
INC_TBC	83.278	82.500	14.604	63.000	109.000	0.224	1.848
COD_NCD	85.956	86.190	2.584	81.600	89.600	−0.197	1.753
ALC_PC	7.075	7.075	0.089	6.933	7.217	0.000	1.793
ALC_PC_FML	2.625	2.625	0.089	2.483	2.767	0.000	1.793
ALC_PC_ML	11.450	11.450	0.178	11.167	11.733	0.000	1.793
MOR_RA	20.601	20.850	0.879	18.880	21.700	−0.609	2.130
CHE_GDP	4.394	4.334	0.385	3.659	5.075	0.057	2.393
CHE_PC	188.770	148.249	138.206	42.354	403.817	0.449	1.602
CHE_PC_PPP	385.326	324.619	229.525	129.500	819.481	0.581	1.969

The mortality rate of children under the age of five has declined from 25.91 per 1000 in the first decade to 12.26 only in the second decade, a significant improvement on this front as well. The improvement in the under-five mortality rate for female children is slightly better compared to male children. The incidence of malaria has also declined from 0.01 per 1000 of the population to 0.003, from the first decade to the second. We may say that China has almost eradicated malaria. The incidence of tuberculosis has also declined from 94.1 to 69.75 per 100,000 of the population, a significant decline of 26% over two decades. However, further efforts are needed to eliminate these diseases from the country.

The mortality rate by non-communicable diseases including cancer, diabetes mellitus, cardiovascular diseases, digestive diseases, skin diseases, musculoskeletal diseases, and congenital anomalies has significantly increased from 84.03 percent in the first decade to 88.36 percent in the second decade. The numbers show that the incidence of deaths by infectious diseases has declined from 16% to 12%. According to descriptive statistics, the consumption of alcohol is one of the weak areas. The numbers show a deteriorating situation. Pure alcohol consumption has significantly increased from 7.008 to 7.16 L per capita.

Interestingly, the alcohol consumption has declined from 2.69 L to 2.54 L for females but for the males it has significantly increased from 11.32 L in first decade to 11.61 L of pure alcohol per capita in the second decade. This is the area which requires government attention because if the present trend continues, the alcohol consumption by males may surpass safe levels and reach the binge level. This will result in alcohol-related diseases and the deteriorating health of men.

The mortality rate from road accidents has significantly declined from 21.25 in the first decade to 19.79 per 100,000 population in the second decade. More efforts are needed to halve the number as per the SDGs by 2030. With the improvement in the economy, spending on current health expenditure has significantly increased from 4.16% of GDP to 4.69% over the period of two decades. Percentage increase in current healthcare expenditure relative to GDP is more vivid in health expenditure per capita which have increased from $80.38 to 324.26, a rise of 303% in nominal terms and current healthcare expenditure per capita in terms of PPP has increased from $211.46 to 602.66, an increase of 185%.

Table 3. Correlation matrix.

	MMR_EST	MMR_NEST	NN_MR	NND_NUMB	MR_U5	MR_U5_FML	MR_U5_ML	INC_MLRA
MMR_EST	1							
MMR_NEST	0.993	1						
NN_MR	0.987	0.974	1					
NND_NUMB	0.989	0.976	1.000	1				
MR_U5	0.986	0.971	1.000	1.000	1			
MR_U5_FML	0.995	0.986	0.997	0.998	0.996	1.000		
MR_U5_ML	0.996	0.987	0.997	0.997	0.996	0.994	1	
INC_MLRA	0.794	0.781	0.715	0.728	0.718	0.741	0.748	1
INC_TBC	0.996	0.983	0.990	0.993	0.990	0.994	0.995	0.786
COD_NCD	−0.998	−0.989	−0.989	−0.992	−0.989	−0.996	−0.997	−0.787
ALC_PC	−0.994	−0.984	−0.976	−0.981	−0.977	−0.985	−0.987	−0.818
ALC_PC_FML	−0.994	−0.984	−0.976	−0.981	−0.977	−0.985	−0.987	0.818
ALC_PC_ML	−0.994	−0.984	−0.976	−0.981	−0.977	−0.985	−0.987	−0.818
MOR_RA	0.945	0.934	0.900	0.911	0.903	0.918	0.922	0.887
CHE_GDP	−0.587	−0.568	−0.470	−0.489	−0.472	−0.519	−0.528	−0.822
CHE_PC	−0.952	−0.947	−0.895	−0.904	−0.895	−0.920	−0.924	−0.909
CHE_PC_PPP	−0.947	−0.939	−0.895	−0.905	−0.896	−0.917	−0.922	−0.891

	INC_TBC	COD_NCD	ALC_PC	ALC_PC_FML	ALC_PC_ML	MOR_RA	CHE_GDP	CHE_PC	CHE_PC_PPP
INC_TBC	1								
COD_NCD	−0.999	1							
ALC_PC	−0.996	0.997	1						
ALC_PC_FML	−0.996	0.997	1.000	1					
ALC_PC_ML	−0.996	0.997	1.000	1.000	1				
MOR_RA	0.950	−0.950	−0.972	−0.972	−0.972	1			
CHE_GDP	−0.573	0.583	0.632	0.632	0.632	−0.758	1		
CHE_PC	−0.945	0.949	0.966	0.966	0.966	−0.984	0.785	1	
CHE_PC_PPP	−0.946	0.949	0.970	0.970	0.970	−0.997	0.784	0.992	1

Table 4. Difference in mean test.

	MMR_EST	MMR_NE	NN_MR	NND_NUMB	MR_U5	MR_U5_FML	MR_U5_ML	INC_MLRA	INC_TBC
2000–09	48.400	44.885	14.870		25.910	25.655	28.845	0.010	94.100
2010–17	29.250	22.950	6.375		12.263	11.481	13.144	0.003	69.750
t stats	7.208 ***	6.967 ***	5.490 ***		5.409 ***	6.261 ***	6.324 ***	5.164 ***	6.525 ***

	COD_NCD	ALC_PC	ALC_PC_FML	ALC_PC_ML	MOR_RA	CHE_GDP	CHE_PC	CHE_PC_PPP
2000–09	84.030	7.008	2.692	11.317	21.250	4.159	80.376	211.463
2010–17	88.363	7.158	2.542	11.617	19.790	4.689	324.262	602.656
t stats	−6.664 ***	−6.802 ***	−6.802 ***	−6.802 ***	6.432 ***	−3.963 ***	−8.371 ***	−7.107 ***

*** Represent statistical significance at 1% level

Table 5 presents the results of a simple linear regression model mentioned in the methodology section. Time is a significant determinant for all the variables used in the study, which implies that different variables that measure the performance of the Chinese healthcare sector have significantly changed over time. The maternal mortality rate, neonatal mortality rate, mortality rate of children under the age of five, the incidence of Malaria, the incidence of tuberculosis, and the road accident mortality rate has declined while deaths as a result of non-communicable diseases and current healthcare expenditure have significantly increased over the sample period. Overall, the healthcare sector of China has shown improvements in the recent past.

Table 5. Simple linear regression.

	MMR_EST	MMR_NE	NN_MR	MR_U5	MR_U5_FML	MR_U5_ML	INC_MLRA
Year	−2.085 ***	−2.383 ***	−0.982 ***	−1.587 ***	−1.587 ***	−1.756 ***	−0.001 ***
	(0.000)	(0.000)	(0.000)	(0.000)	(0.000)	(0.000)	(0.000)
CONS.	4226.855 ***	4821.785 ***	1984.150 ***	3208.157 ***	3206.632 ***	3549.489 ***	1.499 ***
	(0.000)	(0.000)	(0.000)	(0.000)	(0.000)	(0.000)	(0.000)
Adj. R-Square	0.988	0.966	0.949	0.951	0.969	0.973	0.648
	INC_TBC	COD_NCD	MOR_RA	CHE_GDP	CHE_PC	CHE_PC_PPP	
Year	−2.723 ***	0.482 ***	−0.160 ***	0.046 ***	25.004 ***	41.723 ***	
	(0.000)	(0.000)	(0.000)	(0.005)	(0.000)	(0.000)	
CONS.	5553.279 ***	−882.850 ***	342.168 ***	−87.291 ***	−50,032.550 ***	−83,415.830 ***	
	(0.000)	(0.000)	(0.000)	(0.007)	(0.000)	(0.000)	
Adj. R-Square	0.991	0.993	0.942	0.362	0.929	0.942	

*** Represent statistical significance at 1% level. *p* values are given in parentheses.

Beta coefficients of the variables given in Table 5 have been used for extrapolation to forecast. The graphical depiction of the performance of the Chinese healthcare sector and its comparison with the SDGs is presented in Figures 1–7. All the figures provide ex-post and ex-ante information. The ex-post period ranges from 2000 to 2017, and the ex-ante period is from 2018 to 2022. There are 17 SDGs, and goal 3 is about 'Good Health and Well-Being'. Like all other goals, goal 3 also has some targets that the participating nations should achieve before 2030 to make this planet a healthy place. Every figure provides information about the target and how the Chinese healthcare sector has performed against that target.

Figure 1 is about target 3.1, which aims to reduce the maternal mortality ratio below 70 per 100,000 live births. The maternal mortality rate was far below the target of 70 even in the year 2000, both according to national as well as World Bank estimates. As per the national estimates, only 18 women died of maternity-related problems per 100,000 live births. As per the World Bank estimates, the number was only 25 in the year 2017. If the current trend prevails, the maternal mortality rate is expected to drop to 12 as per the national estimates and 14 according to World Bank estimates.

Figure 2 relates to target 3.2, which states that the nations should reduce the neonatal mortality rate to at most 12 per 1000 live births, and the under-five mortality rate should be at least reduced to 25 per 1000 live births. China achieved the target of at most 12 neonatal deaths per 1000 way back in year 2007, and a target of less than 25 deaths of children under the age of five per 1000 live births was achieved in 2005. China recorded the lowest neonatal mortality rate of only 4.7 per 1000 live births in the year 2017, and the mortality rate of children under the age of five per 1000 live births was recorded to be only 9.3. If the current trend continues, the neonatal mortality rate is expected to drop to 2.7 per 1000 live births in the year 2022, and the mortality rate for children under the age of five is expected to drop to 5.8 by the year 2022.

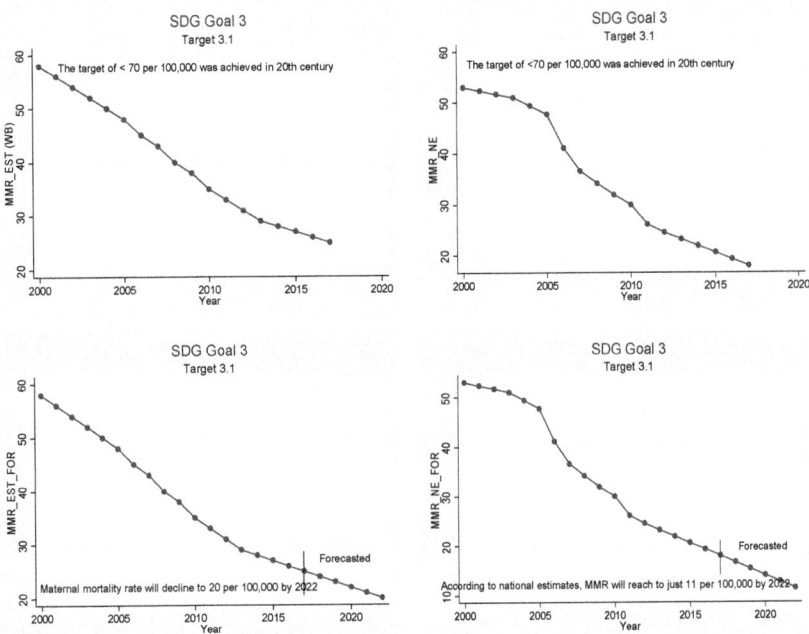

Figure 1. Sustainable development goal 3, target 3.1 (maternal mortality) ex-post and ex-ante.

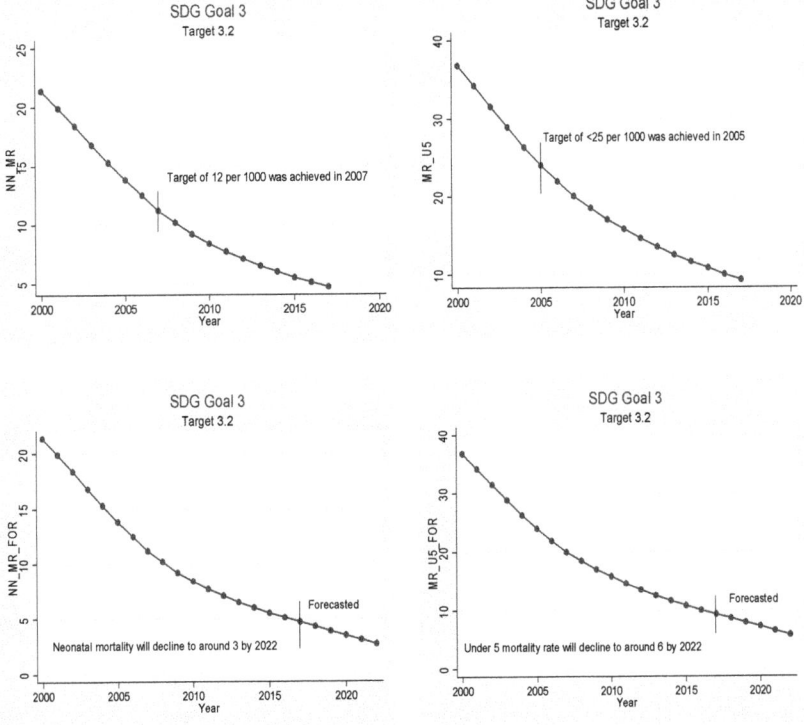

Figure 2. Sustainable development goal 3, target 3.2 (neonatal mortality) ex-post and ex-ante.

Figure 3 is about target 3.3, which states that the countries should end epidemics such as tuberculosis, malaria, and neglected tropical diseases by the year 2030. China has almost succeeded in eliminating malaria and tuberculosis. The incidence of malaria was recorded to be 0.000 patients per 1000 in 2017, and the incidence of tuberculosis was recorded to be only 63 per 100,000 population in 2017. If the current trend continues, malaria will be eliminated by 2022, and only 58 people out of 100,000 are expected to have TB in 2022. The results related to the incidence of tuberculosis seem to contradict the findings of [36] but it is not so. Our findings suggest that tuberculosis will still exist in the future and its incidence rate will be 0.058%, which is low enough to be neglected. The difference between our study and theirs is that their study only focuses on tuberculosis but ours is broader in context as we have studied the healthcare sector as a whole and not only a single disease.

Figure 4 is related to target 3.4, which aims to lower mortality from non-communicable diseases through prevention and treatment. More and more patients are dying of non-communicable diseases rather than communicable diseases. In 2017, 89.6% of deaths were caused by non-communicable diseases, and only 10.4 deaths were caused by communicable diseases. If the current trend continues, 91.1% of deaths will be caused by non-communicable diseases in 2022. This area has been constantly neglected by Chinese health authorities, but it needs immediate consideration by policy-makers [37].

Figure 5 relates to target 3.5, which states that nations should strengthen the prevention and treatment of narcotics use and the harmful use of alcohol. One of the areas that need to be managed carefully in China is alcohol consumption. Pure alcohol consumption in China is on the rise. Each person in China drank 7.22 L of pure alcohol on average in 2017, and pure alcohol consumption has recorded an upward trend. Careful analysis of the numbers reveals that male and female sections of society are behaving totally differently. Alcohol consumption by females is on the decline, and alcohol consumption by males is surging at a very high rate. Females only drank 2.48 L of pure alcohol in the year 2017, while the males drank 11.73 L on average in 2017. Our results still validate the findings of [38] that males' alcohol consumption is many times more than females' consumption. If the current trend continues, females are expected to drink only 2.4 L of pure alcohol in the year 2022. On the other hand, males expected to drink 11.9 L on average; i.e., males will be touching the binge-drinking level by 2022. The binge-drinking level of 6.49 L per year for females and 12.98 L for males is calculated based on standards set by the National Institute on Alcohol Abuse and Alcoholism. This finding supports the results of [39] that the production and consumption of alcohol in China has increased manyfold. Therefore, the government should take measures to encourage the male population to drink alcohol within their limits. Otherwise, the harmful use of alcohol will lead to medical, social, and legal problems.

Figure 6 is about target 3.6, which states that the number of deaths and injuries from road traffic accidents should be halved by the year 2020. Unlike many other targets, this target is to be achieved by 2020 and not 2030, which shows the urgency of the problem. According to statistics, 19.4 deaths are caused by road traffic injuries per 100,000 of the population. The number is comparatively high due to rapid economic growth and increased motorization [40]. So, as per the target, the number should decrease to 9.7 deaths per 100,000 of the population. However, the number only dropped to 18.88 in the year 2017, and if the current trend continues, the number will only drop to 7.58 per 100,000 of population. Therefore, the government must take stringent actions to make roads safer for travelers to halve the number of deaths from traffic injuries by the year 2020. Special attention is needed to improve road safety because according to [41], the death rate from road accidents is three times higher than reported by the police.

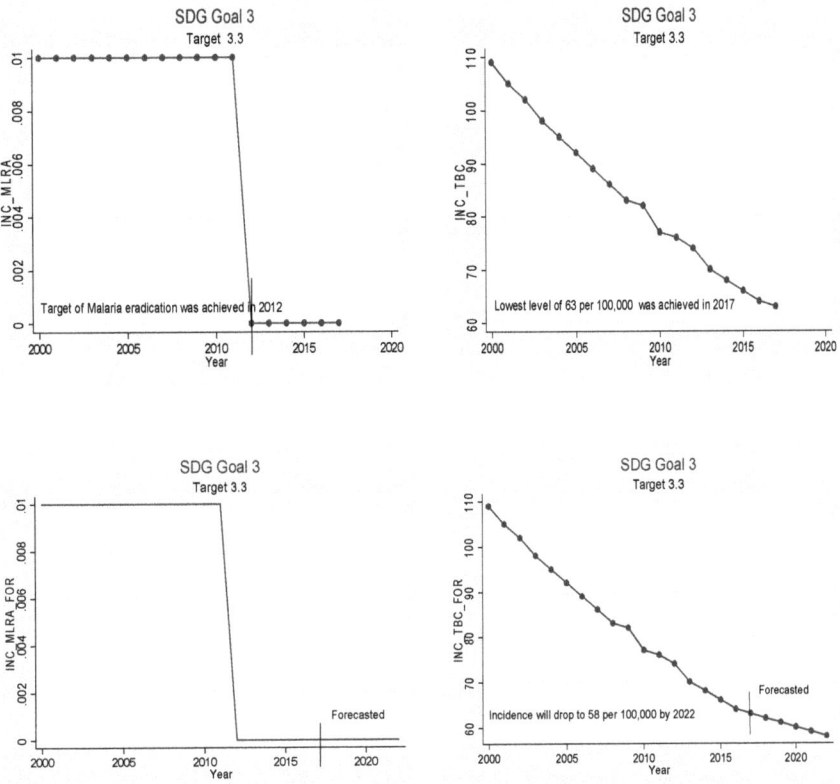

Figure 3. Sustainable development goal 3, target 3.3 (end of tuberculosis, malaria, etc.) ex-post and ex-ante.

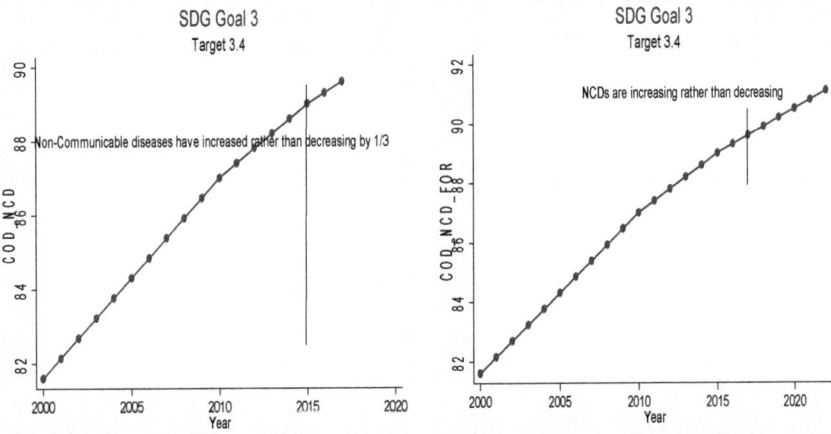

Figure 4. Strategic development goal 3, target 3.4 (mortality from non-communicable diseases) ex-post and ex-ante.

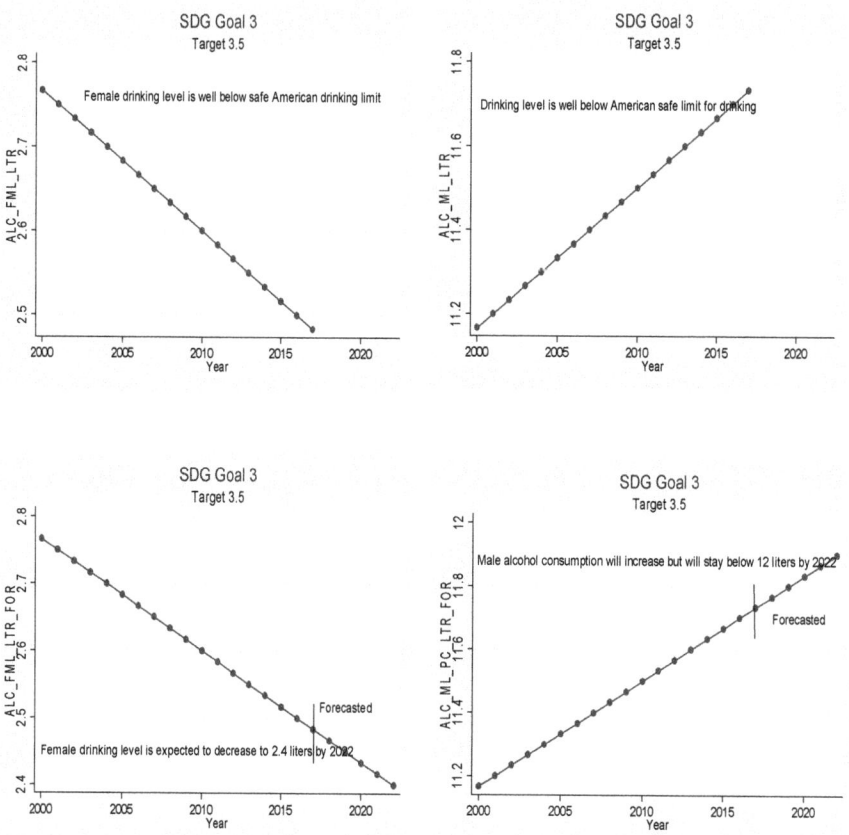

Figure 5. Sustainable development goal 3, target 3.5 (prevention of drugs and alcohol abuse) ex-post and ex-ante.

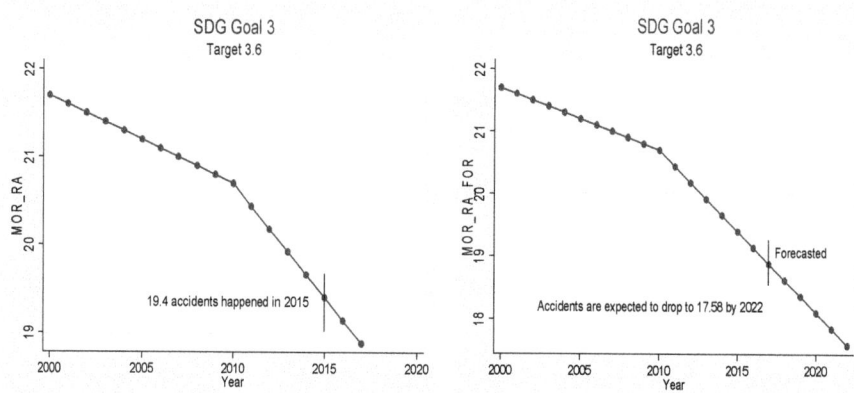

Figure 6. Sustainable development goal 3, target 3.6 (deaths by road accidents) ex-post and ex-ante.

Figure 7 relates to target 3.8, which stresses the importance of healthcare finance. This target is qualitative in nature as it does not provide any target in the form of numbers to achieve. This target suggests that governments should develop the systems so that everyone can have access to quality and affordable healthcare services and medicines. Chinese healthcare expenditure is increasing at a very rapid pace. The current healthcare expenditure is recorded to be 5.08% of the GDP, the highest over the sample period. If the trend continues, this number is expected to reach 5.54% of GDP in 2022. Current healthcare expenditure in terms of nominal as well as PPP terms is also on the rise. If the current trend continues, expenditure on healthcare per capita is expected to reach $431.25 in nominal terms and $1109.44 in PPP terms.

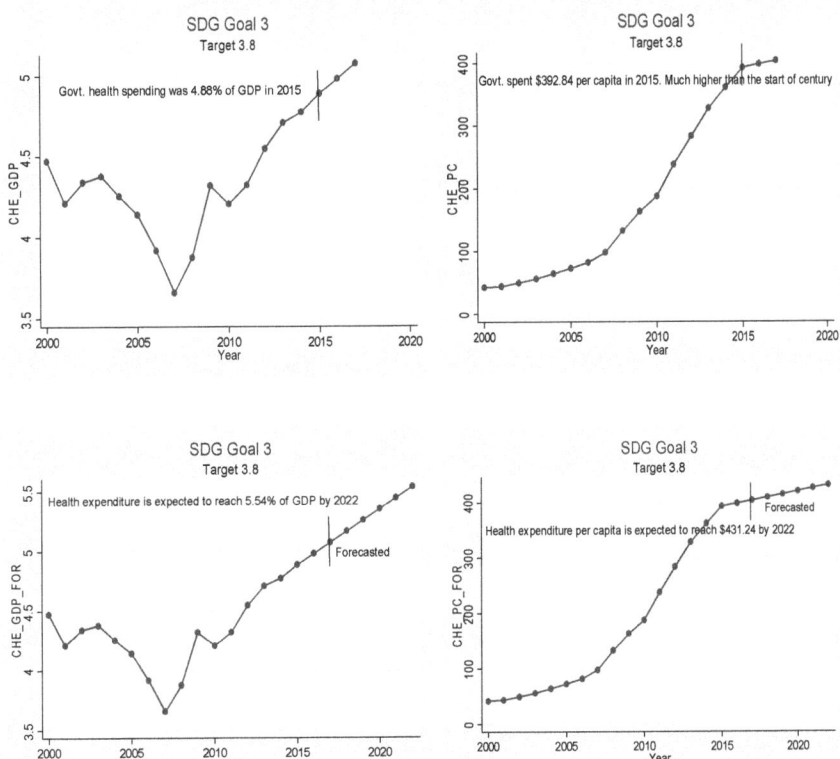

Figure 7. Sustainable development goal 3, target 3.8 (universal health coverage), ex-post and ex-ante.

Based on all the results mentioned above, we may state that China is doing very well regarding improvements in healthcare services as the current healthcare expenditure is increasing, thanks to the higher economic growth over the last three decades. The healthcare expenditure as a percentage of GDP dropped from 4.47% in 2000 to 3.67% in 2007 and rebounded to 4.98% in 2017. At this pace, healthcare expenditure is expected to grow to 5.54% by 2022. The current healthcare expenditure does not include capital health expenditures such as buildings, machinery, IT and stocks of vaccines for an emergency or outbreak.

One of the most important areas where the government of China should pay attention is alcohol consumption in the male population of China. The government must take measures to encourage the male population to drink less alcohol so that many medical, social, and legal problems may be avoided. The second area that needs urgent attention is traffic safety. The authorities must make every possible effort to reduce traffic accidents as soon as possible. The government may do it by educating people and introducing severe penalties for violations. Another area that needs immediate attention is to control the incidence of non-communicable diseases.

4. Conclusions

The study concludes that the Chinese healthcare system has performed very well on many fronts of the sustainable development goals (SDGs). The statistics show significant improvement in healthcare performance in the second decade of the 21st century compared to the first decade. The areas that still need immediate attention include alcohol consumption, road traffic accidents and the incidence of non-communicable diseases. The government should spend resources to curtail the spread of non-communicable diseases along with the prevention of communicable diseases. The government should heavily focus on educating the male population about the harms of alcohol abuse so that they lower alcohol consumption to stay fit and healthy and to protect the society from harm overall. Road accidents are also an area where the government should focus its attention. The number of deaths by road accidents is declining but a lot more is needed to reduce the deaths by half by the year 2020. This could be achieved by educating people about road safety and issuing hefty fines to violators.

Author Contributions: All the authors have contributed substantially to the work reported as follow: Conceptualization, methodology, software, validation, formal analysis, investigation, resources, data curation, writing original draft preparation, writing—review and editing, visualization, supervision, project administration, funding acquisition. All authors have read and agreed to the published version of the manuscript.

Funding: This research was supported by Instituto Politécnico de Lisboa.

Institutional Review Board Statement: Not applicable.

Informed Consent Statement: Not applicable.

Data Availability Statement: The data regarding this study can be assessed at https://databank.worldbank.org/source/health-nutrition-and-population-statistics (accessed on 13 May 2021).

Acknowledgments: We thank Instituto Politécnico de Lisboa for providing funding for this study.

Conflicts of Interest: The authors declare no conflict of interest.

Appendix A

Calculations regarding calculation of alcohol consumption level of Chinese males and females

One alcoholic drink in America = 14 g = $0.01783 \times 5 \times 52$ L= 4.6358 L/year for men

Female $52 \times 7 \times 0.01783 = 6.49$

Male $52 \times 14 \times 0.01783 = 12.98$

https://www.niaaa.nih.gov/alcohol-health/overview-alcohol-consumption/moderate-binge-drinking (accessed on 12 May 2018)

References

1. UN Millennium Project. *Investing in Development: A Practical Plan to Achieve the Millennium Development Goals*; United Nations: New York, NY, USA, 2005.
2. Nilsson, M.; Griggs, D.; Visbeck, M. Present a simple way of rating relationships between the targets to highlight priorities for integrated policy. *Nature* **2016**, *534*, 320–323. [CrossRef] [PubMed]
3. World Health Organization. World Health Statistics, Geneva: World Health Organization. 2015. Available online: https://www.who.int/gho/publications/world_health_statistics/2015/en/ (accessed on 23 December 2018).
4. Horton, R. Offline: Why the Sustainable Development Goals will fail. *Lancet* **2014**, *383*, 2196. [CrossRef]
5. Yamey, G.; Shretta, R.; Binka, F.N. The 2030 sustainable development goal for health. *BMJ* **2014**, *349*, g5295. [CrossRef] [PubMed]
6. Hickel, J. The Problem with Saving the World. *Jacobin*, 8 August 2015. Available online: https://www.jacobinmag.com/2015/08/global-povertyclimate-change-sdgs/ (accessed on 16 July 2016).
7. The 169 Commandments. *The Economist*, 28 March 2015. Available online: http://www.economist.com/news/leaders/21647286-proposed-sustainable-development-goalswould-be-worse-useless-169-commandments (accessed on 16 July 2016).

8. Unsustainable Goals. *The Economist*, 26 March 2015. Available online: http://www.economist.com/news/international/21647307-2015-willbe-big-year-global-governance-perhaps-too-big-unsustainable-goals (accessed on 16 July 2016).
9. Hák, T.; Janoušková, S.; Moldan, B. Sustainable Development Goals: A need for relevant indicators. *Ecol. Indic.* **2016**, *60*, 565–573. [CrossRef]
10. Starfield, B.; Shi, L. Commentary: Primary care and health outcomes: A health services research challenge. *Health Serv. Res.* **2007**, *42*, 2252–2256. [CrossRef] [PubMed]
11. Hung, L.M.; Rane, S.; Tsai, J.; Shi, L. Advancing primary care to promote equitable health: Implications for China. *Int. J. Equity Health* **2012**, *11*. [CrossRef]
12. Sun, D.; Ahn, H.; Lievens, T.; Zeng, W. Evaluation of the performance of national health systems in 2004–2011: An analysis of 173 countries. *PLoS ONE* **2017**, *12*, e0173346. [CrossRef]
13. Asandului, L.; Roman, M.; Fatulescu, P. The Efficiency of Healthcare Systems in Europe: A Data Envelopment Analysis Approach. *Procedia Econ. Financ.* **2014**, *10*, 261–268. [CrossRef]
14. Bitton, A.; Fifield, J.; Ratcliffe, H.; Karlage, A.; Wang, H.; Veillard, J.H.; Schwarz, D.; Hirschhorn, L.R. Primary healthcare system performance in low-income and middle-income countries: A scoping review of the evidence from 2010 to 2017. *BMJ Glob. Health* **2019**, *4*, e001551. [CrossRef]
15. Dixit, S.K.; Sambasivan, M. A review of the Australian healthcare system: A policy perspective. *SAGE Open Med.* **2018**, *6*. [CrossRef]
16. Ibrahim, M.D.; Daneshvar, S. Efficiency Analysis of Healthcare System in Lebanon Using Modified Data Envelopment Analysis. *J. Healthc. Eng.* **2018**, *2018*. [CrossRef] [PubMed]
17. The Lancet. China's health-care reform: An independent evaluation. *Lancet* **2019**, *394*, 1113. [CrossRef]
18. Meng, Q.; Mills, A.; Wang, L.; Han, Q. What can we learn from China's health system reform? *BMJ* **2019**, *365*. [CrossRef] [PubMed]
19. Sang, S.; Wang, Z.; Yu, C. Evaluation of Health Care System Reform in Hubei Province, China. *Int. J. Environ. Res. Public Health* **2014**, *11*, 2262–2277. [CrossRef] [PubMed]
20. Chan, R.; Yao, S. Urbanization and sustainable metropolitan development in China: Patterns, problems, and prospects. *GeoJournal* **1999**, *49*, 269–277. [CrossRef]
21. Zhang, X.; Wu, Z.; Feng, Y.; Xu, P. "Turning green into gold": A framework for energy performance contracting (EPC) in China's real estate industry. *J. Clean. Prod.* **2015**, *109*, 166–173. [CrossRef]
22. Chen, Z. Launch of the health-care reform plan in China. *Lancet* **2009**, *373*, 1322–1324. [CrossRef]
23. Yip, W.; Hsiao, W. Harnessing the privatization of China's fragmented health-care delivery. *Lancet* **2014**, *384*, 805–818. [CrossRef]
24. Yip, W.C.; Hsiao, W.C.; Chen, W.; Hu, S.; Ma, J.; Maynard, A. Early appraisal of China's huge and complex health-care reforms. *Lancet* **2012**, *379*, 833–842. [CrossRef]
25. Blumenthal, D.; Hsiao, W. Privatization and its discontents—The evolving Chinese health care system. *N. Engl. J. Med.* **2005**, *353*, 1165–1170. [CrossRef]
26. Tang, S.; Brixi, H.; Bekedam, H. Advancing universal coverage of healthcare in China: Translating political will into policy and practice. *Int. J. Health Plan. Manag.* **2014**, *29*, 160–174. [CrossRef] [PubMed]
27. Yip, W.C.; Hsiao, W.; Meng, Q.; Chen, W.; Sun, X. Realignment of incentives for health-care providers in China. *Lancet* **2010**, *375*, 1120–1130. [CrossRef]
28. Liu, Y.; Hsiao, W.C.; Eggleston, K. Equity in health and health care: The Chinese experience. *Soc. Sci. Med.* **1999**, *49*, 1349–1356. [CrossRef]
29. Meng, Q.; Yang, H.; Chen, W.; Sun, Q.; Liu, X. Health Systems in Transition. In *the People's Republic of China Health System Review*; WHO Regional Office for the Western Pacific: Manila, Philippines, 2015.
30. World Health Organization. *WHO Global Strategy on People-Centered and Integrated Health Services: Interim Report*; World Health Organization: Geneva, Switzerland, 2015; p. 47.
31. National Health and Family Planning Commission. *China Health and Family Planning Statistical Yearbook 2017*; Peking Union Medical College Press: Beijing, Chaina, 2017.
32. Lozano, R.; Fullman, N.; Abate, D.; Abay, S.M.; Abbafati, C.; Abbasi, N.; Abbastabar, H.; Abd-Allah, F.; Abdela, J.; Abdelalim, A.; et al. Measuring progress from 1990 to 2017 and projecting attainment to 2030 of the health-related Sustainable Development Goals for 195 Countries and territories: A systematic analysis for the Global Burden of Disease Study 2017. *Lancet* **2018**, *392*, 2091–2138. [CrossRef]
33. World Health Organization. *Tobacco in China*; World Health Organization: Geneva, Switzerland, 2018; Available online: http://www.wpro.who.int/china/mediacentre/factsheets/tobacco/en/ (accessed on 23 December 2018).
34. World Bank Group. *World Health Organization, Ministry of Finance, PRC, National Health and Family Planning Commission, PRC and Ministry of Human Resources and Social Security, PRC. Deepening Health Reform in China: Building High-Quality and Value-Based Service Delivery*; World Bank Group: Washington, DC, USA, 2016. Available online: https://openknowledge.worldbank.org/handle/10986/24720 (accessed on 23 December 2018).
35. State Council of the People's Republic of China. *"Healthy China 2030" Planning Outline*; State Council of China: Beijing, China, 2016. Available online: http://www.gov.cn/zhengce/2016-10/25/content_5124174.htm (accessed on 23 December 2018).

36. Zhao, Y.; Xu, S.; Wang, L.; Chin, D.P.; Wang, S.; Jiang, G.; Xia, H.; Zhou, Y.; Li, Q.; Ou, X.; et al. National Survey of Drug-Resistant Tuberculosis in China. *N. Eng. J. Med.* **2012**, *23*, 2161–2170. [CrossRef]
37. Tang, S.; Ehiri, J.; Long, Q. China's biggest, most neglected health challenge: Non-communicable diseases. *Infect. Dis. Poverty* **2013**, *2*, 7. [CrossRef]
38. Wei, H.; Derson, Y.; Shuiyuan, X.; Lingjiang, L.; Yalin, Z. Alcohol consumption and alcohol-related problems: Chinese experience from six area samples, 1994. *Addiction* **1999**, *94*, 1467–1476. [CrossRef]
39. Cochrane, J.; Chen, H.; Conigrave, K.M.; Hao, W. Alcohol use in China. *Alcohol Alcohol.* **2003**, *38*, 537–542. [CrossRef]
40. Wang, S.Y.; Chi, G.B.; Jing, C.X.; Dong, X.M.; Wu, C.P.; Li, L.P. Trends in road traffic crashes and associated injury and fatality in the People's Republic of China, 1951–1999. *Inj. Control Saf. Promot.* **2003**, *10*, 83–87. [CrossRef]
41. Ma, S.; Li, Q.; Zhou, M.; Duan, L.; Bishai, D. Road traffic injury in China: A review of national data sources. *Traffic Inj. Prev.* **2012**, *13* (Suppl. 1), 57–63. [CrossRef]

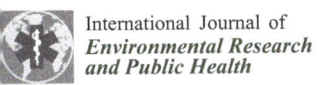

Article

Competency Model for the Middle Nurse Manager (MCGE-Logistic Level)

Alberto González-García [1], Arrate Pinto-Carral [1,*], Jesús Sanz Villorejo [2] and Pilar Marqués-Sánchez [1]

[1] Department of Nursing and Physiotherapy, Leon University, 24071 León, Spain; agong@unileon.es (A.G.-G.); pilar.marques@unileon.es (P.M.-S.)
[2] University Dental Clinic, European University of Madrid, 28045 Madrid, Spain; jesus.sanz@universidadeuropea.es
* Correspondence: arrate.pcarral@unileon.es

Abstract: Healthcare systems are immersed in transformative processes, influenced by economic changes, together with social and health instability. The middle nurse manager plays a fundamental role, since he or she is responsible for translating the strategic vision, values and objectives of the organization. The objective of this study was to propose the model of competencies to be developed by the middle nurse manager in the Spanish healthcare system. Our methodology consisted in the application of the Delphi method in order to reach an agreement on the necessary competencies, and principal component analysis (PCA) was used to determine the construct validity, reducing the dimensionality of the set of data. Fifty-one competencies were identified for the definition of the model, highlighting decision-making, leadership and communication. The PCA pointed out the structural validity of the proposed model through the saturation of the main components (α Cronbach > 0.631). The results show the model of competencies which the middle nurse manager in the Spanish healthcare system must develop. Middle nurse managers may use these as criteria to plan their professional strategies in the context of management. This model of competencies can be applied to establishing selection processes or training programs for the role of middle nurse manager.

Keywords: model of competencies; competency; middle nurse manager; nurse manager; logistic level; health policy; healthcare services; healthcare affordability; Hospital efficiency

Citation: González-García, A.; Pinto-Carral, A.; Villorejo, J.S.; Marqués-Sánchez, P. Competency Model for the Middle Nurse Manager (MCGE-Logistic Level). *Int. J. Environ. Res. Public Health* **2021**, *18*, 3898. https://doi.org/10.3390/ijerph18083898

Academic Editor: Dimitris Zavras

Received: 8 March 2021
Accepted: 7 April 2021
Published: 8 April 2021

Publisher's Note: MDPI stays neutral with regard to jurisdictional claims in published maps and institutional affiliations.

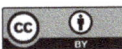

Copyright: © 2021 by the authors. Licensee MDPI, Basel, Switzerland. This article is an open access article distributed under the terms and conditions of the Creative Commons Attribution (CC BY) license (https://creativecommons.org/licenses/by/4.0/).

1. Introduction

Healthcare systems are immersed in processes of global transformation, influenced by economic and social changes, changes in health technology and structural alterations in systems for the provision of healthcare [1–5]. In this uncertain context, nurses are under pressure to improve quality of care [6]. It thus seems logical that nurses should form part of the nucleus of healthcare so that organizations are able to deal with these changes successfully [7–9]. Thus, as highlighted by Witt et al. [10], when the nurse takes part in the healthcare process (management and nursing care) organizations achieve better performances [11,12]. Within health organizations, nurse managers are a key part of any healthcare attention team. Nurse managers are responsible for introducing changes and creating environments in which nurses are able to provide quality attention, at the same time as guaranteeing the achievement of the objectives of the organization under sustainability and efficiency criteria [13–15].

The relationship between economic and sustainability policies with respect to offering quality care in health systems is the starting point and is of interest in justifying the development of managerial competencies, which are related to a higher degree of performance and results [16–19]. In this sense, Yoder-Wise [20] states that that the development of an advanced level of managerial competency is fundamental in achieving the objectives of the organization. Warshawsky [21] highlights that one of the key strategies for the success of health organizations currently resides in the capacity of the nurse manager to develop advanced management skills. This development is achieved through carrying out postgraduate university studies [22]. In this sense, West [23] states that it is possible to observe a difference between nurse managers who have undertaken university programs in management compared to others who have not completed this type of training program. For his part, Herrin [24] points out how master's degree training empowers nurse managers, enabling the effective management of the healthcare process.

Therefore, in order to identify, orient and train nurse managers, managerial competencies are an essential resource [25]. This competency training in management must go beyond the ambit of nursing, for example, including business management, artificial intelligence, technology, etc. [26–28].

Although there is no single definition of management competency [29], we can define it as the correct combination and application of the knowledge, attitudes and skills of middle nurse managers in specific management functions, which are observed and measured as behaviors [30]. New [31] defines managerial competencies as those in which the nurses are able to collaborate with other people, whereast Hudak et al. [32] define them as the skills, knowledge and capacities necessary to achieve quality healthcare.

In healthcare organizations, there is a chain of authority from upper management to the assistance level (Figure 1) [33]. A middle nurse manager (known in Spain as a "supervisora de área de enfermería" or "jefa de área de enfermería") is the person in the intermediate position between the operational level of the nurse manager and the nurse executive [34]. The middle nurse manager is responsible for translating the culture and strategy of the organization to the operational level, as well as managing resources, coordinating nursing care and planning and contributing to the evaluation of services provided, together with supporting and encouraging teamwork in the attention units and implementing innovative practices [33,35–38]. Therefore, the middle nurse manager plays a key position, since they do not only carry out clinical leadership and management, but are also responsible for translating the strategic vision and the values and objectives of the organization's care actions [39,40]. In the Spanish healthcare system, the middle nurse manager is responsible for the management and coordination of a functional area of nursing in a healthcare organization, for example, the surgical area [41].

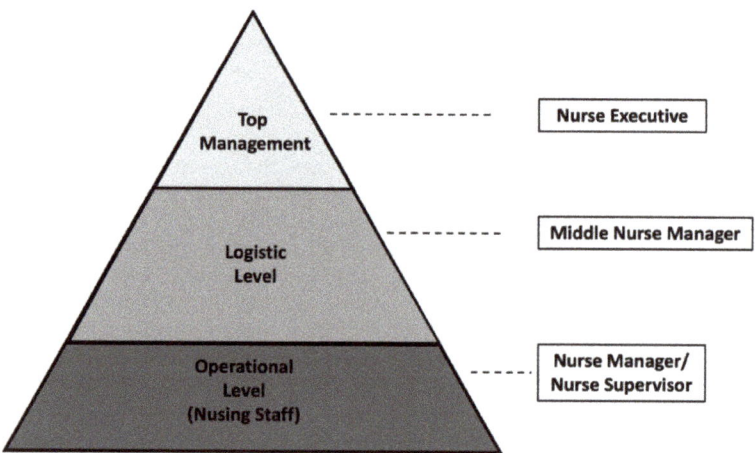

Figure 1. Management levels. Source: own elaboration.

Managerial competencies have been researched from various angles. For example, Chase [41] identified technical, human and conceptual skills, as well as leadership and financial management skills. The American Organization of Nurse Executives (AONE) [36] identified the management of the relationships, communication, leadership, knowledge of the health environment and financial skills as strategic areas in the development of competencies. González García et al. [42] highlighted the management of relationships, communication skills, listening, leadership, conflict management, ethical principles and skills for managing teams as core competencies for nurse managers. Finally, in a brief summary, Pillay [43] highlighted the management of people and organizational capacity, together with strategic thinking, as key competencies.

On the other hand, based on the literature review, it can be deduced that it is necessary to improve the state of knowledge about the role of the middle nurse manager [35,44,45]. The competencies necessary are not usually clearly defined, which would explain this gap in the understanding of the middle nurse managers. This same absence is evident in the Spanish context, as there is no model of competencies for the carrying out of management functions at the logistical level.

For this reason, the main objective of this study was to propose a model of competencies which should be developed by a middle nurse manager in the Spanish healthcare system. For this reason, the following specific objectives were proposed:

- Reach a consensus on the competencies required for a middle nurse manager.
- Establish a consensus on the degree of development of each of the competencies required for a middle nurse manager.
- Achieve consensus about the training required to develop each competency.
- Assess the structural validity of the proposed model.

2. Materials and Methods

2.1. Revision of the Literature

Based on the scoping review [46] of the literature carried out during 2010–2019 to determine the competencies associated with nursing management, electronic databases were used (Web of Science, Scopus, PubMed and CINAHL) to carry out the search, identifying 56 competencies for middle nurse managers. The results of this review provided the basis for carrying out this Delphi study, evaluating the competencies of the positions of the middle nurse manager.

2.2. Delphi Methodology

A four-round Delphi method was employed. The Delphi method focuses on the identification of expert opinion to reach a consensus [47]. The Delphi methodology has been considered the most convenient method when there is a lack of knowledge on a topic. [47,48].

The aim of the first Delphi round was to generate a list of competencies required for middle nurse managers. In the second round, experts were provided with feedback from the first iteration. All participants were invited to reconsider their opinion. In the third round, the experts were asked their opinion on the competencies of the middle nurse manager, in order to reach a consensus. The expert panel also was asked to indicate the training necessary to achieve specific levels of competency (expert, very competent, competent, advanced novice and novice). During round four, experts were provided with feedback from the third round and they were encouraged to rethink their original answers after reviewing the report of the third Delphi round.

2.2.1. Consensus

For this research, consensus was set at 80% or greater agreement (defined as somewhat in agreement–total agreement [score 4–5]) with regard to (I) the proposed competencies; (II) the level of development of the competencies; (III) the training for each competency. Items with less than an 80% response rate were eliminated for the following Delphi round.

2.2.2. Participants

Two categories of experts, consisting of a combined total of 50 experts (Table 1), were established based on the Delphi Technique:

Table 1. Sociodemographic characteristics of the panel experts.

Characteristics	Range/Category	Frequency	Percentage
Age	<40	10	20
	40–50	15	30
	51–60	18	36
	>60	7	14
Sex	Female	32	64
	Male	18	36
Education	Master's degree	34	68
	Ph.D	14	28
Expert group 1	Minister of Health	3	6.1
Expert group 2	Head of the Health Department	5	10
Expert group 3	General Council of Nurses	3	6
Expert group 4	Scientific Association	4	8
Expert group 5	Trade Union	3	6
Expert group 6	General Manager	5	10
Expert group 6	Medical Director	2	4
Expert group 6	Nurse Executive	5	10
Expert group 6	Management Director	1	2
Expert group 7	Middle Nurse manager	2	4.1
Expert group 8	Nursing supervisor	3	6.1
Expert group 9	Nurse	3	6.1
Expert group 9	Doctor	2	4.1
Expert group 9	Assistant Nursing Care Technician	2	4.1
Expert group 10	Nursing Degree Students	2	4.1
Expert group 11	Research/Teaching	4	8.2
Expert group 12	Lawyer	1	1

Source: own elaboration.

Experts in healthcare management. This category of experts represented healthcare from the different hospitals and institutions, and performed management and leadership functions.

Experts in the health environment. This category of experts represented the different fields involved in healthcare and were selected for their specific views on healthcare practices, university training, students and healthcare research.

2.2.3. Variables

The following variables were used:

Sociodemographic variables: to determine the characteristics of the participants, information was collected on age, gender, university degree, university training, postgraduate training, professional role, location of the study, years of national activity, years of management experience, management functions carried out and international experience. Sociodemographic variables were used to establish the profile of the expert panel.

Competencies: the competencies suggested to the experts came from the literature review. The competencies were used to establish the competency model for the middle nurse manager.

2.2.4. Delphi Surveys

Two surveys were developed for the specific purpose of the study.

Competencies necessary for middle nurse managers: Every participant quantified their level of agreement or disagreement with each competence in accordance with the Likert scale from 1 to 5 (1 = disagree totally, 5 = completely in agreement).

Degree of development of the competencies of middle nurse managers: In order to achieve an agreement on the competencies required for each functional level of nurse manager, the level of consensus with each competency was registered in accordance with the Likert scale from 1 to 5 (1 = beginner, 5 = expert), and the type of training required to develop the competencies, in accordance with the Likert scale of 1 to 6 (1 = university extension, 2 = continuous training, 3 = university expert, 4 = diploma in university specialization, 5 = master's degree, 6 = PhD).

2.2.5. Degree of Development

The term "degree of development" was used to indicate the degree of proficiency shown by middle nurse managers in the performance of each competency. Based on Bernner's theory [49], therefore, the level of development was expressed as follows.

- Novice: a middle nurse manager who has no prior experience in a competency associated with a professional role or situation. In many instances, this is the starting point for a nurse manager, as they would be in possession of clinical competencies, yet lack knowledge and skills in management.
- Advanced novice: someone who is able to contribute partial solutions to unknown or complex situations. Although an advanced novice may be able to perform the functions required for the nurse manager position, they may or may not have the ability to understand the context and actions required.
- Competent: implies an adequate understanding of the context and situation. The competent middle nurse manager may be able to cope with situations associated with the nurse executive role, although they may lack analytical skills and an understanding of complex situations.
- Very competent: the middle nurse manager focuses on a comprehensive understanding of situations at every level, and is someone who is able to anticipate problems and make appropriate decisions.
- Expert one who demonstrates the behavior of the model of competencies. The expert nurse manager anticipates problems, understands them at an instinctive level and proposes correct and appropriate solutions [49].

The degree of development must be understood in a progressive and exclusive manner, starting at the level of novice and ending at the level of expert. The degree of development is achieved through assigning the appropriate training to each level.

2.3. Principal Component Analysis

Principal component analysis (PCA) is a technique for the transformation of data [50]. The main purpose is to reduce the dimensionality of a data set by reducing the number of variables and preserving as much relevant information as possible [50]. Factor analyses were performed according to Thurstone's theory [51,52] (3 phases): first, determining if the data are suitable for factor analysis; second, performing the extraction of the factors and, finally, carrying out the rotation and interpretation of the factors.

The Kaiser–Meyer–Olkin (KMO) method was used to determine the suitability of the data for the factorial analysis. The following step was the extraction of the data, using the Kaiser criterion, making the decision based on values higher than 1 [53], and a scree plot, which is a graphical representation transit value [54]. Finally, the rotation interpretation of the factors was made by means of the varimax rotation method and Kaiser standardization to obtain the simplest possible structure that was easy to interpret.

3. Results

3.1. Demographic Data of the Panel of Experts

Fifty experts responded to our invitation to participate and take part in the Delphi study. All of them completed the questionnaires of the Delphi study (100% response rate). The characteristics of the full 50-member Delphi panel are listed in Table 1.

3.2. Model of Competencies for the Middle Nurse Manager

During the first and second Delphi rounds, a consensus was reached (more than 80%) for 51 competencies from the proposed list. The consensus of round 2 details the competencies that make up the model (Table 2) structured into six dimensions, according to the following definitive characteristics: management, communication and technology, leadership and teamwork, knowledge of the healthcare system, nursing knowledge and personality (Figure 2). In round 2, competencies with a consensus of less than 80% were eliminated.

Table 2. Model of competencies for a middle nurse manager.

I. Management
1. Analytical thinking (V. COMP)
2. Decision-making (V. COMP)
3. Innovation (V. COMP)
4. Strategic management (V. COMP)
5. Human resources management (V. COMP)
6. Legal aspects (V. COMP)
7. Organizational management (COMP)
8. Result orientation (V. COMP)
II. Communication and technology
9. Communication skills (V. COMP)
10. Feedback (V. COMP)
11. Evaluation of information and its sources (V. COMP)
12. Listening (V. COMP)
13. Information systems and computers (EXP)
14. Technology (COMP)
15. English medium level of writing (COMP)
III. Leadership and teamwork
16. Relationship management (V. COMP)
17. Leadership (COMP)
18. Career planning (V. COMP)
19. Influence (V. COMP)
20. Change management (V. COMP)
21. Delegation (V. COMP)
22. Conflict management (V. COMP)
23. Ethical principles (V. COMP)
24. Power and empowerment (V. COMP)
25. Critical thinking (EXP)
26. Collaboration and team management skills (V. COMP)
27. Interpersonal relations (EXP)
28. Multi-professional management (V. COMP)
29. Team-building strategies (V. COMP)
30. **Talent management (COMP)**
IV. Knowledge of the healthcare system
31. Care management systems (V. COMP)
32. User care skills (V. COMP)
33. Health policy (COMP)
34. Identification and responsibility with organization (V. COMP)
35. Knowledge of the health environment (V. COMP)
36. Quality and safety (V. COMP)
37. Quality and improvement processes (V. COMP)
V. Nursing knowledge
38. Clinical skills (V. COMP)
39. Standard Nursing Practice (COMP)
40. Nurse Research (COMP)
41. Nursing Theories (COMP)
42. Care Planning (COMP)
43. Nursing training planning (V. COMP)
44. Professionalism (COMP)
VI. Personality
45. Serve as a model (V. COMP)
46. Awareness of personal strengths and weaknesses (EXP)
47. Strategic vision (V. COMP)
48. Personal and professional balance (V. COMP)
49. Compassion (V. COMP)
50. Emotional intelligence (V. COMP)
51. Integrity (EXP)

Source: own elaboration. Legend of the table: EXP = expert. V. COMP = very competent. COMP = competent.

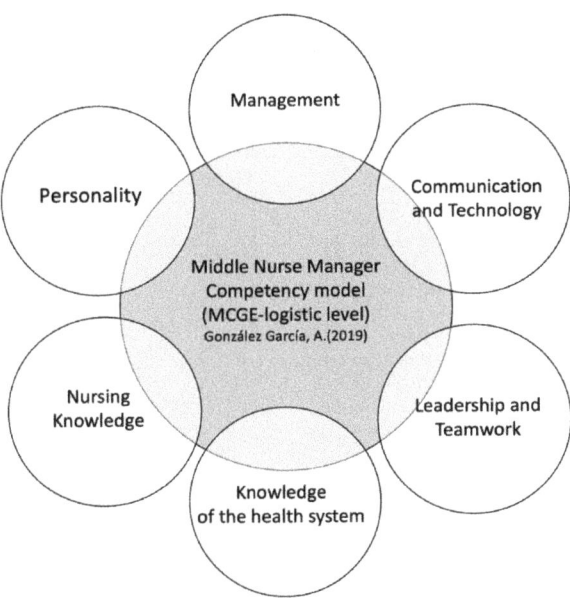

Figure 2. Dimensions of the middle nurse manager executive competency model. Source: own elaboration.

The third and fourth Delphi rounds demonstrated that 51 competencies are necessary for middle nurse managers, with a consensus that the development of these competencies should be at the level of "Expert", "Very competent" and "Competent". A consensus was also reached during rounds 3 and 4 to achieve the level of development of each competency. The final consensus as detailed in Table 2 and makes up the competency model for the middle nurse manager in the Spanish healthcare system.

As regards the training necessary for the development of each of the levels of competency, in Table 3, we can observe the consensus reached for each of the levels of development of the competency.

Table 3. Level of competency development and training.

	Univ. Ext.	Cont. Ed	Univ. Exp.	Univ. Spec. D	Master	Ph.D.
Novice	100%					
Novice Advanced	90%	98%				
Competent		90%	90%	96%		
Very Competent		96%	100%	96%	96%	
Expert					96%	96%

Source: own elaboration. Note: Univ. Ext. = university extension diploma; Cont. Ed = continuing education; Univ. Exp. = university expert; Univ. Spec. D. = university specialization diploma; Master = master's degree; Ph.D. = Ph.D. degree.

3.3. Principal Component Analysis

For the principal component analysis, the competencies were grouped together in dimensions, in accordance with their definitive characteristics. The dimensions of management, communication and technology and leadership and teamwork made up four principal components, the dimensions of knowledge of the healthcare system and the personality dimension comprised two principal components, whereas the nursing knowledge dimension was designated as a single main component (Table 4). The factorial loads of each of the items integrated into each dimension widely exceeded the lower level of 0.4, and the α Cronbach demonstrates the quality of the adjustment (Table 4). From these results it can be deduced that the proposed model is structurally sound.

Table 4. Factor structure of the proposed competency model.

	Management Dimension				
	CP1	CP2	CP3	CP4	
Result orientation	0.789				
Strategic management	0.725				
Innovation	0.710				
Legal aspects		0.936			
Analytical thinking		0.554			
Organizational management			0.968		
Decision-making				0.980	
Explained variance	32.325%	18.075%	12.822%	11.569%	
Eigenvalue	2.263	1.265	0.898	0.810	
α Cronbach					0.631
	Communication and Technology Dimension				
	CP1	CP2	CP3	CP4	
Listening	0.905				
Information systems and computers	0.679				
English medium level of writing		0.874			
Technology		0.636			
Feedback			0.88		
Communication skills			0.589		
Evaluation of information and its sources				0.826	
Explained variance	31.326%	17.341%	16.065%	13.076%	
Eigenvalue	2.193	1.214	1.125	0.915	
α Cronbach					0.6
	Leadership and Teamwork Dimension				
	CP1	CP2	CP3	CP4	
Change management	0.812				
Influence	0.802				
Leadership	0.703				
Delegation	0.696				
Collaboration and team management skills		0.85			
Critical thinking		0.786			
Team-building strategies		0.736			
Career planning		0.707			
Ethical principles			0.885		
Power and empowerment			0.765		
Conflict management				0.936	
Explained variance	46.309%	12.796%	10.286%	8.17%	
Eigenvalue	5.094	1.408	1.131	0.899	
α Cronbach					0.876

Table 4. Cont.

	Management Dimension	
	Knowledge of the Healthcare System	
	CP1	CP2
Quality and safety	0.971	
Quality and improvement processes	0.948	
Identification and responsibility with the organization		0.917
Health policy		0.838
Explained variance	57.954%	29.970%
Eigenvalue	2.318	1.199
α Cronbach		0.749

	Nursing Knowledge
	CP1
Nursing training planning	0.918
Nurse research	0.910
Nursing theories	0.822
Clinical skills	0.777
Explained variance	73.733%
Eigenvalue	2.949
α Cronbach	0.808

	Personality	
	CP1	CP2
Awareness of personal strengths and weaknesses	0.905	
Strategic vision	0.891	
Personal and professional balance	0.836	
Compassion		0.884
Emotional intelligence		0.735
Explained variance	54.76%	21.705%
Eigenvalue	2.738	1.085
α Cronbach		0.809

Source: own elaboration.

4. Discussion

In this study, a competency model for the role of middle nurse manager was developed and validated (In Spain, the middle nurse manager is known as the "supervisora de área de enfermería" or "jefa de área de enfermería") in the context of the Spanish health system. The model of competencies for middle nurse managers in Spain is made up of 51 competencies, structured into six dimensions, according to their defining characteristics—(1) Management, (2) Communication and Technology, (3) Leadership and Teamwork, (4) Knowledge of the Healthcare System, (5) Nursing Knowledge and (6) Personality. These findings are in line with the arguments of McCarthy and Fitzpatrick [55], who state that the competencies of the middle nurse manager should be oriented towards negotiation, the coordination of resources, the monitoring of the activity, negotiation and empowerment. The AONE in its models suggested the need to develop 35 competencies [56], and Pillay described 51 competencies, building on the research carried out by AONE [43]. However, these models differ from our proposal in terms of the weight that has been awarded to some of the competencies that coincide within the models, such as, for example, the relationships with the management of the business.

During the third and fourth Delphi rounds, agreement was achieved among our experts on the development of the competencies. Agreement was reached for the following levels: "competent" levels (this level is achieved when there is a robust demonstration of competency), "very competent" (this level is considered to be achieved when there is a meaningful demonstration of competency) and "expert" (this level is considered to be achieved when the knowledge and skills of the competency model are demonstrated). This proposal coincides with that of AONE, which uses the levels of competent, proficient and expert for the development of competencies, highlighting how these levels are achieved by means of a master's degree or PhD studies [57,58]. For the assessment of its relevance, we must highlight that the studies carried out by Chase [40] are different in some ways compared to our research, in that the levels of development of the competencies are not indicated, centering on the degree (minimally, moderately, significantly and essentially for management) to which they contribute to the role of a nursing manager. The results of our research highlight the importance of the strong development of competencies, in the same manner as Crawford et al. [58] emphasized the need for a high level of expertise and the development of a set of competencies to cope with the functions of a logistics-level manager.

During rounds 3 and 4 of the Delphi method, the panel of experts reached a consensus on the training that the nurse manager should develop at the logistic level in three levels of competency ("expert", "very competent" and "competent"). The "competent" level is achieved by completing continuing education, university expertise and a diploma in university specialization. As regards the "very competent" level, the experts agreed that this is achieved with university expertise, a diploma in university specialization or a master's degree. Finally, the "expert" level is reached by completing a master's degree program and PhD studies. It must be borne in mind that work experience does not prepare the nurse to assume management functions, with training being the factor that most significantly influences the development of the competencies of middle nurse managers [59]. Warshawsky et al. [21] warn of the risks to the organization if the nurses assume management responsibilities without the suitable knowledge and training. In the same way, Rizani et al. [60] and Herrin et al. [24] point out that that the competency of the nurse manager is greater when they have carried out advanced studies (a master's degree or PhD), increasing their level of competency over time to a higher degree than that of the managers who have not carried out advanced training. In this sense, the American Nurses Credentialing Center has made adjustments to the standards of training recommended for all nurse managers, elevating the degree of exigency [61].

The PCA verified the model of competencies for the middle nurse manager, highlighting that the importance of competencies can be defined by three principal components—communication (communication skills, relationship management, conflict management), leadership (leadership skills and team management) and decision-making (decision-making and ethical principles). The eigenvalues demonstrated that the decision-making and ethical principles indicate a strong and significant relationship between these competencies [62]. Furthermore, the eigenvalues also point to the relationship between leadership and work teams [63], and between communication and conflict resolution.

The development of communication skills expected from the middle nurse manager must include the ability to provide critical thinking and stimulate reflection before taking action in nursing teams [35]. It should also provide, for instance, conflict resolution and shared decision-making, which is also associated with team management [64].

5. Conclusions

In this study, consensus was reached on the competencies necessary for establishing a model of competencies for middle nurse managers (MCGE-logistic level) (In Spain: "supervisora de área de enfermería" or "jefa de área de enfermería") adapted to current health policies, economic necessities and the sustainability of the organizations and healthcare in an uncertain environment. In conclusion, this study developed a consensus on 51 competencies necessary for middle nurse managers in Spain, of which the following can be highlighted: communication, leadership and decision-making. The middle nurse manager is accountable for one of the most critical divisions of a healthcare organization, and is essential in the management of nurses and material resources. The quality of the final care provided will depend on their management style. Therefore, a nurse or a nurse manager should not be promoted to the role of middle nurse manager without undertaking advanced programs in management.

The results of our research show the accurate levels of development for each competency for a middle nurse manager. It would be recommendable for the nurse to achieve these competencies before performing the functions of a middle nurse manager.

Any nurse who aspires to carry out the role of a middle nurse manager would be advised to develop the competencies that are set out in the proposed model beforehand.

Furthermore, this study sets out the training necessary to acquire the development of the competencies necessary for the logistical level. Both nurses who wish to be promoted to middle nurse managers and nurse managers who presently work at this level would be advised to follow the education programs that have emerged from our research, in order to adapt their knowledge to the requirements of this role.

Implications for Nursing Management

This model has implications for the Spanish healthcare system, healthcare policies, and for the practices and education related to middle nurse management. The proposed model contributes to the design of the function of the middle nurse manager, to the selection processes and the design of the study plans of the nurse managers in traditional academic institutions and in programs for continuous professional development within organizations. It is probable that a greater understanding of these competencies can serve as the basis for developing interventions, which could improve the working environment of nurses and patient care, as well as ensuring the safety and the productivity of the organization.

Author Contributions: Conceptualization, A.G.-G., P.M.-S. and A.P.-C.; methodology, A.G.-G. and A.P.-C.; software, A.G.-G. validation, A.G.-G., P.M.-S., J.S.V. and A.P.-C.; formal analysis, A.G.-G. and P.M.-S.; investigation, A.G.-G. resources A.G.-G., P.M.-S., J.S.V. and A.P.-C. data curation, A.G.-G., P.M.-S., J.S.V. and A.P.-C.; writing—original draft preparation, A.G.-G.; writing—review and editing, A.G.-G., P.M.-S. and A.P.-C.; visualization, A.G.-G., P.M.-S., J.S.V. and A.P.-C.; supervision, A.G.-G., P.M.-S., J.S.V. and A.P.-C.; project administration, A.G.-G., P.M.-S. and A.P.-C. All authors have read and agreed to the published version of the manuscript.

Funding: This research received no external funding.

Institutional Review Board Statement: Not applicable.

Informed Consent Statement: Informed consent was obtained from all subjects involved in the study.

Data Availability Statement: The data presented in this study are available on request from the corresponding author.

Conflicts of Interest: The authors declare no conflict of interest.

References

1. Leontiou, I.; Merkouris, A.; Papastavrou, E.; Middleton, N. Self-efficacy, empowerment and power of middle nurse managers in Cyprus: A correlational study. *J. Nurs. Manag.* **2021**, *11*, 1–11.
2. Kantanen, K.; Kaunonen, M.; Helminen, M.; Suominen, T. Leadership and management competencies of head nurses and directors of nursing in Finnish social and health care. *J. Res. Nurs.* **2017**, *22*, 228–244. [CrossRef]
3. Cathcart, E.B.; Greenspan, M. A new window into nurse manager development. *J. Nurs. Adm.* **2012**, *42*, 557–561. [CrossRef]
4. Kleinman, S.C. Leadership Roles, Competencies, and Education: How Prepared Are Our Nurse Managers? *J. Nurs. Adm.* **2003**, *33*, 451–455. [CrossRef]
5. Ding, B.; Liu, W.; Tsai, S.B.; Gu, D.; Bian, F.; Shao, X. Effect of patient participation on nurse and patient outcomes in inpatient healthcare. *Int. J. Environ. Res. Public Health* **2019**, *16*, 1344. [CrossRef]
6. Van Dyk, J.; Siedlecki, S.L.; Fitzpatrick, J.J. Frontline nurse managers' confidence and self-efficacy. *J. Nurs. Manag.* **2016**, *24*, 533–539. [CrossRef]
7. Thorne, S. Nursing now or never. *Nurs. Inq.* **2019**, *26*, e12326. [CrossRef]
8. Aiken, L.H.; Cimiotti, J.P.; Sloane, D.M.; Smith, H.L.; Flynn, L.; Neff, D.F. Effects of nurse staffing and nurse education on patient deaths in hospitals with different nurse work environments. *Med. Care* **2011**, *49*, 1047–1053. [CrossRef]

9. Savage, C.; Kub, J. Public health and nursing: A natural partnership. *Int. J. Environ. Res. Public Health* **2009**, *6*, 2843–2848. [CrossRef]
10. Whitt, M.; Baird, B.; Wilbanks, P.; Esmail, P. Tracking decisions with shared governance. *Nurse Lead.* **2011**, *9*, 53–55. [CrossRef]
11. Ho, E.; Principi, E.; Cordon, C.P.; Amenudzie, Y.; Kotwa, K.; Holt, S.; Macphee, M. The Synergy Tool: Making Important Quality Gains within One Healthcare Organization. *Adm. Sci.* **2017**, *7*, 32. [CrossRef]
12. McHugh, G.A.; Horne, M.; Chalmers, K.I.; Luker, K.A. Specialist community nurses: A critical analysis of their role in the management of long-term conditions. *Int. J. Environ. Res. Public Health* **2009**, *6*, 2550–2567. [CrossRef]
13. Seabold, K.; Sarver, W.; Kline, M.; McNett, M. Impact of intensive leadership training on nurse manager satisfaction and perceived importance of competencies. *Nurs. Manag.* **2020**, *51*, 34–42. [CrossRef]
14. Duffield, C.; Gardner, G.; Doubrovsky, A.; Wise, S. Manager, clinician or both? Nurse managers' engagement in clinical care activities. *J. Nurs. Manag.* **2019**, *27*, 1538–1545. [CrossRef]
15. Kodama, Y.; Fukahori, H. Nurse managers' attributes to promote change in their wards: A qualitative study. *Nurs. Open* **2017**, *4*, 209–217. [CrossRef]
16. Boyatzis, R.E. *The Competent Manager: A Model for Effective Performance*; John Wiley & Sons: Toronto, ON, Canada, 1982; ISBN 0-471-09031-X.
17. Groves, K. Talent management best practices: How exemplary health care organizations create value in a down economy. *Health Care Manag. Rev.* **2011**, *3*, 227–240. [CrossRef]
18. Kerfoot, K.M.; Luquire, R. Alignment of the system's chief nursing officer: Staff or direct line structure? *Nurs. Adm. Q.* **2012**, *36*, 325–331. [CrossRef]
19. MacMillan-Finlayson, S. Competency development for nurse executives: Meeting the challenge. *J. Nurs. Adm.* **2010**, *40*, 254–257. [CrossRef]
20. Yoder-Wise, Y.; Scott, E.; Sullivan, D. Expanding leadership capacity: Educational levels for nurse leaders. *J. Nurs. Adm.* **2013**, *43*, 326–328. [CrossRef] [PubMed]
21. Warshawsky, N.E.; Caramanica, L.; Cramer, E. Organizational Support for Nurse Manager Role Transition and Onboarding: Strategies for Success. *J. Nurs. Adm.* **2020**, *50*, 254–260. [CrossRef]
22. Institute of Medicine of the National Academies. The Future of Nursing: Leading change, advancing health. *Rep. Brief* **2010**, *40*, 1–4.
23. West, M. Evaluation of a nurse leadership development programme. *Nurs. Manag.* **2016**, *22*, 1–6. [CrossRef]
24. Herrin, D.; Jones, K.; Krepper, R.; Sherman, R.; Reineck, C. Future nursing administration graduate curricula, Part 2: Foundation and strategies. *J. Nurs. Adm.* **2006**, *36*, 498–505. [CrossRef] [PubMed]
25. Meadows, M.T.; Dwyer, C. AONE continues to guide leadership expertise with post-acute competencies. *Nurse Lead.* **2015**, *13*, 21–25. [CrossRef]
26. Baxter, C.; Warshawsky, N. Exploring the acquisition of nurse manager competence. *Nurse Lead.* **2014**, *12*, 46–59. [CrossRef]
27. Chase, L.K. Are you confidently competent? *Nurs. Manag.* **2012**, *43*, 50–53. [CrossRef]
28. DeOnna, J. Developing and Validating an Instrument to Measure the Perceived Job Competencies Linked to Performance and Staff Retention of First-Line Nurse Managers Employed in a Hospital Setting. Ph.D. Thesis, The Pennsylvania State University, College of Education, State College, PA, USA, 2006.
29. Gunawan, J.; Aungsuroch, Y.; Fisher, M.L.; McDaniel, A.M. Development and Psychometric Properties of Managerial Competence Scale for First-Line Nurse Managers in Indonesia. *SAGE Open Nurs.* **2019**, *5*, 1–12. [CrossRef]
30. Gunawan, J.; Aungsuroch, Y.; Fisher, M.L.; McDaniel, A.M. Managerial Competence of First-Line Nurse Managers in Public Hospitals in Indonesia. *J. Multidiscip. Healthc.* **2020**, *13*, 1017–1025. [CrossRef]
31. New, E.G. Reflections A three-tier model of organizational competencies. *J. Manag. Psychol.* **1996**, *11*, 44–51. [CrossRef]
32. Hudak, R.P.; Brooke, P.; Finstuen, K. Identifying management competencies for health care executives: Review of a series of Delphi studies. *J. Health Adm. Educ.* **2000**, *18*, 213–219.
33. Holden, L.; Roberts, I. The depowerment of European middle managers: Challenges and uncertainties. *J. Manag. Psychol.* **2004**, *19*, 269–287. [CrossRef]
34. Lalleman, P.; Smid, G.; Lagerwey, M.D.; Oldenhof, L.; Schuurmans, M.J. Nurse middle managers' dispositions of habitus a bourdieusian analysis of supporting role behaviors in Dutch and American hospitals. *Adv. Nurs. Sci.* **2015**, *38*, E1–E16. [CrossRef]
35. Scoble, K.B.; Russell, G. Vision 2020, Part I: Profile of the future nurse leader. *J. Nurs. Adm.* **2003**, *33*, 324–330. [CrossRef]
36. AONE. Competencies Assessment. Available online: http://www.aone.org/resources/online-assessments.shtml (accessed on 18 September 2020).
37. Carney, M. Understanding organizational culture: The key to successful middle manager strategic involvement in health care delivery? *J. Nurs. Manag.* **2006**, *14*, 23–33. [CrossRef]
38. Engle, R.L.; Lopez, E.R.; Gormley, K.E.; Chan, J.A.; Charns, M.P.; van Deusen Lukas, C. What roles do middle managers play in implementation of innovative practices? *Health Care Manag. Rev.* **2017**, *42*, 14–27. [CrossRef]
39. Ofei, A.M.A.; Paarima, Y.; Barnes, T. Exploring the management competencies of nurse managers in the Greater Accra Region, Ghana. *Int. J. Afr. Nurs. Sci.* **2020**, *13*, 100248.
40. Chase, L. *Nurse Manager Competencies*; University of Iowa: Iowa City, IA, USA, 2010.
41. González-García, A. *Modelo de Competencias para la Gestora Enfermera*; European University of Madrid: Madrid, Spain, 2019.

42. Gonzalez Garcia, A.; Pinto-Carral, A.; Sanz Villorejo, J.; Marqués-Sánchez, P. Nurse Manager Core Competencies: A Proposal in the Spanish Health System. *Int. J. Environ. Res. Public Health* **2020**, *17*, 3173. [CrossRef]
43. Pillay, R. The skills gap in nursing management in the South African public health sector. *Public Health Nurs.* **2011**, *28*, 176–185. [CrossRef]
44. Meadows, M.T. New Competencies for System Chief Nurse Executives. *J. Nurs. Adm.* **2016**, *46*, 235–237. [CrossRef]
45. Vance, M. Scotland the brave: Statutory supervision transformed. *Pract. Midwife* **2009**, *12*, 16–77.
46. Arksey, H.; O'Malley, L. Scoping studies: Towards a methodological framework. *Int. J. Soc. Res. Methodol. Theory Pract.* **2005**, *8*, 19–32. [CrossRef]
47. Varela-Ruiz, M.; Díaz-Bravo, L.; García-Durán, R. Descripción y usos del método Delphi en investigaciones del área de la salud. *Investig. Educ. Méd.* **2012**, *1*, 90–95.
48. Linstone, H.A.; Turoff, M.; Helmer, O. *The Delphi Method*; Addison-Wesley: Redeading, MA, USA, 1975; ISBN 0-201-04294-0.
49. Shirey, M.R. Competencies and tips for effective leadership: From novice to expert. *J. Nurs. Adm.* **2007**, *37*, 167–170. [CrossRef]
50. Sewell, M. *Principal Component Analysis*; University College London: London, UK, 2008.
51. Thurstone, L.L. *Multiple Factor Analysis*, 5th ed.; University of Chicago Press: Chicago, IL, USA, 1957.
52. Thurstone, L.L. Multiple factor analysis. *Psychol. Rev.* **1931**, *38*, 406–427. [CrossRef]
53. Kaiser, H.F. The Application of Electronic Computers to Factor Analysis. *Educ. Psychol. Meas.* **1960**, *20*, 141–151. [CrossRef]
54. Cattell, R.B. The scree test for the number of factors. *Multivar. Behav. Res.* **1966**, *1*, 245–276. [CrossRef]
55. McCarthy, G.; Fitzpatrick, J.J. Development of a Competency Framework for Nurse Managers in Ireland. *J. Contin. Educ. Nurs.* **2009**, *40*, 346–350. [CrossRef]
56. American Organization of Nurse Executives. *AONE Nurse Manager Competencies*; The American Organization of Nurse Executives: Chicago, IL, USA, 2015.
57. Waxman, K.T.; Roussel, L.; Herrin-Griffith, D.; D'Alfonso, J. The AONE Nurse Executive Competencies: 12 Years Later. *Nurse Lead.* **2017**, *15*, 120–126. [CrossRef]
58. Crawford, C.L.; Omery, A.; Spicer, J. An Integrative Review of 21st-Century Roles, Responsibilities, Characteristics, and Competencies of Chief Nurse Executives: A Blueprint for the Next Generation. *Nurs. Adm. Q.* **2017**, *41*, 297–309. [CrossRef]
59. Kuraoka, Y. The relationship between experiential learning and nursing management competency. *J. Nurs. Adm.* **2019**, *49*, 99–104. [CrossRef]
60. Rizany, I.; Hariyati, R.T.S.; Handayani, H. Factors that affect the development of nurses' competencies: A systematic review. *Enferm. Clin.* **2018**, *28*, 154–157. [CrossRef]
61. American Nurses Credentialing Center. ANCCMagnet Recognition Program. Available online: https://www.nursingworld.org/organizational-programs/%0Dmagnet/ (accessed on 18 September 2020).
62. Loreggia, A.; Mattei, N.; Rossi, F.; Venable, K.B. Preferences and Ethical Principles in Decision Making. In Proceedings of the 2018 AAAI/ACM Conference on AI, Ethics and Society-AIES'18, New York, NY, USA, 2–3 February 2018.
63. Berrios Martos, P.; Lopez Zafra, E.; Aguilar Luzon, M.C.; Auguste, J.M. Relationship between leadership style and attitude toward working groups. *Int. J. Psychol.* **2008**, *43*, 444.
64. Garman, A.N.; Fitz, K.D.; Fraser, M.M. Communication and relations management. *J. Healthc. Manag.* **2006**, *51*, 291–294.

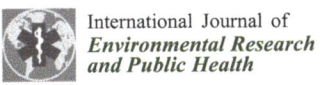

Article

How Do Pharmaceutical Companies Overcome a Corporate Productivity Crisis? Business Diversification into Medical Devices for Growth Potential

Yoonje Euh and Daeho Lee *

Department of Interaction Science, Sungkyunkwan University, Seoul 03063, Korea; yoonje.euh@bd.com
* Correspondence: daeho.lee@skku.edu

Abstract: The purpose of this study was to analyze the performance of pharmaceutical companies' business diversification into medical devices in terms of their technical efficiency (TE) as compared to that of traditional pharmaceutical companies. For a total of 174 externally audited pharmaceutical companies engaged in the drug product business between 2008 and 2019, pharmaceutical companies were classified into two groups according to medical device business diversification. The TE of pharmaceutical companies that diversify the medical device business was lower than that of traditional pharmaceutical companies. However, in terms of the meta-technology ratio (MTR) calculated using meta-frontier analysis, pharmaceutical companies diversified into medical devices showed higher MTR than the traditional pharmaceutical company group. The results imply that the corporate performance growth potential of traditional pharmaceutical companies is lower than that of pharmaceutical companies that have diversified into the medical device business.

Keywords: pharmaceutical company; business diversification; medical device; technical efficiency; meta-frontier analysis

Citation: Euh, Y.; Lee, D. How Do Pharmaceutical Companies Overcome a Corporate Productivity Crisis? Business Diversification into Medical Devices for Growth Potential. *Int. J. Environ. Res. Public Health* **2021**, *18*, 1045. https://doi.org/10.3390/ijerph18031045

Received: 7 December 2020
Accepted: 20 January 2021
Published: 25 January 2021

Publisher's Note: MDPI stays neutral with regard to jurisdictional claims in published maps and institutional affiliations.

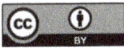

Copyright: © 2021 by the authors. Licensee MDPI, Basel, Switzerland. This article is an open access article distributed under the terms and conditions of the Creative Commons Attribution (CC BY) license (https://creativecommons.org/licenses/by/4.0/).

1. Introduction

Health issues caused by cancer, diabetes, population aging with low birth rate, infectious diseases, etc. are topics of interest to many people. The importance of the medical device and pharmaceutical industries has been emphasized due to infectious diseases such as influenza, Middle East respiratory syndrome, and coronavirus viral disease 2019 (COVID-19). In the case of COVID-19, the virus has serious adverse effects not only on human health but also the social economy. Thus, a diagnostic test device and a vaccine for the disease are being devised and demanded in countries around the world [1–3]. This is because medical devices and medicine for patient treatment are directly connected to each other. However, despite the importance of these industries, pharmaceutical companies are under significant pressure between the consumer associations that demand inexpensive products with good efficacy and investors who pursue high performance and profit [4].

Interestingly, research and projects related to the pharmaceutical industry over the past two decades have been invested in discovering new drugs to generate profit [5]. However, as the cost for basic research and development (R&D) is gradually increased, much research and many projects at pharmaceutical companies were stopped [6]. Furthermore, poor R&D led to a decrease in the pharmaceutical industry's productivity. Specifically, changes in the industrial structure such as the rise of the biotechnology field contributed to the increase in R&D costs of pharmaceutical companies [7]. As productivity declines continue, the pharmaceutical industry is facing unprecedented industrial challenges and surveillance with the extinction of monopoly products and the reduction of pipelines caused by patent expiration [8].

To overcome the crisis of productivity decline, pharmaceutical companies first made an effort to improve the process for finding new drug candidates [9]. When productivity was significantly lowered, R&D through outsourcing was boldly chosen as an alternative to reduce costs [10]. Second, pharmaceutical companies aimed at increasing overall corporate productivity by improving the pharmaceutical manufacturing process [11] and optimizing the supply chain with inventory management [12]. These efforts in internal processes did not lead to improved R&D process for a new drug or higher profit that could raise corporate performance, because the causes of productivity decline in pharmaceutical companies are diverse and complex [13].

Another effort of pharmaceutical companies to overcome the crisis was business diversification [14]. For example, the number of mergers and acquisitions for the pharmaceutical and biotechnology industry in 2018 recorded a total of 1438 and a total volume of $339.6 billion as the highest in the last decade. The medical device industry, which is indicated as a major factor in the decline of the pharmaceutical industry [15], has become a major target of business diversification from pharmaceutical companies. Interestingly, at this time, the number of acquisitions in the healthcare industry (131 cases), including medical devices, was the second highest after acquisitions of the homogeneous sector (449 cases) followed by distribution/logistics (57 cases) and the information and communication sector (30 cases) [16]. Pharmaceutical companies are highly interested in diversifying the medical device business because both medical device and drug are used by patients or doctors as end users for clinical purpose, and the distribution environment of products looks the same. The phenomenon by which multinational medical device companies are gradually developing and launching medical devices that contain medicines can also be attributed to the fact that the business environment is similar [17]. For these reasons, many pharmaceutical companies are expecting to raise overall corporate performance by improving their productivity through the business diversification of medical devices because of the productivity crisis.

However, there are many discussions on how merge and acquisition (M&A) or business diversification will affect corporate performance due to complex factors such as market characteristics of industry and understanding of product, conflicting regulations, organization, etc. as well as additional cost in the process [18–20]. In terms of the pharmaceutical industry, the studies for pharmaceutical companies mainly focused on R&D synergy of M&A with the biotechnology industry [21–23]. The integration of biotechnology with a similar R&D environment also presents various uncertainties regarding the improvement of pharmaceutical companies' performance [23]. When considering these studies, there is still an absence of research on whether the business diversification of pharmaceutical companies into medical devices positively affects their corporate performance in the crisis of productivity.

The pharmaceutical business differs from medical device in the characteristics of the entire business cycle from product R&D through sales. In the traditional pharmaceutical business, when a product is released through a large R&D investment, it continuously generates high profits with improving the supply of raw materials and promoting sales within the protection of patent rights [24]. When compared to pharmaceuticals, the medical device business has a short product life cycle and risk about easy product duplication, so the market competition is overheated due to the low entry barrier and product profits are not very high. Due to these differences, when a pharmaceutical company diversifies its medical device business, the total sales of the company might increase, but the overall performance of the company might decrease. Furthermore, considering additional costs and time, such as new production line, labor, preparation for medical device regulations, and expenses from sales and management, manufacturers should be aware that pharmaceutical and medical device businesses differ not only in their product development and life cycles, but also in the nature of the business and legal factors [25].

This study attempted to determine whether diversifying the medical device business can increase the performance of pharmaceutical companies by analyzing financial data from South Korea. According to the Ministry of Food and Drug Safety (MFDS), the Korean pharmaceutical market in 2019 increased by 5.2% from 2018 (21.24 billion USD) to 22.33

billion USD, ranking 12th in the world (1.6%). Although the Korean pharmaceutical market is growing at a high level as a mature market, overall pharmaceutical companies are facing a decline in corporate performance and a productivity crisis due to the cost of new drug development, patent expiration, regulation, and competition. The phenomenon is common among pharmaceutical companies around the world. For this reason, many pharmaceutical companies in South Korea are expecting to improve corporate performance through diversification of medical device business. South Korea became a country where the trend and phenomenon of pharmaceutical companies that are representatively diversifying medical device business is gradually expanded to overcome the decline in corporate performance and a productivity crisis. For this purpose, this study measured the performance of companies using technical efficiency (TE) indicators. Where sales or productivity is affected by the company size, technical efficiency has the advantage of not being affected by the firm size because it estimates the firm's production function first and measures technical efficiency according to the distance from the production function. Recently Chung et al. [26], Jo et al. [27], Na et al. [28], and many others measured firm performance using technical efficiency in accordance. Because conventional TE has the disadvantage of not being available for comparison between companies using different production functions, we compared pharmaceutical companies that have expanded their business to medical devices with traditional pharmaceutical companies in terms of a firm's TE.

2. Methodology

2.1. Stochastic Frontier Analysis (SFA)

SFA expresses the relationship between input and output factors as a production function and estimates the TE using the frontier production function representing the maximum output from the input. At this time, the TE of a company indicates where the company's technology level is relatively located, when compared to the efficiency technology level of the frontier production function. The farther the technology level of a company is from the frontier production function represents a lower level of efficiency. The production frontier can be estimated through both nonparametric and parametric methods. In this study, the production frontier for the parametric method was estimated using SFA. Also, FRONTIER Version 4.1 software provided by Coelli was used for estimation.

According to Battesse and Coelli [29], the model of the stochastic production frontier is assumed as the following Equation (1) to reflect the change of time in efficiency.

$$Y_{it} = f(x_{it}, \beta)e^{V_{it}-U_{it}}, \ i = 1, 2, \ldots, N, \ t = 1, 2, \ldots, T \tag{1}$$

At this time, Y_{it} is the output of company i at time t, x_{it} is the input vector of company i at time t, f is the production function, β is a vector containing the parameters of the production function, V_{it} is independent of U_{it} with a random error with a distribution of $N(0, \sigma_v^2)$, and U_{it} is a nonnegative random variable representing the TE of company i at time t. If V_{it} is the general random error of the regression equation, then U_{it} represents the company's inefficiency. To show that it is always inefficient, U_{it} itself is not negative and this study assumed that U_{it} follows a half-normal distribution. Because data from 2008 to 2019 were used, T is 12.

From Equation (1), the efficiency, TE_{it}, of company i at time t is given by Equation (2) below.

$$TE_{it} = e^{-U_{it}} = \frac{Y_{it}}{f(X_{it}, \beta)e^{V_{it}}}, \ i = 1, 2, \ldots, N, \ t = 1, 2, \ldots, T \tag{2}$$

In general, the Cobb–Douglas function and the translog function are the most widely used SFA production functions. However, in the case of Cobb and Glass, there is a tendency to oversimplify it because the output variable is seen as a linear combination of input variables. Therefore, in this study, we used the translog function. In particular, a random-effects, time-varying production model was used. When assuming a translog type of production function, Equation (1) can be expressed as Equation (3) below.

$$\ln Y_{it} = \beta_0 + \sum_{m=1}^{3} \beta_m \ln x_{mit} + \sum_{m=1}^{3}\sum_{k\geq m}^{3} \beta_{mk} \ln x_{mit} \ln x_{kit} + V_{it} - U_{it} \qquad (3)$$

where x_{1it} represents the amount of capital (K) of the i-th company at time t, x_{2it} represents the cost (M) of the i-th company at time t, and x_{3it} is the number of workers (L) who receive a salary from the i-th company at time t. The total assets for K, the number of employees for L, and the cost of revenue for M are used as input variables, and net sales (Y) are used as an output variable in this study.

2.2. Meta-Frontier Analysis

Since the TE of a specific company is difficult to compare with other companies using different technologies, comparisons of technological efficiency between each group cannot be performed through traditional SFA. Therefore, to compare the efficiency levels of different groups operating under different technical conditions, we used the meta-frontier production function that wraps the production functions of all groups [30]. From Battese, Rao, and O'Donnell [31], the meta-frontier production function model is defined as follows.

$$Y_{it}^* = f(x_{it}, \beta^*) = e^{x_{it}\beta^*}, \; i = 1, 2, \ldots, N, \; N = \sum_{i=1}^{R} N_j, \; t = 1, 2, \ldots, T, \text{ s.t. } x_{it}\beta^* \geq x_{it}\beta_{(j)} \text{ for all } j \qquad (4)$$

In this case, $\beta_{(j)}$ is a vector composed of the parameters of the j-th group's production function and j indicates each group. In this study, the two groups are traditional pharmaceutical companies that have only produced medicines ($j = 1$) and diversified pharmaceutical companies that also produce medical devices ($j = 2$). β^* is a vector of unknown variables of the meta-frontier function that satisfies the following equation. From Equation (4) above, the graph of the meta-frontier production function is positioned above the graph of the production frontier function of each group for all periods. The meta-frontier production function becomes an envelope of the frontier functions of each group based on the same technology. For simplicity, if we assume that function f in Equation (1) is $e^{X_{it}\beta_{(j)}}$, Equation (1) can be divided as shown in Equation (5).

$$Y_{it} = e^{-U_{it(j)}} \times \frac{e^{x_{it}\beta_{(j)}}}{e^{x_{it}\beta^*}} \times e^{x_{it}\beta^* + V_{it(j)}} \qquad (5)$$

Dividing both sides of Equation (5) by $e^{x_{it}\beta^* + V_{it(j)}}$ yields the following.

$$\frac{Y_{it}}{e^{x_{it}\beta^* + V_{it(j)}}} = e^{-U_{it(j)}} \times \frac{e^{x_{it}\beta_{(j)}}}{e^{x_{it}\beta^*}} \qquad (6)$$

In Equation (6) above, the right side, $e^{-U_{it(j)}}$ is the technical efficiency (TE) of Group j and the second is the j group frontier for the meta-frontier function. It is expressed as a ratio of a function, which is called the Technical Gap Ratio or Meta-Technology Ratio (MTR). TE^*, representing TE in the meta-frontier function, is calculated by multiplying TE by MTR and can be expressed as Equation (7).

$$TE_{it}^* = \frac{Y_{it}}{e^{x_{it}\beta^* + V_{it(j)}}} = TE_{it} \times TGR_{it} \qquad (7)$$

There are two methods of measuring the parameters of a meta-frontier function: Linear Programming (LP) and Quadratic Programming (QP). LP is a method of minimizing the sum of the absolute deviation values, and QP is a method of minimizing the sum of the squares of deviations. According to Battese, Rao, and O'Donnell [31], LP and QP are defined as following Equations (8) and (9).

$$\text{LP}: \min_{\beta^*} L^* = \sum_{t=1}^{T}\sum_{i=1}^{N}\left|x_{it}\beta^* - x_{it}\hat{\beta}_{(j)}\right|, \ x_{it}\beta^* \geq x_{it}\hat{\beta}_{(j)} \qquad (8)$$

$$\text{QP}: \min_{\beta^*} L^* = \sum_{t=1}^{T}\sum_{i=1}^{N}\left(x_{it}\beta^* - x_{it}\hat{\beta}_{(j)}\right)^2, \ x_{it}\beta^* \geq x_{it}\hat{\beta}_{(j)} \qquad (9)$$

Matlab 7.1 software was used to measure the parameters of the meta-frontier function using LP and QP.

3. Estimation Results

In this study, actual corporate financial data were secured from the KIS-VALUE database of the National Information and Credit Evaluation. Based on the information from the South Korean Ministry of Food and Drug Safety (MFDS), pharmaceutical companies are divided into traditional pharmaceutical companies and diversified pharmaceutical companies for medical devices according to their import certifications and licenses to manufacture medical device products. Specifically, the number of externally audited Korean pharmaceutical companies that acquire approval to manufacture and import medical devices for general treatment and surgery from the MFDS has increased rapidly since 2008. Because of a novel influenza outbreak in 2009, Korean pharmaceutical companies expanded to new businesses that manufacture, import, and distribute various types of medical devices, from advanced medical devices to diagnostic test kits and instrument. Thus, a total of 174 externally audited pharmaceutical companies in South Korea were identified for the period between 2008 and 2019.

One hundred three traditional pharmaceutical companies that only conducted pharmaceutical business and 71 pharmaceutical companies that diversified into the medical device business were separated into two groups. The total number of samples with fiscal data used in the study was 1028 for traditional pharmaceutical companies and 728 for pharmaceutical companies diversified into medical devices. Table 1 contains details regarding the samples.

Table 1. Sample statistics.

	Traditional Pharmaceutical Companies	Pharmaceutical Companies Diversified into the Medical Device Business
Revenue (unit: KRW)	56,448,976,777.2374 (62,455,618,526.1714)	157,844,096,262.3630 (224,171,430,459.2680)
Total cost of sales (unit: KRW)	30,811,491,241.2451 (35,513,449,329.7149)	92,076,225,212.9121 (146,325,067,289.8940)
Total Asset (unit: KRW)	83,909,168,301.5564 (100,265,820,064.0890)	209,512,446,516.4840 (293,839,417,481.1320)
Total Wage (unit: KRW)	7,478,634,065.1751 (10,223,940,758.3186)	19,322,657,708.7912 (21,378,708,878.6833)
Number of firms	103	71
Number of samples	1028	728

Note: Numbers in the parenthesis are standard deviations. 1 USD is 1,105.0 KRW (Korean Won) as of 25 January 2021.

FRONTIER 4.1 was used for SFA and meta-frontier analysis (MFA) with MATLAB 7.1 was carried out to verify corporate efficiency. Table 2 shows the estimated frontier production function for each group with meta-frontier production function parameters optimized through LP and QP methods.

Table 2. Estimation results of group and meta-frontier production functions.

	Traditional Pharmaceutical Companies	Pharmaceutical Companies Diversified into the Medical Device Business	Meta-Frontier	
	Estimate (t-Value)	Estimate (t-Value)	LP	QP
Constant	5.9381 (1.3361)	−4.9398 *** (−2.9994)	8.8697	12.3158
$\ln x_1$	1.6171 *** (6.1998)	2.1117 *** (7.9280)	1.7413	0.5321
$\ln x_2$	−0.5390 (−1.3407)	−0.3842 (−1.3342)	−0.3704	−0.7483
$\ln x_3$	−0.4458 (−1.3457)	−0.2718 (−1.0542)	−1.0931	0.3011
$(\ln x_1)^2$	−0.0157 *** (−4.0087)	0.0836 *** (11.1918)	0.0949	0.0428
$(\ln x_2)^2$	0.0178 (1.0392)	−0.0400 ** (−2.0595)	0.0072	0.0026
$(\ln x_3)^2$	−0.0179 (−1.0271)	0.0440 *** (3.3018)	0.0715	0.0427
$\ln x_1 \times \ln x_2$	0.0357 *** (−3.0172)	−0.0281 (−1.0409)	−0.0731	0.0173
$\ln x_2 \times \ln x_3$	0.0285 (0.9297)	0.1421 *** (5.6209)	0.0847	0.0180
$\ln x_3 \times \ln x_1$	0.0297 * (1.9506)	−0.2101 *** (−11.0269)	−0.1683	−0.1045

Note: *, **, and *** mean $p < 0.1$, $p < 0.05$, $p < 0.01$ respectively.

Table 3 shows the results of the TE for each group and the value of TE* in the meta-frontier production function with the MTR by using the estimates of the group frontier production function and meta-frontier production function.

Table 3. SFA estimates of technical efficiencies and meta-technology ratios.

		Traditional Pharmaceutical Companies	Pharmaceutical Companies Diversified into the Medical Device Business
TE	average	0.7628	0.5911
	stdev	0.1645	0.1019
	min	0.0452	0.2446
	max	0.9847	0.9848
MTR_LP	average	0.8039	0.9454
	stdev	0.1296	0.0650
	min	0.0004	0.4129
	max	1.0000	1.0000
MTR_QP	average	0.7667	0.8882
	stdev	0.1153	0.0816
	min	0.0071	0.5257
	max	1.0000	1.0000
TE*_LP	average	0.6097	0.5559
	stdev	0.1492	0.0814
	min	0.0002	0.1989
	max	0.9195	0.8365
TE*_QP	average	0.5817	0.5223
	stdev	0.1389	0.0825
	min	0.0068	0.1846
	max	0.8570	0.8513

As a result, traditional pharmaceutical companies (76.28%) showed higher TE values when compared to diversified pharmaceutical companies for medical devices (59.11%). However, as mentioned earlier, comparisons between groups using different production functions are meaningless. Therefore, the TE of the two groups using different production functions should be compared through MTR. Conversely, a group of diversified pharmaceutical companies for medical devices showed a higher MTR value both with LP and QP (MTR_LP: 94.54%, MTR_QP: 88.82%) when compared to the group of traditional pharmaceutical companies (MTR_LP: 80.39%, MTR_QP: 76.67%).

4. Discussion

Traditional pharmaceutical companies have pursued high corporate efficiency through continuous research on pharmaceutical business models in diverse fields such as patents, regulations, distribution, R&D, and manufacturing innovation. With recent advances in marketing strategies and technologies, the pharmaceutical industry has been trying to overcome the decline in productivity by maximizing profits for many years [32–34].

Nevertheless, unlike increasing their market size, the problem of decreasing productivity has not yet been solved. For the pharmaceutical industry, this is expected to be a complex cause of the already mature business model, excessive market competition, regulation, and competition with similar businesses such as the biotechnology and medical device industries. Companies might seek to integrate with homogeneous firms to improve performance and expect corporate synergy through the combination and expansion of heterogeneous industries. The pharmaceutical industry is also making an effort to reinforce their business portfolio through mergers and acquisitions and business diversification due to the efficiency decline and low productivity. As mentioned in the introduction, in 2018, a total of 1438 transactions with a total volume of $339.6 billion in global mergers and acquisitions in the pharmaceutical and bio-industry industries were recorded. The number of acquisitions in the healthcare industry including medical devices (131 cases) was the highest after homogeneous industry acquisitions (449) [16].

As mentioned earlier, pharmaceutical companies expect to improve overall productivity by reinforcing R&D pipelines between homogeneous industries [35], while expecting to improve corporate performance through business expansion into different industries. Globally, pharmaceutical companies' business expansion of the healthcare business including medical devices has gradually increased, and Korean pharmaceutical companies, which are diversifying into the medical device business, also had a total of 31 (17.8%) in 2008. Currently, a total of 71 (40.8%) pharmaceutical companies have gradually increased their number to diversify their medical device business. Thus, the importance of research on how the medical device business affects the performance of pharmaceutical companies has been raised in South Korea.

As a result of this study, the MTR of the pharmaceutical company group that conducted business diversification was higher than that of the traditional pharmaceutical company group. This higher MTR of the diversified group means that the group's frontier production function is located closer to the meta-frontier production function. The frontier production function is determined by the technology used by the companies in the group and is the set of maximum outputs that the companies can produce. Therefore, the fact that the MTR of the pharmaceutical group that diversified into the medical device business is higher than the MTR of the traditional pharmaceutical group means that the maximum output that can be produced through the same input is higher, that is, it has a higher potential. Interestingly, in the MFA, which is the same production function, both TE* calculated with LP and QP showed higher results than traditional pharmaceutical companies diversifying their medical device business. As described above, TE* can be calculated as the multiplication of TE and MTR. In traditional pharmaceutical companies, although the MTR was lower than that of the pharmaceutical company group that diversified into the medical device business, the TE was much higher than that of the group. Thus, the TE* was higher. This means that traditional pharmaceutical companies are exhibiting higher efficiency under the current production function, but their potential is lower than that of pharmaceutical companies that have diversified into the medical device business.

Based on research results, policy makers and corporate decision makers as well as future study should consider the following implications of this study for sustainable management in the pharmaceutical industry and the medical device industry.

First, in terms of theoretical implications, while most of the existing studies for decades focused mainly on improving the R&D process of the pharmaceutical industry, the industry has been establishing diverse strategies to grow the productivity and performance potential of companies such as the business diversification of medical device. Future studies should be able to fill the blanks in these relevant research topics and provide new perspectives to improve the performance of pharmaceutical companies.

Second, in terms of practical implications, the interaction between doctors and pharmaceutical companies is known to influence the prescription of medicines [36]. Although doctors are users, they have a large portion of the patents for medical devices [37]. Since they have already been involved from the earliest stages of development in clinical trials [38], doctors are interested in not only medicines but also medical devices. Furthermore, since the trend of the treatment process is rapidly changing due to the development of medical devices, the direction of drug development and productivity can be flexibly modified. This is the reason why medicines and medical technology are complementary to each other and technology advancement is simultaneously progressing. Therefore, business diversification into medical devices seems to increase the potential for corporate performance by improving the technological efficiency of pharmaceutical companies.

Third, in terms of policy implications, policy makers considering and reviewing business promotion of the pharmaceutical industry should be encouraged to review diversified business models to improve corporate performance and potential. Furthermore, R&D for new drugs must be continuously conducted by promoting corporate policy with business portfolio expansion of medical device with complicated crisis of productivity.

5. Conclusions

The medical device business clearly differs from the pharmaceutical business in terms of the product production cycle from R&D to product launch and follow-up management. However, when we examined the two businesses from the perspective of healthcare providers and users, not from manufacturers or regulatory agencies, medical devices and medicines in treatment are complementarily connected. In other words, both products are developed and used for the purpose of treatment based on the interaction between the doctor and patient. In conclusion, when compared to traditional pharmaceutical companies, pharmaceutical companies diversified into the medical device business are dominating the traditional pharmaceutical companies in the trends of treatment process and the contact point of customers with market changes. Therefore, these advantages appear to improve overall corporate performance growth potential.

As the pharmaceutical industry may experience a decline affected by major developments in the medical device industry and the biotechnology industry, it is necessary to take insights on multiple businesses and have a view of political decision for pharmaceutical industry promotion. Policy makers should not encourage companies to carry out one business and a similar industry as their conservative general policy.

This study has the following limitations. First, since this study used data from externally audited companies for the period between 2008 and 2019, smaller companies with low total assets were excluded from the group. Second, different variables that could affect the TE of pharmaceutical companies were not considered as well as business diversification. Third, the study is insufficient to provide global implications because it analyzed data only from Korean pharmaceutical companies. Therefore, future research could provide additional implications for the pharmaceutical industry if it continuously expands its importance by using worldwide data and considering other variables that can affect technological efficiency.

Author Contributions: Conceptualization, Y.E. and D.L.; Analysis, D.L.; Writing, Y.E. and D.L. All authors have read and agreed to the published version of the manuscript.

Funding: This research was supported by the Ministry of Education of the Republic of Korea and the NRF (No. 2020S1A5A8045556, 2020R1F1A1048202).

Institutional Review Board Statement: Not applicable.

Informed Consent Statement: Not applicable.

Data Availability Statement: Restrictions apply to the availability of these data. Data was obtained from KIS-VALUE and are available from https://www.kisvalue.com/web/index.jsp with the permission of KIS-VALUE.

Conflicts of Interest: The authors declare no conflict of interest.

References

1. Binnicker, M.J. Emergence of a novel coronavirus disease (COVID-19) and the importance of diagnostic testing: Why partnership between clinical laboratories, public health agencies, and industry is essential to control the outbreak. *Clin. Chem.* **2020**, *66*, 664–666. [CrossRef]
2. Lamprou, D.A. Emerging technologies for diagnostics and drug delivery in the fight against COVID-19 and other pandemics. *Expert Rev. Med. Devices* **2020**, *17*, 1007–1012. [CrossRef]
3. Le, T.T.; Andreadakis, Z.; Kumar, A.; Román, R.G.; Tollefsen, S.; Saville, M.; Mayhew, S. The COVID-19 vaccine development landscape. *Nat. Rev. Drug Discov.* **2020**, *19*, 305–306. [CrossRef]
4. Baxendale, I.R.; Hayward, J.J.; Ley, S.V.; Tranmer, G.K. Pharmaceutical Strategy and Innovation: An Academics Perspective. *Chem. Med. Chem.* **2007**, *2*, 268–288. [CrossRef]
5. Sams-Dodd, F. Is poor research the cause of the declining productivity of the pharmaceutical industry? An industry in need of a paradigm shift. *Drug Discov. Today* **2013**, *18*, 211–217. [CrossRef]
6. Cockburn, I. Is the pharmaceutical industry in a productivity crisis? In *Innovation Policy and the Economy*; Jaffe, A., Lerner, J., Stern, S., Eds.; MIT Press: Cambridge, MA, USA, 2006; Volume 7, pp. 1–32.
7. Cockburn, I. The Changing Structure of the Pharmaceutical Industry. *Health Aff.* **2004**, *23*, 10–22. [CrossRef]
8. Khanna, I. Drug Discovery in Pharmaceutical Industry: Productivity Challenges and Trends. *Drug Discov. Today* **2012**, *17*, 1088–1102. [CrossRef] [PubMed]
9. Munos, B.H.; Chin, W.W. How to Revive Breakthrough Innovation in the Pharmaceutical Industry. *Sci. Transl. Med.* **2011**, *3*, 89cm16. [CrossRef]
10. Higgins, M.J.; Rodriguez, D. The Outsourcing of R&D through Acquisitions in the Pharmaceutical Industry. *J. Financ. Econ.* **2006**, *80*, 351–383.
11. Chowdary, B.V.; George, D. Improvement of manufacturing operations at a pharmaceutical company: A lean manufacturing approach. *J. Manuf. Technol. Manag.* **2012**, *23*, 56–75. [CrossRef]
12. Uthayakumar, R.; Priyan, S. Pharmaceutical supply chain and inventory management strategies: Optimization for a pharmaceutical company and a hospital. *Oper. Res. Health Care* **2013**, *2*, 52–64. [CrossRef]
13. Ruffolo, R.R. Why has R&D productivity declined in the pharmaceutical industry? *Expert Opin. Drug Discov.* **2006**, *1*, 99–102. [PubMed]
14. Rusu, A.; Kuokkanen, K.; Heier, A. Current trends in the pharmaceutical industry-A case study approach. *Eur. J. Pharm. Sci.* **2011**, *44*, 437–440. [CrossRef]
15. Burgess, L.J.; Terblanche, M. The future of the pharmaceutical, biological and medical device industry. *J. Clin. Trials* **2011**, *3*, 45–50.
16. SamjongKPMG. Samjong INSIGHT Vol. 65. Available online: https://assets.kpmg/content/dam/kpmg/kr/pdf/2019/kr-insight65-ma-in-pharmaceutical-industry-20190424.pdf (accessed on 20 May 2020).
17. Schorn, I.; Malinoff, H.; Anderson, S.; Lecy, C.; Wang, J.; Giorgianni, J.; Papandreou, G. The Lutonix® drug-coated balloon: A novel drug delivery technology for the treatment of vascular disease. *Adv. Drug Deliv. Rev.* **2017**, *112*, 78–87. [CrossRef]
18. Orlando, B.; Renzi, A.; Sancetta, G.; Cucari, N. How does firm diversification impact innovation? *Technol. Anal. Strateg. Manag.* **2017**, *30*, 391–404. [CrossRef]
19. Rozen-Bakher, Z. Comparison of merger and acquisition (M&A) success in horizontal, vertical and conglomerate M&As: Industry sector vs. services sector. *Serv. Ind. J.* **2017**, *38*, 492–518.
20. Sohl, T.; Vroom, G.; McCann, B.T. Business model diversification and firm performance: A demand-side perspective. *Strateg. Entrep. J.* **2020**, *14*, 198–223. [CrossRef]
21. Hsieh, S.-F.; Wu, C.-S.; Wu, C.-F. Observations of Biotech and Pharmaceutical Industry Merger and Acquisition Acquired In-Process Research and Development Impairment Indicators. *SSRN Electron. J.* **2016**. [CrossRef]
22. Schweizer, L. Organizational Integration of Acquired Biotechnology Companies into Pharmaceutical Companies: The Need for a Hybrid Approach. *Acad. Manag. J.* **2005**, *48*, 1051–1074. [CrossRef]
23. Danzon, P.M.; Epstein, A.; Nicholson, S. Mergers and Acquisitions in the Pharmaceutical and Biotech Industries. *Manag. Decis. Econ.* **2007**, *28*, 307–328. [CrossRef]
24. Kneller, R. The importance of new companies for drug discovery: Origins of a decade of new drugs. *Nat. Rev. Drug Discov.* **2010**, *9*, 867–882. [CrossRef] [PubMed]
25. Food and Drug Administration. Guidance for Industry Presenting Risk Information in Prescription Drug and Medical Device Promotion. Available online: https://www.fda.gov/regulatory-information/search-fda-guidance-documents/presenting-risk-information-prescription-drug-and-medical-device-promotion (accessed on 15 April 2020).
26. Chung, W.Y.; Jo, Y.; Lee, D. Where should ICT startup companies be established? Efficiency comparison between cluster types. *Telemat. Inform.* **2020**, *56*, 101482. [CrossRef]
27. Jo, Y.; Chung, W.Y.; Lee, D. The capability-enhancing role of government-driven industrial districts for new technology-based firms in South Korea. *Asia Pac. Policy Stud.* **2020**, *7*, 306–321. [CrossRef]
28. Na, C.; Lee, D.; Hwang, J.; Lee, C. Strategic groups emerged by selecting R&D collaboration partners and firms' efficiency. *Asian J. Technol. Innov.* **2020**. [CrossRef]
29. Battese, G.E.; Coelli, T.J. Frontier production functions, technical efficiency and panel data: With application to paddy farmers in India. *J. Prod. Anal.* **1992**, *3*, 153–169. [CrossRef]

30. Battesse, G.E.; Rao, D.S.P. Technology gap, efficiency, and a stochastic metafrontier function. *Int. J. Bus. Econ.* **2002**, *1*, 87–93.
31. Battesse, G.E.; Rao, D.S.P.; O'Donnell, C.J. A metafrontier production function for estimation of technical efficiencies and technology gaps for firms operating under different technologies. *J. Prod. Anal.* **2004**, *21*, 91–103. [CrossRef]
32. Masood, I.; Ibrahim, M.I.M.; Hassali, M.A.; Ahmed, M. Evolution of marketing techniques, adoption in pharmaceutical industry and related issues: A review. *J. Clin. Diagn. Res.* **2009**, *3*, 1942–1952.
33. Roberts, P.W. Product innovation, product-market competition and persistent profitability in the U.S. pharmaceutical industry. *Strateg. Manag. J.* **1999**, *20*, 655–670. [CrossRef]
34. Scherer, F.M. Pricing, Profits, and Technological Progress in the Pharmaceutical Industry. *J. Econ. Perspect.* **1993**, *7*, 97–115. [CrossRef]
35. Danzon, P.M.; Nicholson, S.; Pereira, N. Productivity in Pharmaceutical-Biotechnology R&D: The Role of Experience and Alliances. *J. Health Econ.* **2005**, *24*, 317–339. [PubMed]
36. Fickweiler, F.; Fickweiler, W.; Urbach, E. Interactions between physicians and the pharmaceutical industry generally and sales representatives specifically and their association with physicians' attitudes and prescribing habits: A systematic review. *BMJ Open* **2017**, *7*, e016408. [CrossRef] [PubMed]
37. Chatterji, A.K.; Fabrizio, K.R.; Mitchell, W.; Schulman, K.A. Physician-industry cooperation in the medical device industry. *Health Aff.* **2008**, *27*, 1532–1543. [CrossRef] [PubMed]
38. Baim, D.S.; Donovan, A.; Smith, J.J.; Feigal, D.; Briefs, N.; Geofferion, R.; Kaplan, A.V. Medical Device Development: A Balanced Approach to Managing Conflicts of Interest Encountered by Physicians. *Catheter. Cardiovasc. Interv.* **2007**, *69*, 655–664. [CrossRef]

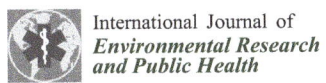

Article

Studying Healthcare Affordability during an Economic Recession: The Case of Greece

Dimitris Zavras

Department of Public Health Policy, School of Public Health, University of West Attica, 11521 Athens, Greece; dzavras@uniwa.gr

Received: 18 August 2020; Accepted: 22 October 2020; Published: 24 October 2020

Abstract: The significant deterioration of economic prosperity in Greece during the economic crisis decreased patients' ability to pay. Thus, the objective of this study is to determine the factors affecting healthcare affordability in Greece during an economic recession. This study used data from the European Union Statistics on Income and Living Conditions (EU-SILC) 2016. The sample consisted of 18,255 households. Healthcare affordability was regressed on geographic characteristics as well as several variables that refer to the households' financial condition. Region of residence, ability to make ends meet, and capacity to cope with unexpected financial expenses were found to be statistically significant. Using sample sizes of 1000 and 1096 adults, respectively, the European Quality of Life Surveys (EQLS) of 2007 and 2016 were also used as data sources. Economic crisis was expressed with a dummy variable: (1) 0: 2007, and (2) 1: 2016. Difficulty in responding to healthcare costs was regressed on survey year and several demographic, socioeconomic, and health characteristics, revealing that individuals were more likely to face difficulties in responding to healthcare costs during the economic crisis. These results confirm the mechanism on the basis of which economic crises affect healthcare access: primarily through the effects of demand-side barriers.

Keywords: healthcare affordability; economic crisis; ability to make ends meet; capacity to cope with unexpected financial expenses; geographic characteristics; socioeconomic characteristics; epidemiologic characteristics; demand-side barriers; supply-side barriers

1. Introduction

Healthcare affordability, or, in other terms, "financial access", is among the main dimensions of healthcare access and relates the healthcare services' prices and providers' insurance or deposit demands to users' income, capacity to pay, and existing health insurance coverage [1]. Healthcare affordability may depend on a ratio of healthcare expenditure to non-healthcare expenditure with a consideration for budget constraints and other sourced elements of coverage [2]; the term "affordability" has no clear meaning in economics [3].

Thus, the operationalization of the concept of affordability requires: (i) informative data on household incomes; (ii) knowledge of the commodity price, and (iii) a definition of "unreasonable burden" [4]. However, there is a consensus that affordability is a subjective concept [5,6].

Healthcare affordability refers to financial and incidental costs [7] imposing barriers to access [8,9] and resulting in unmet healthcare needs [10], i.e., situations in which an individual needs healthcare but does not receive it [11]. Because both supply factors and demand factors result in unmet healthcare needs [12], unmet healthcare needs are a function of the healthcare system features or associated with the personal circumstances of those seeking healthcare [13]. In other words, unmet healthcare needs may be a consequence of limited availability of health services but may also arise, among others, from individual accessibility issues, such as cost [14].

The variables presented below are the key demand-side determinants of healthcare affordability, as they have been identified in the international bibliography.

By definition, healthcare affordability looks at prices of services as they relate to patients' income and capacity to pay [15]. As such, affordability is associated with dimensions of poverty [16], as poverty directly negates access to material resources [17].

Since income and, to a lesser extent, occupation determine the resources of individuals [18], limited income, unemployment and lack of health insurance coverage are strongly related to affordability barriers [19]. That is, higher income as an indicator of the disposable financial means of individuals [20] directly increases healthcare affordability [21], while those with lower incomes often have restricted access to healthcare services [22]. Additionally, unemployment puts individuals at risk of poverty and because of its influence on material circumstances, it can impair financial healthcare access [23]. In addition to drastic income reduction, job loss is often linked to a loss of health insurance [24], especially in Bismarck-type social security schemes, although this is not the case in all healthcare systems. On the other hand, the existence of health insurance coverage can nearly eliminate the negative influence of limited income on healthcare access and by decreasing out-of-pocket payments, makes healthcare more affordable for lower income individuals [25], providing access that would be otherwise unaffordable [26].

Research shows that healthcare expenditures often compete with other expenses in family budgets. According to Kushel et al. (2006) [27], housing instability, i.e., difficulties in paying rent, mortgage, or utility bills, is considered a risk factor for reduced access to healthcare services. Thus, because high housing costs reduce disposable income and impede families' capacity to account for other necessities [28], they constitute a risk factor for the postponement of healthcare services [29,30], which in essence translates to less overall investment in healthcare [31].

The relationship between health status, poverty and access to care is complex and confounded by several biologic as well as social determinants of health. Individuals with poor health often face unaffordable healthcare costs [32] due to their greater need for healthcare (more intense and more frequent use of healthcare), but also due to their low socioeconomic status. Poor health can result in fewer labor market opportunities and lower income as a result of lower productivity [33]. It is also well documented in social epidemiology that lower socioeconomic status and less disposable income force individuals to make life choices that lead to lower health status, creating a vicious cycle of increasingly poor health that leads to poor income and vice versa.

Age is another important variable in this discussion. In general, younger individuals are healthier than older adults but are more likely to be uninsured [34], and thus they face financial barriers in accessing healthcare [35] when they need it. However, the effect of age on healthcare affordability requires special analysis, since the probability of an individual being in poverty decreases from childhood to adulthood and then increases again with advanced age over one's own life cycle [36].

Research on gender differences shows that females have more difficulty affording healthcare than males [37], because females are more vulnerable to gaps in medical insurance coverage [38], but also because they have less access to material resources as compared to males [39]. In addition, females are more likely to develop numerous chronic health conditions resulting in high costs [38], but also are more vulnerable to reduced incomes and unemployment, as mentioned above.

Place of residence is one more variable that is important in the analysis between income, healthcare affordability and access. Healthcare affordability is found to be reduced for residents of rural areas [40], perhaps because rural populations are poorer, earn less at work, and work in industries with lower levels of employer-sponsored healthcare insurance coverage [41].

In summary, healthcare affordability depends on health systems features, such as financing [42], but it also depends on the population characteristics. Specifically, demographic (age and gender) and socioeconomic characteristics (income and occupation), health-related characteristics (health status, existence of a chronic health disease) and structural characteristics (health insurance coverage) affect healthcare affordability (Figure 1). Although demand-side factors such as those mentioned above are the main determinants of healthcare affordability at the individual level, the interrelation of these factors with the healthcare system should not be neglected. However, the causal relationship between healthcare systems with health and wealth-two of the most important determinants of healthcare affordability-is not clear cut and not easily measurable [43].

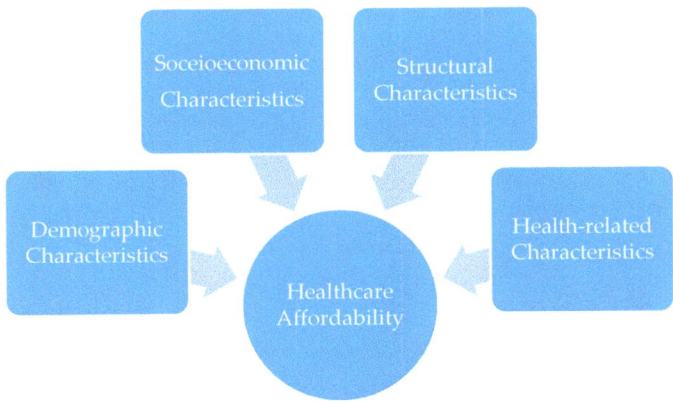

Figure 1. Main demand-side factors affecting healthcare affordability.

As mentioned above, healthcare access depends not only on individual or population characteristics, but also on healthcare system characteristics [44]. Access to care issues as a function of the characteristics of particular healthcare systems must also be studied. For example, exemptions and low-income protection in several healthcare systems guarantee access to certain vulnerable groups of the population, such as those in poor health, older individuals, children or adolescents, women, and low-income individuals [45]. That is, the factors that affect access are related to healthcare system design.

Although in theory most of the European countries provide universal or nearly universal population coverage, research shows that low-income individuals, those in poor health, those between 20 and 30 years old, the unemployed, and women have a higher probability of feeling unable to access care. That is, the most financial disadvantaged groups of the population are the most likely to feel that they will be unable to access needed care [46].

Indeed, it is evident that people in the lowest income quintile are almost three times more likely to forgo healthcare for financial reasons versus richer individuals. In most member countries of the Organization for Economic Co-operation and Development (OECD), healthcare is less affordable for households with a low income than those with a high income [47]. The same figure also stands for developing countries: the poor face more financial difficulties to access healthcare [48].

Among the countries facing the economic crisis of 2008, Greece experienced the most severe economic recession. Several fiscal measures and structural reforms were implemented after May 2010 and triggered high unemployment and a considerable reduction in disposable income.

Greece's healthcare system is a mixed system in terms of both funding and provision-that is, a national health service type of system that coexists with a compulsory work-related social insurance system and a private healthcare sector. The National Organization for the Provision of Health Services (EOPYY) was established in 2011 after merging four large health insurance funds and was both a provider and purchaser of care. It covers the insured and their dependents. Since 2014, EOPYY has acted only as purchaser of care for the vast majority of the insured.

Insured individuals can access all public primary and secondary healthcare services free of charge; they also have access, on a case-by-case cost-sharing basis, to certain private providers contracted with EOPYY. In the case of private healthcare providers not contracted with EOPYY, insured individuals have to pay the entire cost by themselves (out-of-pocket payments) or through private insurance. Public healthcare coverage by EOPYY has been ensured since 2016 for uninsured citizens [49].

The significant deterioration of economic prosperity in Greece during the economic crisis decreased patients' ability to pay [50]. Thus, a substantial percentage of the Greek population could not afford healthcare [51]. The abovementioned evidence reflects the fact that private spending is one of the main sources of healthcare funding in Greece; the other two are taxation and social insurance. That is, not only could few Greeks afford private healthcare [52], but a significant percentage of insured individuals also limited their use of the EOPYY units because they could not afford co-payments [53].

Based on the previous points, the objective of this study is to determine the factors affecting the affordability of healthcare services in Greece during an economic recession. A second goal is to determine the characteristics of those considering healthcare affordability as a reason for unmet healthcare needs. A third goal is to study the impact of the economic crisis on individuals' ability to respond to their healthcare costs.

2. Materials and Methods

2.1. Data Sources

In this study, healthcare affordability was operationalized as households' perceived ability to respond to the healthcare costs.

In order to study healthcare affordability, three different models were fitted. The first model, which attempts to determine the factors affecting the affordability of healthcare services in Greece during an economic recession, used data at the household level from the EU-SILC 2016. The second model, which attempts to determine the characteristics of those considering healthcare affordability as a reason for unmet healthcare needs, used data at the individual level from the EU-SILC 2016. The third model, which attempts to study the impact of the economic crisis on individuals' ability to respond to the healthcare costs, used data at the individual level from the EQLS 2007 and 2016.

As mentioned above, in the first model and second model, data from the EU-SILC 2016 were used (Source: Hellenic Statistical Authority, EU-SICL 2016). The survey used a two-stage stratified sampling. The sample selection strata were based on the 2011 Census of the Hellenic Statistical Authority and were defined by region based on the Nomenclature of Territorial Units for Statistics II (NUTS II) and urbanity status. The sample size was 18,255 households. A total of 37,850 interviews were completed. All household members aged 16 years and over were selected for an interview. A personal interviewing technique was used for data collection. The data collection took place between May 2016 and November 2016.

In addition, in order to study the effect of the economic crisis on individuals' ability to respond to the healthcare costs (third model), we used data from the EQLS of 2007 and 2016 (Source: United Kingdom Data Archive (UKDA), EQLS 2003–2016) [54]. EQLS 2007 used a multi-stage, stratified, and clustered design with a "random walk" procedure for the selection of the households at the last stage. The sample size was 1000 adults. A face-to-face interviewing technique was used for the data collection. The data collection took place between September 2007 and November 2007. EQLS 2016 used a multi-stage, stratified, random sampling design. The sample size was 1096 adults. A face-to-face interviewing technique was used for the data collection. The data collection took place between September 2016 and February 2017. Economic crisis was expressed with a dummy variable: (1) 0: 2007, and 1: 2016. The analysis was not based on weighted data because the weighting methods of EQLS 2007 and EQLS 2016 were different (Eurofound, 2020).

2.2. Dependent and Independent Variables Used in the Three Models

Potential predictors in the analysis were considered that: (a) are dependent on the economic crisis; and (b) have been identified in the international bibliography as determinants of healthcare affordability, unmet healthcare needs, and individuals' ability to respond to the healthcare costs. An additional criterion of independent variable selection was variable availability. For example, health insurance coverage was not available in the EU-SILC 2016, EQLS 2007, and EQLS 2016 surveys.

2.2.1. Variables Used in the First Model

The dependent variable in the first model was households' perceived ability to afford to pay for healthcare or households' perceived ability to respond to the healthcare costs; the question under study was asked as follows: "is your household able to afford to pay for health care services provided for all household members?", with answers: (1) with great difficulty; (2) with difficulty; (3) with some difficulty; (4) fairly easily; (5) easily, and (6) very easily. That is, perceived ability to afford to pay for healthcare corresponds to a single item concerning the household as a whole. The question was asked to the person responding to the household questionnaire.

In several studies, the ability to pay for healthcare is used as a synonym of healthcare affordability [55–58]. This specific ability interacts with direct, indirect, and opportunity costs in order to generate access. Thus, affordability reflects the economic capacity for people to spend resources and time to use services [59].

The outcome was dichotomized [60]: 0 to denote difficulty (great difficulty; difficulty; or some difficulty; and 1 ease (fairly easily; easily; or very easily) [61]. Health care spending is identified as unaffordable if costs exceed a relative threshold determined by a family's income or, more appropriately, a fraction of a family's available resources [62]. The existence of the affordability threshold justifies the use of a dichotomous variable. In addition, several studies have focused on the presence or absence of financial barriers [63–65]. Furthermore, the ability to pay may be approached by a dichotomous variable [66]. Thus, a logistic regression model was fitted to determine the factors associated with the degree of cost-related difficulty facing Greek households with regard to healthcare use. The potential predictors used in the first model are presented in Table 1.

Table 1. Potential predictors (1st model).

Variable	Categories
Region	1: Attica 2: Islands of Aegean and Crete 3: Northern Greece 4: Central Greece
Population Density	1: Thinly Populated Areas 2: Intermediate Populated Areas 3: Densely Populated Areas
Total Household Disposable Income	Continuous Variable
Ability to Make Ends Meet	1: With Great Difficulty 2: With Difficulty 3: With Some Difficulty 4: Fairly Easily 5: Easily 6: Very Easily
Capacity to Cope with Unexpected Financial Expenses	0: No 1: Yes
Being in Arrears on Utility Bills During the Last 12 Months	1: No 2: Yes, Once 3: Yes, Twice or More
Financial Burden Induced from Total Housing Cost	1: A Heavy Burden 2: Somewhat of a Burden 3: Not a Burden at All

Densely populated areas are defined as those areas with at least 50% of people living in contiguous grid cells of 1 km^2 with a density of at least 1500 inhabitants per km^2 and a minimum population of 50,000. Intermediate density areas are defined as areas with clusters of contiguous grid cells of 1k^2 with a density of at least 300 inhabitants per k^2 and a minimum population of 5000. Thinly-populated areas are defined as areas with more than 50% of the population living in rural grid cells outside urban clusters (Eurostat, 2020).

2.2.2. Variables Used in the Second Model

As mentioned above, data at the individual level (data source: EU-SILC 2006) were also analyzed. Specifically, each household member was asked two questions in terms of their healthcare use. The first question was, "was there any time during the past 12 months when you really needed medical examination or treatment (excluding dental) for yourself?" The potential answers to the first question were (1) no and (2) yes, at least one occasion. The 2nd question was "did you have a medical examination or treatment each time you really needed?" The potential answers to the second question were (1) yes (I had a medical examination or treatment each time I needed) and (2) no (there was at least one occasion when I did not have a medical examination or treatment). The respondents were then asked the question: "what was the main reason for not having a medical examination or treatment? with answers: (1) could not afford it (too expensive or there was no insurance coverage; (2) waiting list; (3) could not take time because of work, care for children, or for others, etc.; (4) too far to travel or no means of transportation; (5) fear of medical doctors, hospitals, examination, or treatment; (6) wanted to wait and see if the problem got better on its own; (7) did not know any good medical doctor; and (8) other reasons. This was dichotomized as: (a) 1: could not afford it (too expensive or there was no insurance coverage) and (b) 0: all the remaining reasons. Thus, a logistic regression model was performed, using the derived variable as the outcome. The potential predictors used in the second model are presented in Table 2.

Table 2. Potential predictors (2nd model).

Variable	Categories
Gender	0: Women
	1: Men
Age	1: 17–24
	2: 25–34
	3: 35–44
	4: 45–54
	5: 55–64
	6: 65–74
	7: 75+
Self-Rated Health	1: Very Bad
	2: Bad
	3: Moderate
	4: Good
	5: Very Good
Existence of a Chronic Health Condition	0: No
	1: Yes
Income	Continuous Variable
Education	1: Less than Primary Education
	2: Primary Education
	3: Lower Secondary Education
	4: Upper Secondary Education
	5: Post-Secondary, Non-Tertiary Education
	6: Short Cycle Tertiary Education
	7: Bachelor or Equivalent
	8: Master or Equivalent
	9: Doctorate or Equivalent

Table 2. *Cont.*

Variable	Categories
Occupation	1: Employee Working Full-time and Self-employed Working Full-time (Including Family Worker) 2: Employee Working Part-time and Self-Employed Working Part-Time (Including Family Worker) 3: Unemployed 4: Pupil, Student, in Compulsory Military Community or Service, Further Training, Unpaid Work Experience 5: In Retirement or in Early Retirement or Has Given Up Business 6: Permanently Disabled or/and Unfit to Work 7: Fulfilling Domestic Tasks and Care Responsibilities 8: Other Inactive People

2.2.3. Variables Used in the Third Model

In order to study the effect of the economic crisis on individuals' ability to respond to the healthcare costs, we used data from the EQLS of 2007 and 2016. The respondents were asked the question, "thinking about the last time you needed to see or be treated by a General Practitioner (GP), family doctor, or health center, to what extent did any of the following make it difficult or not for you to do so?" With regard to the option "cost of seeing the doctor", the answers were: (1) very difficult; (2) a little difficult, and (3) not difficult at all. This variable (the outcome) was dichotomized as follows: (1) 0 was not difficult at all, and 1 was a little difficult and very difficult. The rationale of dichotomization is as mentioned above, but it also was driven by the need for comparability with previous results. Since the outcome was dichotomized, a logistic regression model was fitted. The potential predictors used in the third model are presented in Table 3. Income was not used as a potential predictor due to the high percentage of missing values (19.37%).

Table 3. Potential predictors (3rd model).

Variable	Categories
Degree of Urbanity (Subjective)	1: The Open Countryside 2: A Village/Small Town 3: A Medium to Large Town 4: A City or City Suburb
Year	0: 2007 1: 2016
Age	Continuous Variable
Gender	0: Women 1: Men
Family Size	Continuous Variable
Self-Rated Health	1: Very Bad 2: Bad 3: Moderate 4: Good 5: Very Good
Existence of a Chronic Health Condition	0: No 1: Yes
Education	1: Primary 2: Secondary 3: Tertiary

Table 3. Cont.

Variable	Categories
Occupation	1: At Work as Employee or Employer/Self-Employed 2: Employed, on Childcare Leave 3: Employed, on Other Special Leave (e.g., Sickness; Not Holiday) 4: In Receipt of Retirement Pension and At Work as Employee or Employer/Self-Employed 5: At work as Relative Assisting on Family Business or Farm 6: Unemployed Less Than 12 Months 7: Unemployed 12 Months or More 8: Unable to Work Due to Long-Term Illness or disability 9: Retired 10: Full-Time Homemaker/Fulfilling Domestic Tasks 11: In Education (at School, University, etc.)/Student 12: Other
Ability to Make Ends Meet	1: Very Easily 2: Easily 3: Fairly Easily 4: With Some Difficulty 5: With Difficulty 6: With Great Difficulty

2.3. Independent Variables' Coding

Helmert coding was applied to the ordinal variables (a) 1st model: population density, ability to make ends meet, being in arrears on utility bills during the last 12 months, financial burden induced by total housing cost; (b) 2nd model: age, self-rated health, education and (c) 3rd model: degree of urbanity(subjective), self-rated health, education, ability to make ends meet). Helmert contrast compares each category (except the last) with the differences from the balanced mean of subsequent levels. Indicator coding was applied to the nominal variables (a) 1st model: region; (b) 2nd model: occupation and (c) 3rd model: occupation). Indicator contrast compares the reference category of a nominal variable with the remaining categories. Binary variables (a) 1st model: capacity to cope with unexpected financial expenses; (b) 2nd model: gender, existence of a chronic health condition and (c) 3rd model: year, gender, existence of a chronic health condition) were treated as such.

2.4. Multicollinearity

Multicollinearity was tested through the variance inflation factor (VIF) and the tolerance. The VIF should not be greater than 10, and the tolerance should not be less than 0.1. Multicollinearity was not present (in each model, VIF < 10 for all predictors, and tolerance > 0.1 for all predictors).

2.5. Fitting Process

The fitting process for all three models is as follows: although, the sample sizes of both EU-SILC 2016 and EQLS 2007 and 2016 surveys were large, the variable selection was based on a univariate model for each explanatory variable. Any variable with $p < 0.25$ was considered to be a candidate for the multivariate model. Once the variables were identified, a model containing all of the selected variables was fitted [67]. The healthcare affordability model had $p < 0.25$ for all potential predictors in the univariate analysis. For the unmet need due to affordability issues model, the existence of a chronic health disease had $p > 0.25$ ($p = 0.873$) in the univariate analysis. The remaining variables had $p < 0.25$. In the individuals' ability to respond to the healthcare costs model, age ($p = 0.371$), occupation ($p = 0.526$), and subjective urbanity status ($p = 0.336$) had $p > 0.25$ in the univariate analysis. The other variables had $p < 0.25$. The models only included the statistically significant covariates (significance level was set to a = 0.05).

The calibration of the models was tested with the calibration belt test [68]. In addition, the models were tested for specification error through the link test [69]. McFadden's R^2 [70] was then calculated.

The STATA 14 statistical software package was used for the analysis. More specifically, the commands desmat [71], collin (Author: Ender P. B.), logistic, linktest, calibrationbelt [72], and fitstat [73] tests were used.

3. Results

3.1. First Model

Most (71.25%) Greek households used healthcare services during the last 12 months. In addition, 89.52% of the Greek households made a payment (either fully or partially) for healthcare services during the last 12 months. Furthermore, a substantial percentage of the Greek population (31.97%) reported facing great difficulty in responding to healthcare costs, while a similar percentage (34.70%) reported facing difficulty (Table 4).

Table 4. Healthcare affordability.

Responding to Healthcare Cost	Percent (%)
With Great Difficulty	31.97
With Difficulty	34.70
With Some Difficulty	22.72
Fairly Easily	7.67
Easily	2.58
Very Easily	0.36

According to the logistic regression model (first model), healthcare affordability depends on the region of residence, the ability to make ends meet, and the capacity to face unexpected financial expenses. Residents of Attica found it easier to respond to the cost of healthcare versus residents of other regions. In the same vein, financially comfortable households and households that could face unexpected financial expenses reported a lower likelihood of cost-related difficulties with regard to healthcare use (Table 5).

Table 5. First model (logistic regression model).

Variable	OR	p	95% Confidence Interval	
Region		<0.001		
Islands of Aegean and Crete	0.45	<0.001	0.34	0.58
Northern Greece	0.58	<0.001	0.47	0.72
Central Greece	0.56	<0.001	0.44	0.70
Making Ends Meet		<0.001		
Making Ends Meet with Great Difficulty vs. Subsequent Levels	0.04	<0.001	0.03	0.05
Making Ends Meet with Difficulty vs. Subsequent Levels	0.04	<0.001	0.03	0.06
Making Ends Meet with Some Difficulty vs. Subsequent Levels	0.07	<0.001	0.04	0.11
Making Ends Meet Fairly Easily vs. Subsequent Levels	0.29	<0.001	0.15	0.57
Making Ends Meet Easily vs. Subsequent Level	0.57	0.377	0.16	2.00
Capacity to Cope with Unexpected Expenses	2.20	<0.001	1.80	2.69
Constant	0.40	<0.001	0.30	0.53

The link test indicates that the model does not suffer from specification error (Table 6).

In addition, McFadden's $R^2 = 0.30$ indicates a perfect fit [70]. Furthermore, the calibration belt test ($p = 0.096$) indicates good calibration.

Table 6. Link test (first model).

Variable	Coefficient	p	95% Confidence Interval	
h	0.94	<0.001	0.83	1.05
h^2	−0.02	0.198	−0.06	0.01
Constant	0.01	0.899	−0.12	0.14

3.2. Second Model

With respect to unmet healthcare needs, 14.40% of the respondents did not receive needed healthcare during the last 12 months at least once. Most respondents (83.15%) reported unmet healthcare needs due to affordability issues (Table 7).

Table 7. Reasons for unmet medical need.

Reasons for Unmet Medical Need	Percent (%)
Could not Afford	83.15
Waiting List	6.13
Could not Take Time Because of Work, Care for Children or for Others etc.	2.56
Too Far to Travel or No Means of Transportation	1.37
Fear of Medical Doctors, Hospitals, Examination, or Treatment	1.22
Wanted to Wait and See if Problem got Better on its Own	4.84
Did not Know Any Good Medical Doctor	0.14
Other Reasons	0.59

According to the logistic regression model (second model), the unmet healthcare need due to affordability issues depends on self-rated health, education, and occupation. Specifically, individuals with lower education are more likely to report unmet healthcare needs due to affordability issues. The same also holds for the unemployed, pupils, students, those in compulsory military or community service, those in further training or in unpaid work experience, and those fulfilling domestic tasks and care responsibilities relative to those working full-time. However, those rating their health as very bad and those rating their health as good are less likely to report an unmet healthcare need due to affordability issues versus the subsequent levels. Those rating their health as fair are more likely to report an unmet healthcare need due to affordability issues (Table 8).

Table 8. Second model (logistic regression model).

Variable	OR	p	95% Confidence Interval	
Education		<0.001		
Less than Primary Education vs. Subsequent Levels	2..19	<0.001	1.44	3.34
Primary Education vs. Subsequent Levels	2.33	<0.001	1.61	3.39
Lower Secondary Education vs. Subsequent Levels	3.15	<0.001	1.96	5.05
Upper Secondary Education vs. Subsequent Levels	2.38	<0.001	1.49	3.80
Post-Secondary Non-Tertiary Education vs. Subsequent Levels	1.58	0.173	0.82	3.03
Short Cycle Tertiary Education vs. Subsequent Levels	4.47	0.022	1.24	16.14
Bachelor or Equivalent vs. Subsequent Levels	3.48	0.007	1.40	8.67

Table 8. Cont.

Variable	OR	p	95% Confidence Interval	
Master or Equivalent vs. Subsequent Level	3.61	0.150	0.63	20.71
Occupation		<0.001		
Employee Working Part-Time and Self-Employed Working Part-Time (Including Family Worker)	1.70	0.058	0.98	2.93
Unemployed	3.69	<0.001	2.63	5.17
Pupil, Student, in Compulsory Military or Community Service, Further Training, Unpaid Work Experience	2.35	0.007	1.26	4.37
In Retirement or in Early Retirement or Has Given up Business	0.79	0.115	0.60	1.06
Permanently Disabled or/and Unfit to Work	1.78	0.084	0.93	3.43
Fulfilling Domestic Tasks and Care Responsibilities	1.67	0.001	1.23	2.27
Other Inactive People	2.10	0.169	0.73	6.02
Self-Rated Health		<0.001		
Very Bad vs. Subsequent Levels	0.57	0.004	0.39	0.84
Bad vs. Subsequent Levels	1.27	0.091	0.96	1.68
Fair vs. Subsequent Levels	1.45	0.003	1.14	1.85
Good vs. Subsequent Level	0.61	0.001	0.46	0.82
Constant	2.32	<0.001	1.71	3.14

The link test indicates that the model does not suffer from a specification error (Table 9).

Table 9. Link test (second model).

Variable	Coefficient	p	95% Confidence Interval	
h	1.21	<0.001	0.72	1.70
h^2	−0.07	0.364	−0.22	0.08
Constant	−0.13	0.500	−0.51	0.25

McFadden's $R^2 = 0.066$ indicates a poor fit [70]. However, the calibration belt test ($p = 0.083$) indicates good calibration. Both models have a good fit based on the diagnostic tests.

3.3. Third Model

According to the EQLS 2007 and 2016 data, in 2007, the percentage of those facing difficulty in responding to the healthcare costs was 46.22%. This percentage was 64.85% in 2016 (Table 10).

Table 10. Difficulty in responding to healthcare cost.

Difficulty in Responding to Healthcare Cost	2007	2016
Very Difficult	17.40	27.44
A little Difficult	28.82	37.41
Not Difficult at All	53.79	35.15

According to the logistic regression model (third model) (Table 11), individuals were more likely to face difficulties in responding to the healthcare costs during the crisis (year = 2016). In addition, women were more likely to face difficulties in responding to the healthcare costs. However, those making ends meet very easily, easily, fairly easily, and with some difficulty were less likely to face difficulties in responding to the healthcare costs than those making ends meet with higher levels of difficulty.

Table 11. Third model (logistic regression model).

Variable	OR	p	95% Confidence Interval	
Year	1.74	<0.001	1.44	2.10
Gender	0.83	0.049	0.69	1.00
Ability to Make Ends Meet		<0.001		
Very Easily vs. Subsequent Levels	0.30	0.003	0.13	0.66
Easily vs. Subsequent Levels	0.58	0.001	0.42	0.79
Fairly Easily vs. Subsequent Levels	0.43	<0.001	0.33	0.58
With Some Difficulty vs. Subsequent Levels	0.58	<0.001	0.47	0.72
With Difficulty vs. Subsequent Level	0.88	0.360	0.66	1.16
Constant	0.78	0.016	0.64	0.95

According to the link test (Table 12), the model does not suffer from specification error. McFadden's $R^2 = 0.057$ indicates a poor fit [70]. However, the calibration belt test ($p = 0.192$) indicates good calibration.

Table 12. Link test (third model).

Variable	Coefficient	p	95% Confidence Interval	
h	0.95	<0.001	0.77	1.13
h^2	0.18	0.188	−0.09	0.44
Constant	−0.05	0.419	−0.18	0.07

4. Discussion

Affordability is commonly referred to as the "degree of fit" between the full costs (the price of service at the point of delivery as well as other direct or indirect costs) and the users' capacity to pay within the framework of their budget and other demands on that budget [74].

As mentioned in the introduction, healthcare affordability is a subjective concept [75]. We note that uncertainty constitutes a source of subjectivity with regard to healthcare affordability because prices in the healthcare market are uncertain [76,77], and the same holds for both the health and the effectiveness of medical treatment [78]; thus, the price and quantity of medical services are not initially known [79]. The uncertainty surrounding the decision-making process-the process with regard to healthcare use [80]-refers to limited knowledge and involves subjectivity [81]. Furthermore, self-perceived affordability constitutes a subjective assessment [82].

At this point, we note that affordability is considered a subjective concept not only at the level of individual judgment but also at the level of political judgment [83].

Although several demographic, socioeconomic, structural, and health-related factors influence healthcare affordability, interpreting the effect of geographic characteristics in a consistent health economics framework requires considering both the economic characteristics of the areas under study and the regional distribution of healthcare services.

Thus, the area of residence can have a negative effect on healthcare affordability and may be partially explained by the fact that, in Greece, the best situation with regard to the risk of poverty is observed in Attica (Source: Eurostat, 2020). On the other hand, Greek resources are largely concentrated in Athens [84]. Because supply-side issues play an important role in limiting access [85], it is obvious that people who live further from healthcare services are likely to face higher costs related to the use of medical care than those living closer [86]. It is also evident that a substantial percentage of the Greek population cannot even afford the cost of transportation to healthcare services [87]; thus, accessibility influences the choice of services available and the costs-both monetary and non-monetary-that users must pay to gain access [88]. These findings justify the results of a survey conducted in northern and western Greece indicating that the financial means of a substantial percentage of these areas' residents were not sufficient for them to afford healthcare [89].

The improvements in affordability in Greece requires interventions at the national level in terms of resource allocation, because accessibility overlaps with availability and includes affordability [90]; poor geographic availability of healthcare services impacts affordability [91].

The effect of the remaining variables that were found to be statistically significant is somewhat obvious. The ability to make ends meet is one of the dimensions of living standards [92] and is directly related to healthcare affordability [93]. It is obvious that the inability to make ends meet constitutes the primary determinant of relinquished healthcare due to cost in many countries [94]. That is, greater household capacity to meet economic needs lowers forgone medical care due to cost [95]. Those struggling to make ends meet do not have extra money to pay for unexpected illnesses [96]. Thus, access to affordable healthcare is a great concern for those struggling to make ends meet [97].

According to the bibliography, which is limited, individuals that cannot cope with unexpected expenses face higher healthcare costs [98]. A probable reason is that this group is likely to be in poor health [99]. Because households' poor economic condition implies a burden in terms of healthcare access, those with limited capacity to face unexpected financial expenses are more inclined to report unmet healthcare needs due to cost [100]. On the other hand, the unpredictability of illness exposes individuals to unexpected expenses [101,102].

According the analysis, the results obtained from EU-SILC 2016 justify the results obtained from EQLS 2007 and 2016.

The empirical findings demonstrate a dramatic worsening of the living and welfare standards of many Greeks over the years of recession and austerity [103]. The reduction in economic prosperity during the crisis decreased the patients' capacity to pay and therefore negatively impacted their ability to afford healthcare services [104,105]. On the other hand, as the state reduced its overall financial responsibility in healthcare, a substantial part of the cost was shifted to households and individuals [53]. Thus, while the Greek population is universally covered, healthcare remains unaffordable [106]. This situation justifies the effect of both demand-side and supply-side barriers to healthcare access [107].

What was described in the results section is quite similar to subsequent years, with the exemption of 2017. In 2017, among households that reported unmet healthcare needs, 74.66% cited cost as the main reason for not using needed healthcare. This percentage was 81.65% and 81.40% in 2018 and 2019, respectively. Nevertheless, the percentage of unmet healthcare needs increased compared to that of 2016 (2017: 24.50%; 2018: 23.34%, and 2019: 21.28%) (Source: Hellenic Statistical Authority, EU-SILC 2017, EU-SILC 2018, EU-SILC 2019). These findings confirm the argument that cost is a critical factor driving healthcare-seeking behavior [108].

The results of this study are consistent with a significant strand of the literature, not only with regard to the factors affecting healthcare affordability but also with regard to the characteristics of those reporting unmet healthcare needs due to affordability issues. Indeed, females (OR = 2.20), individuals suffering from at least one chronic disease (OR = 1.41), individuals with poor health (OR = 2.90), individuals with low income (OR for the first quintile = 2.67 and OR for the second quintile = 2.02), people facing economic difficulties (OR for the frequency of economic problems = 1.99 and OR for the degree of economic difficulties = 1.86) and individuals without a paid job (OR = 1.02) are more likely to report unmet healthcare needs for financial reasons. In addition, individuals of higher education (OR = 0.77), and older individuals (OR = 0.97) are less likely to report unmet healthcare needs for financial reasons [109–111].

Based on the results of this study, healthcare costs are a significant barrier for healthcare access in Greece.

This finding is also justified by the data of Eurobarometer 91.2 [112]. According to this survey, 42% of Greek respondents identified more affordable treatments as a way to improve healthcare access for all Europeans. This percentage is much higher than the European Union average (33%).

However, the results of this survey are somewhat surprising because this percentage is too high in countries such as the Netherlands (69%), where affordability-especially for those in a more financially difficult position-is considered to be very good [113]. In addition, this percentage is 29% in United

Kingdom, operating a Beveridge healthcare system, while France's Bismarck healthcare model has 30%. However, with regard to affordability, the United Kingdom is ranked first, while France is ranked second [114]. A similar percentage was reported in Germany (29%), where healthcare is considered to be quite affordable [115].

A probable reason for these inconsistencies may be that the question was not country-specific. That is, according to Mooney (2009) [116], the community's judgement with regard to access barriers is based on putting themselves in the position of those facing these barriers. However, Mooney does not refer to financial barriers, because they apply to all. We argue that that this is not the case in this specific question because the respondents should consider the whole European population.

In the case of Greece, the results are in line with the fact that 48% of the respondents declared unemployment as one of the two essential issues dealing with the country, while 45% declared the economic situation to be one of the two essential issues dealing with the country. Nevertheless, only 12% declared health and social security to be an issue.

However, the EU-SILC 2016 data confirm findings from the literature. Specifically, in the Netherlands, 4.3% of respondents reported great difficulty affording healthcare costs, while 10.4% and 12.5% reported difficulty and some difficulty affording healthcare costs, respectively. Furthermore, in the United Kingdom, the percentage of respondents reporting great difficulty, difficulty, and some difficulty affording healthcare costs was 1.9%, 3.2%, and 7.4%, respectively. In addition, in France, 2.3% of respondents reported great difficulty affording healthcare costs, while 7% and 12.5% reported difficulty and some difficulty affording healthcare costs, respectively. Finally, in Germany, the percentage of respondents reporting great difficulty, difficulty, and some difficulty affording healthcare costs was 2.4%, 4.3%, and 9.3%, respectively [117].

The economic crisis adversely affected a substantial percentage of the Greek population and negatively affected their capacity to satisfy healthcare needs. Indeed, the data from EU-SILC 2007 (Source: Hellenic Statistical Authority) indicate that the percentage of unmet health needs before starting the economic crisis, i.e., 2007, was 6.69%. In addition, among those reporting an unmet healthcare need, 68.98% declared affordability issues.

The economic crisis of 2008 affected the EU Member States in different ways. Taxation revenue decreased and borrowing costs increased in several member states. In some countries where healthcare is financed primarily through health insurance contributions from employees and employers, resources also decreased because of reduced wages and increasing unemployment rates. In addition, public expenditure increased because of an increase in take-up benefits such as unemployment benefits. In order to balance their budgets, many EU governments cut public expenditure including health expenditures. However, the crisis adversely impacted access to healthcare services not only because of budget cuts. Access to healthcare for households also reduced because disposable income decreased [118].

The mechanism on the basis of which economic crisis affected healthcare access is as follows: in combination with budget cuts, household income and wealth reduction led to a reduced ability to pay out of pocket. In countries with a work-related insurance system, job losses led to a loss of coverage. These in turn led to limited healthcare access [119].

Several high-and low-income countries in Europe, North America and Africa constitute examples of the abovementioned point [120–124].

Identifying the factors influencing healthcare affordability is particularly important because certain policies based on these factors can be applied during a period of recession especially for the more disadvantaged. However, this is not an easy task because affordability depends not only on the individuals' characteristics but also on the characteristics of the healthcare system and their interrelation. In addition, as previously mentioned, healthcare affordability is a subjective concept.

The main limitations of this study are: (1) the lack of information with regard to insurance coverage; (2) the fact that the analysis of EQLS 2007 and EQLS 2016 was not based on weighted data, and (3) that the study almost exclusively focused on households' and individuals' characteristics.

Except for the information on geographic characteristics, no information is available with regard to the health system (type of services, availability, etc.).

5. Conclusions

Access to healthcare in Greece presents challenges in terms of affordability, leading to high levels of unmet healthcare needs particularly among financially disadvantaged groups [125]. This point is of great importance because "the proof of access is use of service not simply the presence of a facility" [126].

However, because a large part of the world's population has limited access to affordable healthcare [127], we argue that facing cost-related difficulties with regard to healthcare use is a global phenomenon. All people should have equal financial access to medical care [128], because the accessibility of appropriate and affordable healthcare is vital to improving health outcomes and reducing health disparities [129].

The provision of affordable healthcare services is definitely a challenge that is increasingly difficult. Due to the healthcare system complexities, investigating the utilization and costs of healthcare services is key to informed decision-making [130]. Policy makers must address a diverse array of issues to reduce health disparities by making healthcare more affordable and accessible [131] because achieving equity in health access and outcomes is one of the goals of health policy [132].

If we accept that access may be defined as freedom from barriers to healthcare [133], then understanding the full range of barriers for vulnerable populations such as the poor is important to optimizing healthcare and health outcomes [134].

Thus, there is a need for more research while considering the influence of healthcare systems and patient characteristics [59].

The results of this study confirm that healthcare affordability is a critical issue for the Greek population. Access improvement in Greece requires interventions with regard to healthcare system inefficiencies, but also improvements in living standards, meaning that several factors should be addressed. That is, a multi-factorial health, social, and economic policy approach is required.

The well-documented negative effect of the economic crisis on health outcomes can be partially attributed to the unaffordability of the healthcare services and the healthcare system characteristics.

Funding: This research received no external funding.

Acknowledgments: The authors wish to thank Jason Zavras, 3rd year college student at Dartmouth College, for his work as research assistant in this project.

Conflicts of Interest: The author declares no conflict of interest.

References

1. Penchansky, R.; Thomas, J.W. The Concept of Access: Definition and Relationship to Consumer Satisfaction. *Med. Care* **1981**, *19*, 127–140. [CrossRef] [PubMed]
2. Rosenberg, M.A.; Johnson, P.H., Jr.; Duncan, I.G. Perspectives Articles: Exploring Stakeholder Perspectives on What Is Affordable Health Care. *Risk Manag. Insur. Rev.* **2010**, *13*, 251–263. [CrossRef]
3. Culyer, A.J. *The Dictionary of Health Economics*, 3rd ed.; Edward Elgar: Cheltenham, UK; Northhampton, MA, USA, 2014.
4. Niëns, L.; Van de Poel, E.; Cameron, A.; Ewen, M.; Laing, R.; Brouwer, W. Practical Measurement of Affordability: An Application to Medicines. *Bull. World Health Organ.* **2012**, *90*, 219–227. [CrossRef] [PubMed]
5. McLean, W.J.; Applegate, M. *Economics and Contemporary Issues*, 9th ed.; South-Western Cengage Learning: Mason, OH, USA, 2013.
6. Reinhardt, U.E.; Hussey, P.S.; Anderson, G.F. U.S. Health Care Spending in an International Context. *Health Aff.* **2004**, *23*, 10–25. [CrossRef]
7. Saurman, E. Improving Access: Modifying Penchansky and Thomas's Theory of Access. *J. Health Serv. Res. Policy* **2016**, *21*, 36–39. [CrossRef]

8. Chuma, J.; Okungu, V.; Ntwiga, J.; Molyneux, C. Towards Achieving Abuja Targets: Identifying and Addressing Barriers to Access and Use of Insecticides Treated Nets among the Poorest Populations in Kenya. *BMC Public Health* **2010**, *10*, 137. [CrossRef]
9. Goudge, J.; Gilson, L.; Russell, S.; Gumede, T.; Mills, A. Affordability, Availability and Acceptability Barriers to Health Care for the Chronically Ill: Longitudinal Case Studies from South Africa. *BMC Health Serv. Res.* **2009**, *9*, 75. [CrossRef]
10. Corscadden, L.; Levesque, J.F.; Lewis, V.; Strumpf, E.; Breton, M.; Russell, G. Factors Associated with Multiple Barriers to Access to Primary Care: An International Analysis. *Int. J. Equity Health* **2018**, *17*, 1–10. [CrossRef]
11. Herr, M.; Arvieu, J.-J.; Aegerter, P.; Robine, J.-M.; Ankri, J. Unmet Health Care Needs of Older People: Prevalence and Predictors in a French Cross-Sectional Survey. *Eur. J. Public Health* **2014**, *24*, 808–813. [CrossRef]
12. Dewar, D.M. *Essentials of Health Economcis*; Jones & Bartlett Pub: Sudbury, MA, USA, 2010.
13. Sanmartin, C.; Houle, C.; Tremblay, S.; Berthelot, J.-M. Changes in Unmet Health Care Needs. *Health Rep.* **2002**, *13*, 15–21.
14. Chen, J.; Hou, F. Unmet Needs for Health Care. *Health Rep.* **2002**, *13*, 23–34. [PubMed]
15. Kullgren, J.T.; McLaughlin, C.G.; Mitra, N.; Armstrong, K. Nonfinancial Barriers and Access to Care for U.S. Adults. *Health Serv. Res.* **2012**, *47 Pt 2*, 462–485. [CrossRef]
16. Thomas, B. Health and Health Care Disparities: The Effect of Social and Environmental Factors on Individual and Population Health. *Int. J. Environ. Res. Public Health* **2014**, *11*, 7492–7507. [CrossRef] [PubMed]
17. McAreavey, R.; Brown, D.L. Comparative Analysis of Rural Poverty and Inequality in the UK and the US. *Palgrave Commun.* **2019**, *5*. [CrossRef]
18. Lynch, J.; Kaplan, G. Socioeconomic Position. In *Social Epidemiology*; Berkman, L.F., Kawachi, I., Eds.; Oxford University Press: New York, NY, USA, 2000; pp. 13–35.
19. Edward, J.; Hines-Martin, V. Examining Perceived Barriers to Healthcare Access for Hispanics in a Southern Urban Community. *JHA* **2016**, *5*, 102. [CrossRef]
20. Galobardes, B.; Shaw, M.; Lawlor, D.A.; Lynch, J.W.; Davey Smith, G. Indicators of Socioeconomic Position (Part 1). *J. Epidemiol. Community Health* **2006**, *60*, 7–12. [CrossRef]
21. Law, J.; VanDerslice, J. Proximal and Distal Determinants of Access to Health Care among Hispanics in El Paso County, Texas. *J. Immigr. Minority Health* **2011**, *13*, 379–384. [CrossRef] [PubMed]
22. Vuong, Q.-H.; Ho, T.-M.; Nguyen, H.-K.; Vuong, T.-T. Healthcare Consumers' Sensitivity to Costs: A Reflection on Behavioural Economics from an Emerging Market. *Palgrave Commun.* **2018**, *4*, 1–10. [CrossRef]
23. Adams, M.; Augustyns, N.; Janssens, H.; Vriesacker, B.; Van Hal, G. What Socio-Demographic Factors Influence Poverty and Financial Health Care Access among Disabled People in Flanders: A Cross-Sectional Study. *Arch. Public Health* **2014**, *72*, 5. [CrossRef]
24. Salm, M. Does Job Loss Cause Ill Health? *Health Econ.* **2009**, *18*, 1075–1089. [CrossRef]
25. Bourne, P.A. Impact of Poverty, Not Seeking Medical Care, Unemployment, Inflation, Self-Reported Illness, and Health Insurance on Mortality in Jamaica. *N. Am. J. Med. Sci.* **2009**, *1*, 99–109. [PubMed]
26. Nyman, J.A. The Value of Health Insurance. In *The Elgar Companion to Health Economics*; Jones, A.M., Ed.; Edward Elgar: Cheltenham, UK; Northampton, MA, USA, 2006; pp. 95–103.
27. Kushel, M.B.; Gupta, R.; Gee, L.; Haas, J.S. Housing Instability and Food Insecurity as Barriers to Health Care among Low-Income Americans. *J. Gen. Intern. Med.* **2006**, *21*, 71–77. [CrossRef] [PubMed]
28. Bratt, R.G. Housing and Family Well-Being. *Hous. Stud.* **2002**, *17*, 13–26. [CrossRef]
29. Ortiz, S.E.; Johannes, B.L. Building the Case for Housing Policy: Understanding Public Beliefs about Housing Affordability as a Key Social Determinant of Health. *SSM Popul. Health* **2018**, *6*, 63–71. [CrossRef]
30. Meltzer, R.; Schwartz, A. Housing Affordability and Health: Evidence from New York City. *Hous. Policy Debate* **2016**, *26*, 80–104. [CrossRef]
31. McConnell, E.D. Who Has Housing Affordability Problems? Disparities in Housing Cost Burden by Race, Nativity, and Legal Status in Los Angeles. *Race Soc. Probl.* **2013**, *5*, 173–190. [CrossRef] [PubMed]
32. Almgren, G.R.; Lindhorst, T. *The Safety-Net Health Care System: Health Care at the Margins*; Springer Pub: New York, NY, USA, 2012.
33. Bender, K.A.; Theodossiou, I. Controlling for Endogeneity in the Health-Socioeconomic Status Relationship of the Near Retired. *J. Socio Econ.* **2009**, *38*, 977–987. [CrossRef]

34. Fortuna, R.J. Ambulatory Care among Young Adults in the United States. *Ann. Intern. Med.* **2009**, *151*, 379–385. [CrossRef]
35. Bonnie, R.J.; Stroud, C.; Breiner, H. (Eds.) *Committee on Improving the Health, Safety, and well-being of young adults, Investing in the Health and Well-Being of Young Adults*; Board on Children, Youth, and Families; Institute of Medicine: Washington, DC, USA; National Research Council: Washington, DC, USA; The National Academies Press: Washington, DC, USA, 2014.
36. Radner, D.B. The Economic Status of the Aged. *Soc. Secur. Bull.* **1992**, *55*, 3–23.
37. Saenz, C. Affordability of Health Care: A Gender-Related Problem and a Gender-Responsive Solution. *IJFAB Int. J. Fem. Approaches Bioeth.* **2011**, *4*, 144–153. [CrossRef]
38. Fitzgerald, T.; Cohen, L.; Hyams, T.; Sullivan, K.M.; Johnson, P.A. Women and Health Reform: How National Health Care Can Enhance Coverage, Affordability, and Access for Women (Examples From Massachusetts). *Women's Health Issues* **2014**, *24*, e5–e10. [CrossRef] [PubMed]
39. Qureshi, H. Obligations and Support within Families. In *The New Generational Contract*; Walker, A., Ed.; Routledge: New York, NY, USA, 1996; pp. 100–119.
40. Ramsey, P.; Edwards, J.; Lenz, C.; Odom, J.E.; Brown, B. Types of Health Problems and Satisfaction with Services in a Rural Nurse-Managed Clinic. *J. Community Health Nurs.* **1993**, *10*, 161–170. [CrossRef]
41. Douthit, N.; Kiv, S.; Dwolatzky, T.; Biswas, S. Exposing Some Important Barriers to Health Care Access in the Rural USA. *Public Health* **2015**, *129*, 611–620. [CrossRef]
42. Evans, D.B.; Hsu, J.; Boerma, T. Universal Health Coverage and Universal Access. *Bull. World Health Organ.* **2013**, *91*, 546–546A. [CrossRef]
43. Figueras, J.; Lessof, S.; McKee, M.; Durán, A.; Menable, N. Health Systems, Health, Wealth and Societal Well-Being: An Introduction. In *Health Systems, Health, Wealth and Societal Well-Being*; Figueras, J., McKee, M., Eds.; McGraw Hill; Open University Press: Berkshire, UK, 2012.
44. Gulzar, L. Access to Health Care. *Image J. Nurs. scholarsh.* **1999**, *31*, 13–19. [CrossRef]
45. Mossialos, E.; Wenzl, M.; Osborn, R.; Sarnak, D. (Eds.) *2015 International Profiles of Health Care Systems*; The Commonwealth Fund: New York, NY, USA, 2016.
46. Cylus, J.; Papanicolas, I. An Analysis of Perceived Access to Health Care in Europe: How Universal is Universal Coverage? *Health Policy* **2015**, *119*, 1133–1144. [CrossRef]
47. OECD. *Health for Everyone? Social Inequalities in Health and Health Systems. OECD Health Policy Studies*; OECD Publishing: Paris, France, 2019. [CrossRef]
48. Peters, D.H.; Garg, A.; Bloom, G.; Walker, D.G.; Brieger, W.R.; Hafizur Rahman, M. Poverty and Access to Health Care in Developing Countries. *Ann. N. Y. Acad. Sci.* **2008**, *1136*, 161–171. [CrossRef]
49. Ziomas, D.; Konstantinidou, D.; Capella, A. ESPN Thematic Reporto on Inequalities in Access to Healthcare-Greece. European Commission: Brussels, 2018. Available online: https://ec.europa.eu/social/BlobServlet?docId=20363&landId=en (accessed on 17 September 2020).
50. Kyriopoulos, I.; Nikoloski, Z.; Mossialos, E. The Impact of the Greek Economic Adjustment Programme on Household Health Expenditure. *Soc. Sci. Med.* **2019**, *222*, 274–284. [CrossRef] [PubMed]
51. Hadjimichalis, C. *Crisis Spaces, Structures, Struggles and Solidarity in Southern Europe*, 1st ed.; Routledge: New York, NY, USA, 2018.
52. Kritikos, A.S.; Hafenstein, M. The Greek Crisis, a Tragedy without Catharsis? *Vierteljahrsh. Wirtsch.* **2015**, *84*, 195–209. [CrossRef]
53. Petmesidou, M.; Pavolini, E.; Guillén, A.M. South European Healthcare Systems under Harsh Austerity: A Progress-Regression Mix? *South Eur. Soc. Polit.* **2014**, *19*, 331–352. [CrossRef]
54. European Foundation for the Improvement of Living and Working Conditions. *European Quality of Life Survey Integrated Data File, 2003–2016. [Data Collection]*, 3rd ed.; SN: 7348; UK Data Service: London, UK, 2018. [CrossRef]
55. Strogatz, D.S. Use of Medical Care for Chest Pain: Differences between Blacks and Whites. *Am. J. Public Health.* **1990**, *80*, 290–294. [CrossRef] [PubMed]
56. Russell, S. Ability to Pay for Health Care: Concepts and Evidence. *Health Policy Plan.* **1996**, *11*, 219–237. [CrossRef] [PubMed]
57. Jeon, Y.-H.; Essue, B.; Jan, S.; Wells, R.; Whitworth, J.A. Economic Hardship Associated with Managing Chronic Illness: A Qualitative Inquiry. *BMC Health Serv. Res.* **2009**, *9*, 182. [CrossRef] [PubMed]

58. Kuhlthau, K.A.; Nipp, R.D.; Shui, A.; Srichankij, S.; Kirchhoff, A.; Galbraith, A.A.; Park, E.R. Health Insurance Coverage, Care Accessibility and Affordability for Adult Survivors of Childhood Cancer: A Cross-Sectional Study of a Nationally Representative Database. *J. Cancer Surviv.* **2016**, *10*, 964–971. [CrossRef]
59. Levesque, J.-F.; Harris, M.F.; Russell, G. Patient-Centred Access to Health Care: Conceptualising Access at the Interface of Health Systems and Populations. *Int. J. Equity Health* **2013**, *12*, 18. [CrossRef]
60. Ahmed, S.M.; Lemkau, J.P.; Nealeigh, N.; Mann, B. Barriers to Healthcare Access in a Non-Elderly Urban Poor American Population. *Health Soc. Care Community* **2001**, *9*, 445–453. [CrossRef]
61. Fusco, A. The Dynamics of Perceived Financial Difficulties. *J. Happiness Stud.* **2016**, *17*, 1599–1614. [CrossRef]
62. Briesacher, B.A.; Ross-Degnan, D.; Wagner, A.K.; Fouayzi, H.; Zhang, F.; Gurwitz, J.H.; Soumerai, S.B. Out-of-Pocket Burden of Health Care Spending and the Adequacy of the Medicare Part D Low-Income Subsidy. *Med. Care* **2010**, *48*, 503–509. [CrossRef]
63. Appiah, J.O.; Agyemang-Duah, W.; Fordjour, A.A.; Adei, D. Predicting Financial Barriers to Formal Healthcare Utilisation Among Poor Older People under the Livelihood Empowerment Against Poverty Programme in Ghana. *GeoJournal* **2020**. [CrossRef]
64. Bellettiere, J.; Chuang, E.; Hughes, S.C.; Quintanilla, I.; Hofstetter, C.R.; Hovell, M.F. Association between Parental Barriers to Accessing a Usual Source of Care and Children's Receipt of Preventive Services. *Public Health Rep.* **2017**, *132*, 316–325. [CrossRef]
65. Dyer, K.E.; Dumenci, L.; Siminoff, L.A.; Thomson, M.D.; Lafata, J.E. The Contribution of Body Mass Index to Appraisal Delay in Colorectal Cancer Diagnosis: A Structural Equation Modelling Study. *Br. J. Cancer* **2017**, *116*, 1638–1642. [CrossRef] [PubMed]
66. Kalmijn, M. Longitudinal Analyses of the Affects of Age, Marriage, and Parenthood on Social Contacts and Support. *Adv. Life Course Res.* **2012**, *17*, 177–190. [CrossRef]
67. Hosmer, D.W.; Lemeshow, S. *Applied Logistic Regression*; Wiley: New York, NY, USA, 1989.
68. Nattino, G.; Finazzi, S.; Bertolini, G. A New Test and Graphical Tool to Assess the Goodness of Fit of Logistic Regression Models. *Statist. Med.* **2016**, *35*, 709–720. [CrossRef]
69. Hilbe, J.M. *Logistic Regression Models*; CRC Press: New York, NY, USA, 2009.
70. McFadden, D. Quantitative Methods for Analysing Travel Behaviour of Individuals: Some Recent Developments. In *Behavioural Travel Modelling*; Hensher, D.A., Stopher, P.R., Eds.; Croom Helm: London, UK, 1979; pp. 279–318.
71. Hendrickx, J. *Stata Technical Bulletin-52, Using Categorical Variables in Stata*; Stata Press Publication, Stata Corp LP: College Station, TX, USA, 1999; pp. 2–8.
72. Nattino, G.; Lemeshow, S.; Phillips, G.; Finazzi, S.; Bertolini, G. Assessing the Calibration of Dichotomous Outcome Models with the Calibration Belt. *Stata J.* **2017**, *17*, 1003–1014. [CrossRef]
73. Long, J.S.; Freese, J. *Regression Models for Categorical Dependent Variables Using Stata*, 3rd ed.; Stata Press Publication, Stata Corp LP: College Station, TX, USA, 2014.
74. Mcintyre, D.; Thiede, M.; Birch, S. Access as a Policy-Relevant Concept in Low- and Middle-Income Countries. *HEPL* **2009**, *4*, 179–193. [CrossRef]
75. Polikowski, M.; Santos-Eggimann, B. How Comprehensive Are the Basic Packages of Health Services? An International Comparison of Six Health Insurance Systems. *J. Health Serv. Res. Policy* **2002**, *7*, 133–142. [CrossRef] [PubMed]
76. Cronin, C.J. Insurance-Induced Moral Hazard: A Dynamic Model of Within-Year Medical Care Decision Making Under Uncertainty. *Int. Econ. Rev.* **2019**, *60*, 187–218. [CrossRef]
77. Knowles, J.C. Research Note: Price Uncertainty and the Demand for Health Care. *Health Policy Plan.* **1995**, *10*, 301–303. [CrossRef]
78. Dardanoni, V.; Wagstaff, A. Uncertainty and the Demand for Medical Care. *J. Health Econ.* **1990**, *9*, 23–38. [CrossRef]
79. Santerre, R.E.; Neun, S.P. *Health Economics: Theories, Insights, and Industry Studies*; South-Western Cengage Learning: Mason, OH, USA, 2010.
80. Abraham, J.; Sick, B.; Anderson, J.; Berg, A.; Dehmer, C.; Tufano, A. Selecting a Provider: What Factors Influence Patients' Decision Making? *J. Healthc. Manag.* **2011**, *56*, 99–114. [CrossRef]
81. Marchau, V.A.W.J.; Walker, W.E.; Bloemen, P.J.T.M.; Popper, S.W. *Introduction in: Decision Making under Deep Uncertainty*; Springer: Berlin/Heidelberg, Germany; New York, NY, USA, 2019.

82. Zallman, L.; Nardin, R.; Malowney, M.; Sayah, A.; McCormick, D. Affordability of Health Care under Publicly Subsidized Insurance after Massachusetts Health Care Reform: A Qualitative Study of Safety Net Patients. *Int. J. Equity Health* **2015**, *14*, 1–7. [CrossRef]
83. Pauly, M.V. Medical Spending Reform and the Fiscal Future of the United States, 2011. Available online: https://faculty.wharton.upenn.edu/wp-content/uploads/2012/01/MEDICAL-SPENDING-REFORM-AND-THE-FISCAL-FUTURE-OF-THE-UNITED-STATES_Rice-University_NOVEMBER-14-REVISION.pdf (accessed on 27 June 2020).
84. Davaki, K.; Mossialos, E. Financing and Delivering Health Care. In *Social Policy Developments in Greece*; Petmesidou, M., Mossialos, E., Eds.; Ashgate: Aldershot, UK; Hants, UK; Burlington, VT, USA, 2006; pp. 286–318.
85. Larson, S.L.; Fleishman, J.A. Rural-Urban Differences in Usual Source of Care and Ambulatory Service Use: Analyses of National Data Using Urban Influence Codes. *Med. Care* **2003**, *41*, III-65–III-74. [CrossRef] [PubMed]
86. Lankila, T.; Näyhä, S.; Rautio, A.; Rusanen, J.; Taanila, A.; Koiranen, M. Is Geographical Distance a Barrier in the Use of Public Primary Health Services among Rural and Urban Young Adults? Experience from Northern Finland. *Public Health* **2016**, *131*, 82–91. [CrossRef]
87. Burgi, N. The Downsizing and Commodification of Healthcare: The Appalling Greek Experience Since 2010. In *Living under Austerity: Greek Society in Crisis*; Doxiadis, E., Placas, A., Eds.; Berghahn Books: New York, NY, USA, 2018.
88. Gulliford, M.; Morgan, M. (Eds.) *Access to Health Care*; Routledge: New York, NY, USA, 2003.
89. Siati, G.; Monokrousou, M.; Konstantakopoulos, O.; Galanis, P.; Kaitelidou, D.; Theodorou, M. Living with Chronic Diseases in Greece: Investigating Health Services Utilization Patterns and Economic Consequences. *Value Health* **2017**, *20*, A671. [CrossRef]
90. Yamin, A.E.; Carmalt, J.C. The United States: Right to Health Obligations in the Context of Disparity and Reform. In *Advancing the Human Right to Health*; Zuniga, J.M., Marks, S.P., Gostin, L.O., Eds.; Oxford University Press: Oxford, UK, 2013.
91. Thiede, M.; Akweongo, P.; McIntyre, D. Exploring the Dimensions of Access. In *The Economics of Health Equity*; McIntyre, D., Mooney, G.H., Eds.; Cambridge University Press: Cambridge, UK; New York, NY, USA, 2007; pp. 103–123.
92. Paskov, M.; Madia, J.E.; Goedemé, T. Iddle and Below Living Standards: What Can We Learn from Beyond Income Measures of Economic Well-Being? In *Generating Prosperity for Working Families in Affluent Countries*, 1st ed.; Nolan, B., Ed.; Oxford University Press: Oxford, UK, 2018; pp. 282–311.
93. Leyfman, Y. Washington County, PA-A Case Study to Improve the Obesity Epidemic and Enhance Healthcare Access at the Patient-, Community- and Health System Level. *J. Addict. Res. Treat.* **2019**, *1*, 101.
94. Litwin, H.; Sapir, E.V. Forgone Health Care Due to Cost among Older Adults in European Countries and in Israel. *Eur. J. Ageing* **2009**, *6*, 167–176. [CrossRef] [PubMed]
95. Tur-Sinai, A.; Litwin, H. Forgone Visits to the Doctor due to Cost or Lengthy Waiting Time among Older Adults in Europe. In *Ageing in Europe: Supporting Policies for an Inclusive Society*; Börsch-Supan, A., Kneip, T., Eds.; Walter de Gruyter: Boston, UK, 2015; pp. 291–300.
96. Zaw, N.L.; Pepper, M. Poverty and Health in Contemporary Burma. *Indep. J. Burmese Scholarsh.* **2016**, *1*, 169–186.
97. Saunders, P. *Down and Out: Poverty and Exclusion in Australia*; The Policy Press Portland: Portland, OR, USA, 2011.
98. Salganicoff, A. Diagnosing Women's Health Care. *Natl. Counc. Jewish Women J.* **2006**, *29*, 1–4.
99. Mazeikaite, G.; O'Donoghue, C.; Sologon, D.M. The Great Recession, Financial Strain, and Self-Assessed Health in Ireland. *Eur. J. Health Econ.* **2019**, *20*, 579–596. [CrossRef]
100. Fiorillo, D. Reasons for Unmet Needs for Health Care: The Role of Social Capital and Social Support in Some Western EU Countries. *Int. J. Health Econ. Manag.* **2020**, *20*, 79–98. [CrossRef]
101. Marzban, S.; Rajaee, R.; Gholami, S. Study of Out-of-Pocket Expenditures for Outpatient Imaging Services in Imam-Khomeini Hospital in 2014. *Electron. Physician* **2015**, 1183–1189. [CrossRef]
102. Maruotti, A. Fairness of the National Health Service in Italy: A Bivariate Correlated Random Effects Model. *J. Appl. Stat.* **2009**, *36*, 709–722. [CrossRef]

103. Papanastasiou, S.; Papatheodorou, C. The Greek Depression: Poverty Outcomes and Welfare Responses. *East-West J. Econ. Bus.* **2018**, *XXI*, 205–222.
104. Dassiou, X. Greece in Economic Crisis: The Case of Health and Education. *Vierteljahrsh. Wirtsch.* **2015**, *84*, 145–164. [CrossRef]
105. Kyriopoulos, I.-I.; Zavras, D.; Skroumpelos, A.; Mylona, K.; Athanasakis, K.; Kyriopoulos, J. Barriers in Access to Healthcare Services for Chronic Patients in Times of Austerity: An Empirical Approach in Greece. *Int. J. Equity Health* **2014**, *13*, 54. [CrossRef]
106. Latsou, D.; Geitona, M. The Effects of Unemployment and Economic Distress on Depression Symptoms. *Mater. Socio-Med.* **2018**, *30*, 180. [CrossRef]
107. Kyei-Nimakoh, M.; Carolan-Olah, M.; McCann, T.V. Access Barriers to Obstetric Care at Health Facilities in Sub-Saharan Africa—A Systematic Review. *Syst. Rev.* **2017**, *6*, 110. [CrossRef]
108. Reschovsky, J.D. Do HMOs Make a Difference? Access to Healthcare. *Inquiry* **1999**, *36*, 390–399.
109. Zavras, D.; Naoum, P.; Athanasakis, K.; Kyriopoulos, J.; Pavi, E. Unmet Healthcare Needs due to Financial Reasons in Times of Austerity. *Value Health* **2017**, *20*, PA510–PA511. [CrossRef]
110. Lucevic, A.; Péntek, M.; Kringos, D.; Klazinga, N.; Gulácsi, L.; Fernades, O.B.; Boncz, I.; Baji, P. Unmet Medical Needs in Ambulatory Care in Hungary: Forgone Visits and Medications from a Representative Population Survey. *Eur. J. Health Econ.* **2019**, *20* (Suppl. 1), S71–S78. [CrossRef]
111. Baeten, R.; Spasova, S.; Vanhercke, B. Access to Healthcare in the EU: An Overall Positive Trend but Important Inequalities Persist. *Revue Belge de Sécurité Sociale* **2019**, *1E*, 199–219.
112. European Commission. *Special Eurobarometer 486. Report. Europeans in 2019*; Publications Office of the European Union: Luxembourg, 2019. [CrossRef]
113. Cornish, D.M.; Wolters, B.; Harskamp, M.; Kroomshof, H. Healthcare for Refugees in the Netherlands: The Stepped-Care Model. In *Refugee Migration and Health. Challenges for Germany and Europe*; Krämer, A., Fischer, F., Eds.; Springer: Cham, Switzerland, 2019.
114. Or, Z.; Cases, C.; Lisac, M.; Vrangbæk, K.; Winblad, U.; Bevan, G. Are Health Problems Systemic? Politics of Access and Choice under the Beveridge and Bismarck Systems. *Health Econ. Policy Law* **2010**, *5*, 269–293. [CrossRef]
115. van de Ven, W.P.; Beck, K.; Buchner, F.; Schokkaert, F.T.; Schut, E.; Shmueli, A.; Wasem, J. Preconditions for Efficiency and Affordability in Competitive Healthcare Markets: Are they Fulfilled in Belgium, Germany, Israel, the Netherlands and Switzerland? *Health Policy.* **2013**, *109*, 226–245. [CrossRef]
116. Mooney, G. *Challenging Health Economics*; Oxford University Press: Oxford, UK, 2009.
117. Eurostat. *2016 EU-SILC Module "Access to Services"*, 2018. Available online: https://ec.europa.eu/eurostat/documents/1012329/8088300/LC+22118+EN+Module+2016+assessment.pdf/82b23b36-9e04-4905-ab74-9a07f1223637 (accessed on 18 August 2020).
118. Eurofound. *Access to Healthcare in Times of Crisis*; Publications Office of the European Union: Luxemburg, 2014.
119. Hou, X.; Velényi, V.; Yazbeck, A.S.; Iunes, R.F.; Smith, O. (Eds.) *Learning from Economic Downturns*; The World Bank: Washington, DC, USA, 2013.
120. De Falco, R. Access to Healthcare and the Global Financial Crisis in Italy: A Human Rights Perspective. *E-Cad. CES* **2019**. [CrossRef]
121. Legido-Quigley, H.; Karanikolos, M.; Hernandez-Plaza, S.; de Freitas, C.; Bernardo, L.; Padilla, B.; Sá Machado, R.; Diaz-Ordaz, K.; Stuckler, D.; McKee, M. Effects of the Financial Crisis and Troika Austerity Measures on Health and Health Care Access in Portugal. *Health Policy* **2016**, *120*, 833–839. [CrossRef] [PubMed]
122. Kiernan, F. What Price Austerity-A Nation's Health? The Effect of Austerity on Access to Health Care in Ireland. *Eur. J. Public Health.* **2014**, *24*, cku165-110. [CrossRef]
123. Lusardi, A.; Schneider, D.; Tufano, P. The Economic Crisis and Medical Care Use: Comparative Evidence from Five High-Income Countries. *Soc. Sci. Q.* **2015**, *96*, 202–213. [CrossRef]
124. Mensah, J. The Global Financial Crisis and Access to Health Care in Africa. *Afr. Today* **2014**, *60*, 35–54. [CrossRef]
125. OECD. European Observatory on Health Systems and Policies. In *Greece: Country Health Profile 2017*; State of Health in the EU; OECD: Paris, France, 2017. [CrossRef]

126. Donabedian, A. *Aspects of Medical Care Administration: Specifying Requirements for Health Care*; Published for the Commonwealth Fund by Harvard University Press: Cambridge, UK, 1973.
127. Godbole, P.; Kurian, M. Models of Healthcare in Developed and Developing Countries. In *Hospital Transformation. From Failure to Success and Beyond*; Burke, D., Godbole, P., Cash, A., Eds.; Springer: Cham, Switzerland, 2019.
128. Feldstein, P.J. *Health Care Economics*, 7th ed.; Delmar Cengage Learning: Clifton Park, NY, USA, 2012.
129. Whitley, E.M.; Samuels, B.A.; Wright, R.A.; Everhart, R.M. Identification of Barriers to Healthcare Access for Underserved Men in Denver. *J. Men's Health Gend.* **2005**, *2*, 421–428. [CrossRef]
130. Steinwachs, D.M.; Hughes, R.G. Health Services Research: Scope and Significance. In *Patient Safety and Quality: An Evidence-Based Handbook for Nurses*; Hughes, R.G., Ed.; Advances in Patient Safety; Agency for Healthcare Research and Quality (US): Rockville, MD, USA, 2008.
131. Bhattacharya, J.; Hyde, T.; Tu, P. *Health Economics*; Palgrave Macmillan: Houndmills, UK; Basingstoke, UK; Hampshire, NH, USA; New York, NY, USA, 2014.
132. Yamada, T.; Chen, C.-C.; Murata, C.; Hirai, H.; Ojima, T.; Kondo, K.; Iii, J. Access Disparity and Health Inequality of the Elderly: Unmet Needs and Delayed Healthcare. *IJERPH* **2015**, *12*, 1745–1772. [CrossRef]
133. Holloman, J.L.S., Jr. *Access to Health Care. 1983. Securing Access to Health Care. A Report on the Ethical Implications of Differences in the Availability of Health Services*; Report. U.S. Government Printing Office: Washington, DC, USA, 1983; Volume 1.
134. Larson, C.O.; Schlundt, D.; Patel, K.; McClellan, L.; Hargreaves, M. Disparities in Perceptions of Healthcare Access in a Community Sample. *J. Ambul. Care Manag.* **2007**, *30*, 142–149. [CrossRef] [PubMed]

Publisher's Note: MDPI stays neutral with regard to jurisdictional claims in published maps and institutional affiliations.

© 2020 by the author. Licensee MDPI, Basel, Switzerland. This article is an open access article distributed under the terms and conditions of the Creative Commons Attribution (CC BY) license (http://creativecommons.org/licenses/by/4.0/).

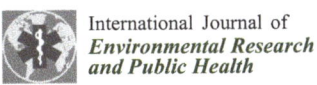

Article

Global Challenges vs. the Need for Regional Performance Models under the Present Pandemic Crisis

Romeo-Victor Ionescu [1], Monica Laura Zlati [2] and Valentin Marian Antohi [3,4,*]

1. Administrative Sciences and Regional Studies, Faculty of Juridical, Social and Political Sciences, Dunarea de Jos University, 111th, Domneasca Street, 800201 Galati, Romania; ionescu_v_romeo@yahoo.com
2. Accounting, Faculty of Economics, Administration and Business, Stefan cel Mare University, Universitatii Street, no. 13, 720229 Suceava, Romania; sorici.monica@usm.ro
3. Business Administration, Faculty of Economics and Business Administration, Dunarea de Jos University, Nicolae Balcescu Street, no. 59-61, 800001 Galati, Romania
4. Finance, Accounting and Economic Theory, Faculty of Economic Sciences and Business Administration, Transylvania University, Colina Universitatii Street, no. 1, 500036 Brasov, Romania
* Correspondence: valentin_antohi@yahoo.com

Abstract: The present study uses the analysis of the EU's regional performance structure based on clusters to test the versatility of the regional administrative capacity in relation to three disruptive global phenomena: the economic crisis, the coronavirus epidemic and the phenomenon of refugee migration to Europe. We defined a regional performance model based on maintaining sustainability indicators in the 240 EU regions. The objectives of the study are aimed primarily at a structured assessment of regional administrative capacity in the initial version, based on statistical indicators, and in the current version, after the outbreak of the pandemic, based on quantifying the impact of the disturbing factors. Secondly, the objectives of the study are to evaluate the reaction of the administrative units according to their ability to respond to the economic problems in the region, in the sense of improving the performance of the regional economies. The methods used in this paper will be empirical (the study of the specialized literature), analytical and will contain econometric modelling and statistical processing of the data. The results of the study will allow the identification of the necessary traits to train a leader in regional performance, traits that will be useful to European decision makers in adjusting the EU regional policy. Moreover, the need to redefine the EU in terms of performance will be substantiated once again. The study is current and is based on the latest Eurostat information, pertinent tables and diagrams.

Keywords: European administrative capacity; econometric model; European regional development; COVID-19; population migration; economic crisis

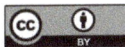

1. General Approach

The current context is an atypical one, in which disturbing factors are manifested both from the social and economic point of view. From the social point of view, regional development is directly influenced by the spread of the new virus (COVID-19), whose effects have manifested in all EU Member States. To this end, we have built a statistical database for the period 2006–2002, using Eurostat information [1].

From the regional point of view, the evolution in the most-affected Member States reflects that the regional character is typical of this disturbing phenomenon. Additionally, the regional specificity of the spread of the disease is manifested in Romania.

Overall, it is noted that three EU-representative economies are placed in the top 12 worldwide in terms of total COVID cases' impact in September 2021: France (6th place), Spain (11th place) and Italy (12th place). The UK has left the EU, but is ranked 4th overall. All European countries are currently facing social and economic crises amid dissent over anti-counterfeiting protective measures [2].

From the economic point of view, the direct impact estimated by the national statistical systems at the level of the four above analysed countries consists of a decrease in GDP.

In this context, the population from the other EU Member States established in areas strongly affected by COVID-19, such as France, Italy or Germany, had the possibility to return massively to their countries of origin, favouring the spread of the virus and generating social problems and economic difficulties for their country of origin. In addition to the restriction of the health system and the increasing need for equipment, medicines and medical staff compared to the planned need, this phenomenon had to provide measures to quarantine the population that returned to the country, as well as to ensure the social protection of the population that lost their places of work during the pandemic. This migration phenomenon is strictly induced by the global pandemic, but Europe is also facing another migration phenomenon of the African, Arab and East Asian populations, which raises issues for European forums regarding ensuring social protection and integrating migrants into a system already incapacitated by the outbreak of the pandemic. The traffic restrictions imposed as a measure to control of the spread of the virus reduced the EU's economic activity and generated financial blockages of those companies which were virtually taken into account when forecasting the budgets of the EU Member States.

These three aggravating factors (pandemic, migration under different aspects and overstretching of economic activity) are significant premises for estimating a serious economic crisis, which will affect global society.

In this context, we aim to develop a regional performance model in the sense of the regional administrative capacity's versatility in relation to these aforementioned phenomena.

The novelty of the present scientific approach lies in identifying and managing a regional leader in terms of socio-economic performance. Moreover, our approach achieves a unified vision of EU regional policy, by standardizing and building on the literature on the subject. Another new element is the emphasis on the need to redefine the EU in performance-related terms.

The paper proceeds as follows. Section 2, Literature Review, discusses relevant models for the topic. It is followed by Section 3, Data and Methodology, in which we highlight the NUTS 2 regional efficiency indicators able to evaluate on a 5-step scale the administrative efficiency data, models and results. This is followed by an analysis of the results in Section 4. An overview in Sections 5 and 6 discusses the results and concludes the paper.

2. Literature Review

Since December 2019, global society has been facing unfavourable conditions regarding economic growth against the background of the COVID-19 pandemic and the necessary global measures to limit the spread of the pandemic.

Although up to this date, the global economy was on an upward slope with normal fluctuations induced by business cycles, the effect of the pandemic downturn has been to freeze the upward slope, as global society is currently facing a significant economic downturn, in the form of short-circuiting the traditional mechanisms of financial, social and security balance of the global market. The factor perpetuating the effects of the pandemic is population migration, which, in this case, contributed to the amplification of the pandemic's effects, generating the multiplication of COVID-19 outbreaks in multiple global regions, from the initial Wuhan centre to Europe, via Italy and America, where the most disastrous effects of the pandemic are currently manifesting.

Faced with the economic downturn, the states of the world have been confronted with an atypical situation against which the traditional models developed by specialists over time and the efforts of sustainable economic growth are annihilated, both in terms of their effects and the expected economic results. In this context, there is a need for a new approach to address the vulnerabilities of classical theories due to the disregard of the exaggerated values of the pandemic, the social and economic risk of disturbing factors which can act on the global economy at a given time. The effect of this action constitutes the global economic crisis itself.

In this gear, several factors related to the specificities of the global economy, namely transactions in financial markets, the role of single currencies, the mechanism of global financing and the interconnection between national economies through multinational companies, are introduced.

From the regional point of view, there is a direct induced reflection of the global economic crisis on regional autonomy by destabilizing the financial equilibrium levers that highlight the difficulty of the regional territorial administrative units and which weaken the effects of the social protection and the sustainable development programs that they had in the usual course.

A summary of the previous research on the effects of the disturbing factors on economic growth, as well as the expiration of the previous models through the effect of disturbing factors, is presented in Table 1.

The analysis of the specialized literature on all the major disturbing aspects that are the subject of the present study supports the opportunity to draw up in the current context a new integrated model for analysing the regional performance of the administrative capacity through the indicators with an essential impact on the disturbance.

Table 1. Literature review.

No.	Authors	Model's Characteristics	Criticism	Proposals/Solutions
1.	Iamsiraroj, S., 2016 [3]	The author analyses the connection between FDI and economic growth based on extensive statistics for a number of 124 states during 1971–2010, according to the following scheme:	The model proposed by the author could not anticipate the effect of the evolution of the disturbing factors on economic growth. As a result, the value of the β coefficients is estimated as positive while, in our opinion, the correct approach for β is $\beta \gtreqless 0$.	Economic growth can be approached from an inter-disciplinary perspective, provided the β coefficients are correctly estimated. In our study, the economic growth is approached both at the regional level (as a factor of the coefficients' diversification) and in terms of connections with other macro indicators (migration, population at risk of poverty, etc.).
2.	Meyer, D. and Shera, A., 2017 [4]	The authors have developed an econometric model regarding the effect of the disturbing factors on economic growth. These factors are attributed to the FDI decrease, migration from less developed countries to developed countries and the transactions' cost due to technological progress. There is an impact on the economic growth at the level of the GDP due to the value of the exchange rate, the debt increase and the aging of the population.	The model benefits from an unjustified optimism regarding the calculation of the positive impact of the increase in schooling rate and of household consumption. A rigid curve influenced in the sense of flattening the regional development's differences is reached in the sense of less significant factors than those affecting today's global economic development.	We believe that economic growth based mainly on consumption is not able to ensure a balanced and sustainable development of the economy. For this reason, our proposed model is not predominantly based on consumption demand, but on sustainable development objectives able to make the economic growth curve more flexible and sustainable, with beneficial effects on the whole economic system.
3.	Pradhan, R.P., Arvin, M.B., Hall J.H. and Nair M., 2016 [5]	The authors used a self-regressive vector to highlight the interdependencies between the financial innovation and the economic development in 18 Euro area countries during 1961–2013. The model based on the scenario method (5 scenario) takes into account a significant growth of the economy during the analysed period in net value at a significance rate of 5% in all scenarios, in the context of the manifestation of the limited growth conditions of the patents/inhabitant and of the financial composite index of the development.	This model indicates that the long-term economic growth is stable, but does not highlight the disruptive effect of situations such as the pandemic and economic crisis.	We consider that this model must be adjusted to more eloquently reproduce the influence of the autoregressive vectors presented during the model.
4.	Bloom, D.E., Canning, D., Kotschy, R., Prettner, K. and Schunemann, J.J., 2019 [6]	The authors developed a directional model for evaluating the effects of population health on economic growth. There is a direct quantifiable impact of population health on economic state based on a classical production function, transformed by the authors.	Some variables such as the effort to maintain the population's proper state of health during the pandemic and the efforts to prevent and update medical systems slow down economic growth at least equal to the disease output as an effect of the pandemic, expressed as a percentage of the base population of the analysed region.	We consider that the presented model should be adjusted, and the curve in the image depreciated with the value of the disturbing impact factors.
5.	Atkeson, A., 2020 [7]	The author, although correctly sensing the impact of the pandemic on the population's health status and indirectly on the economy's state as a whole, based on a model related to the Markov chains, is limited to using the scenario method only to quantify the effect of the pandemic over different exposure times, establishing a set of coefficients based on which the pandemic evolution curves are modelled.	The author's conclusions support the need for economic analyses regarding the consequences of COVID-19 on the economy as a whole and on the public health segment. The proposed analysis is only an intermediate step in evaluating the general disturbing picture of economic growth.	From our point of view, our proposed model is more efficient and competitive and is able to quantify economic performance and to anticipate regional economic developments at least in the short term. The model can be improved by accumulating socio-economic influences on growth, which is also taken into account by our model.

Table 1. *Cont.*

No.	Authors	Model's Characteristics	Criticism	Proposals/Solutions
6.	Gilchrist, S., Schoenle, R., Sim, J. and Zakrajsek, E., 2017 [8]	With relevant available data, the authors performed a pertinent analysis of the disturbing factors' impacts, such as inflation of the global economy during the economic crisis. Thus, the authors correctly conclude that the financial disturbances influence the unjustified increase in the prices, having significant financial adverse effects on the stocks' demand, affecting the liquidity and limiting the access to external financing. These factors act as markers of the growth curve's flattening.	The model needs to be adjusted with the collateral effects of the need for financing due to the measures to combat the pandemic, and the need for financing due to social protection measures and economic recovery.	The issue of economic recovery financing is also treated by us through the prism of the investment process, which is affected by the allocations dedicated to the anti-pandemic fight, which is also reflected in our proposed model.
7.	Adrian, T., Fleming, M., Shachar, O. and Vogt, E., 2017 [9]	[9] The authors developed a detailed study of the financial market in the post-economic crisis period using data over a 25-year period, which included the economic crisis from 2007 to 2009. There was a disturbance on the financial markets within the financial crisis, able to change the trend of the capitalized assets, decelerating their growth under the impact of the financial crisis. The transactions' volatility was presented as a peak during the crisis period, which subsequently tended to reach the values with a delay of 150% compared to the previous period. Thus, in order to calm the volatility, a period of 1.5 times greater than the period preceding the crisis is needed (6 years compared to 4 years). In this research, the debt security positions and the expected returns suffer a minor adjustment to the repayments of placements curve, which reinforces the concept of pessimism that the researchers have pointed out in the article. They also make a financial projection for 2 and 10 years of the effects of the economic crisis.	The model is a relevant one, which realistically captures the impact of the economic crisis on the global economy through the financial markets. The practical example is the situation in China since February 2020, when, in the midst of the economic crisis, the corporate bonds worth about 30% of their capitalized value were traded. These transactions were made in favour of the Chinese state.	We estimate that the occurrence of aggravating factors such as the COVID-19 pandemic and the exacerbation of financial consumption are able to amplify the pessimism of this model. The model can be improved by quantifying the social effect of the pandemic, as well as by quantifying the financial effect of fighting and preventing the disease, which directs a large proportion of economic resources to the medical field, leaving other economic areas uncovered and thus vulnerable (tourism, education, etc.).
8.	Kreichauf, R., 2018 [10]	The author analyses the phenomenon of refugee migration through a socio-spatial model elaborated in order to quantify the results of the measures of the refugees' social inclusion and to accommodate them into the new European socio-economic environment, including the quantification of the asylum austerities' impact and the offered conditions in the refugee campuses in order to strengthen the norms of life safety on a sustainable basis.	There is pressure on asylum seekers that slows the social absorption of the asylum seekers and their integration into the new European socio-economic environment. The aspects invoked by the author must be assimilated into an impact study.	From our point of view, the socio-spatial model is not sufficient to achieve the research objectives proposed in the author's study.

Table 1. Cont.

No.	Authors	Model's Characteristics	Criticism	Proposals/Solutions
9.	Hangartner, D., Dinas, E., Marbach, M., Matakos, K. and Xefteris D., 2018 [11]	The authors conducted a study on the impact of the refugee crisis. The study was conducted on the basis of the information collected by the authors, modelled through the TSLS regression, observing, after modelling, the exacerbation of antisocial behaviour of the natives in the analysed territories in relation to migrants. The favouring factors of the normalized behavioural model are represented by the strengthening of border protection, the measures regarding the prevention of terrorist attacks and social protection measures. The study was conducted across 3 regions of Greece, Italy and Spain, of which Greece represents about 80% of the migrant waves.	The model aims to solve specific issues regarding the affectation of the native population by the migrants' waves, on the basis of the cluster methodology. The unilateral approach is inferior to integrating information in a complex model based on the congruent evaluation of several disturbing factors with a long-term effect on the regional population.	In the current context of the crisis in Afghanistan, this model can be improved with the logistical and economic components which derive from the crisis situation created punctually by the withdrawal of troops from Afghanistan. This information can be a source for adjusting the indicators of the proposed model to predict the downstream and upstream economic dimension of migrant wave absorption.
10.	Harteveld, E., Schaper, J., De Lange, S.L. and Van Der Brug, W., 2017 [12]	The authors investigate how the refugee crisis affects the administrative capacity and the public opinion regarding the exercise of administrative attributes of governmental bodies on levels of influence. The Euroscepticism, as transpired from this study, was found to be directly proportional to the media phenomenon (the refugee crisis). The results of the study show that the polarization of the Europeans' attitude in relation to this phenomenon of migration has the effect of lowering the support measures regarding the integration of new migrants into the European socio-economic life.	The authors analyse the dynamics of the mechanisms in relation to some secondary variables (for example, the media), which could have been replaced by an impact analysis of the socio-economic measures in relation to some primary aggravating factors such as those mentioned at the 9th point of Table 1.	In line with the current situation, we believe that improvements can be made both to the social and economic items as well as to the management and logistical strategy components of the refugee crisis.
11.	Danielli, S. Patria, R., Donnelly, P., Ashrafian, H., Darzi, A., 2020 [13]	The paper presented by the authors analyses the economic intervention to ameliorate the impact of COVID-19 on the economy and the health system through an international comparison, by which the European countries (Spain, Sweden, France, UK, Germany and Italy) appear with the most significant allocations of GDP in terms of fiscal measures in order to combat the effects of COVID-19. The structure of the package of measures (according to the authors) differs from state to state, with the caveat that tax cuts and the adoption of population support measures is an almost general pattern in the states analysed.	The authors manage to centralize some fiscal actions that may lead to certain action profiles during the pandemic, but the comparison between these profiles is weak. The results of the analysis can be further explored to draw more relevant conclusions.	The study is of interest, but needs to be deepened from the comparative analysis point of view as well as from the creating relevant conclusions point of view. In our study, we showed that some European countries (France, Spain, Italy and the UK) faced a significant economic impact, this rationale being the premise for developing working hypotheses leading to conclusive results in terms of regional performance under the impact of COVID-19.

Table 1. *Cont.*

No.	Authors	Model's Characteristics	Criticism	Proposals/Solutions
12.	Umar, M., Xu, Y. and Mirza, S.S., 2021 [14]	The authors address the impact of the COVID-19 crisis on the labour market by analysing the impact of the pandemic on the GIG economy.	The results of the study show that, as far as the labour market is concerned, the degree of its affectation was in the closed economy area where many companies temporarily or permanently ceased their activity. At the same time, there have been online platforms where labour supply and demand could meet and generate a promising impact on "OLI filled jobs".	Although it is an interesting study, the authors approach the effect of digitization on the labour market too optimistically, creating the premises for a positive effect of the transfer of labour supply from the real to the virtual environment. The analysis can be adjusted with additional correction factors on the economic contribution of telework productivity, even if some effects on pollution and social impact seem to confirm the hypotheses of the authors' study. There are some sectors for which the positive impact can be quantified (services), but not in the productive sectors.
13.	Asahi K, Undurraga EA, Valdés R, Wagner R., 2021 [15]	The authors analyse in an interesting way the effect of COVID-19 on the economy in the context of lockdown. The method of analysis is the study of VAT collection in Chile during the lockdown and before the COVID-19 crisis in 170 municipalities.	The picture presented is relevant and proves that the pandemic has a profound disruptive effect on the affected economies. There is both a temporary and a geographical effect, with some regions having more manageable profiles than others.	We believe that the study can be improved by collecting the social components and the measures of prevention and control of the disease in order to highlight a general picture of action and effects during the pandemic period.
14.	Vitenu-Sackey, P.S. and Barfi, R., 2021 [16]	The authors analyse the global impact of the pandemic through a study in which they address both uncertainty and poverty alleviation in relation to economic growth. They point out that the COVID-19 pandemic far surpassed any other global pandemic produced between 1996 and 2020. The social component of the support measures reflects disparities in global economic development.	The model proposed by the authors' aims to quantify the impact of the pandemic on the global economy and poverty alleviation. The model shows interesting composite variables such as the human development index (HDI) reported by the UN. The second composite indicator is the stringency index, which quantifies the impact of school closures, telecommuting and restrictions on free movement on society. These indicators in relation to GDP/capita and COVID'S monitoring indicators of illness and death are fed into a correlation matrix, showing that the pandemic is affecting economic growth and efforts to reduce the risk of poverty.	The study is topical, of interest and demonstrates the societal component as being of utmost importance in the pandemic equation.
15.	Khurshid, A. and Khan, K., 2020 [17]	The authors analyse the impact of COVID-19 on the environment and the economy, making projections up to 2032, based on dynamic modelling. The model takes into account the shock wave theory and is based on the indicators of energy consumption, population, GDP and climate change.	Long-term forecasting in an unpredictable global economy has little chance of verifying the forecasting model ("negative spike will decline the GDP by USD 6313.76 million in 2026").	The scenario method may improve the conclusions of the study, which we find interesting. An increase in the number of indicators per economic segment can better substantiate the presented projections, increasing the reliability of the presentation.

3. Data and Methodology

In order to achieve the major objective of the research, namely the analysis of regional performance according to the versatility of administrative capacity in relation to disturbing factors (the COVID-19 crisis, the induced economic crisis and the migration from Europe manifested in recent years), we proceeded to interrogate the Eurostat database in order to obtain a series of data on NUTS 2 regional efficiency indicators, such as:

I1. Investment share of GDP by institutional sectors, predicted as % of GDP total investment, Eurostat code: 0sdg_08_11
I2. Early leavers from education and training by sex, predicted as % of population aged 18 to 24, Eurostat code: 0sdg_04_10
I3. Gross domestic expenditure on R&D by sector, predicted as % of GDP, Eurostat code: 0sdg_09_10
I4. Employment in high- and medium-high-technology manufacturing and knowledge-intensive services, predicted as % of total employment, Eurostat code: 0sdg_09_20
I5. People at risk of poverty or social exclusion, predicted as percentage, Eurostat code: 0sdg_01_10
I6. People at risk of income poverty after social transfers, predicted as percentage, Eurostat code: 0sdg_01_20
I7. People living in households with very low work intensity, predicted as percentage of total population aged less than 60, Eurostat code: 0sdg_01_40
I8. Share of renewable energy in gross final energy consumption by sector, predicted as % Renewable energy sources, Eurostat code: 0sdg_07_40
I9. Real GDP per capita, predicted as chain-linked volumes (2010), EUR per capita, Eurostat code: 0sdg_08_10 GDP
I10. Long-term unemployment rate by sex, predicted as % of active population, Eurostat code: 0sdg_08_40
I11. R&D personnel by sector, predicted as % of active population, Eurostat code: 0sdg_09_30
I12. Patent applications to the European Patent Office (source: EPO), predicted as number, Eurostat code: 0sdg_09_40
I13. Employment rates of recent graduates by sex, predicted as % of population aged 20 to 34 with at least upper secondary education, Eurostat code: 0sdg_04_50
I14. Energy import dependency by products, predicted as % of imports in total energy consumption, Eurostat code: 0sdg_07_50

These indicators have been selected from specific statistical indicators used by Eurostat in its sustainability analysis (https://ec.europa.eu/eurostat/web/sdi/indicators (accessed on 2 March 2021)). The selection of indicators was based on the relevance of the data to the topic under analysis.

For the assessment of the initial regional administrative capacity (before manifesting the disturbing factors potentiated by the COVID-19 epidemic), the authors proceeded to evaluate on a 5-step scale the administrative efficiency. The scale was adjusted to the values reported by Eurostat for the aforementioned indicators and allowed by using the mean, the median and the module to classify each NUTS 2 region for the 14 indicators on one of the 5 steps of the scale, as defined in Figure 1.

After comparing the data series, a 14-step efficiency chart was obtained for each of the 240 NUTS 2 regions of the EU. This picture, resulting from the application of the individual arithmetic mean to the region, allowed the calculation on the aforementioned scale of basic regional administrative capacity on a performance structure unaffected by the 3 disruptive factors. The graphical centralization of the performance is presented in Figure 2, where due to space restrictions the legend does not show all the regions. These are detailed in the Appendix A (Figure A1).

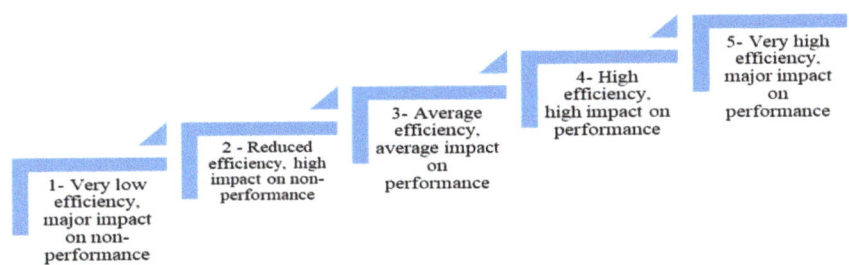

Figure 1. The 5-step scale for administrative efficiency.

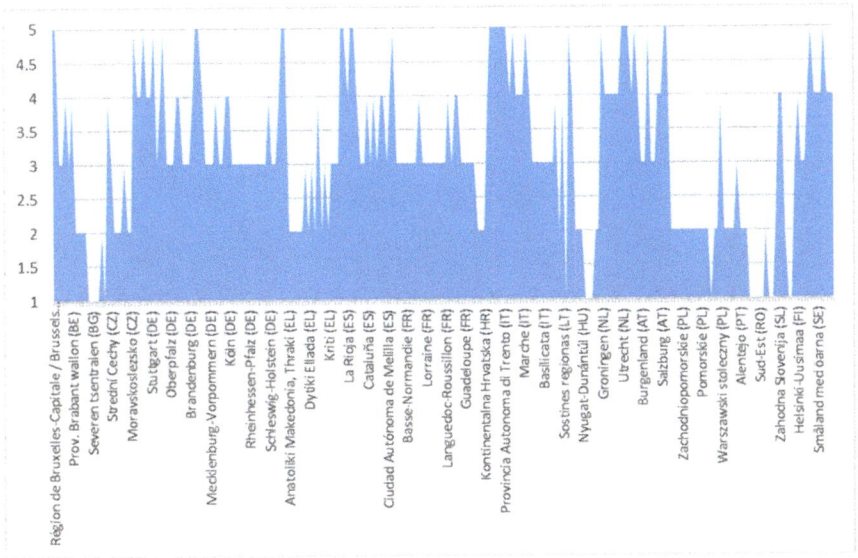

Figure 2. Regional efficiency chart on NUTS 2 regions.

From Figure 2, it appears that the overall distribution is one in favour of medium efficiency, with a medium impact on performance. There are some situations (8 out of 10 regions) where the scalar level of the reliability indicator is very low, denoting a major impact on non-performance. These regions are located in the east of the EU.

The calculation of the coefficients was performed according to the formula:

$$\text{If } \lim_{t \to \infty} \left(\frac{\frac{\sum_{t=1}^{15} I_{i,t}}{\sum_{t=1}^{15} t}}{\frac{\sum_{i=1}^{240} \left(\sum_{t=1}^{15} I_{i,t} \right)}{\sum_{t=1}^{15} t * \sum_{i=1}^{240} i}} \right) \to min \text{ , than } P_{r_{i,t}} = 1 \qquad (1)$$

$$\text{If } \lim_{t \to \infty} \left(\frac{\frac{\sum_{t=1}^{15} I_{i,t}}{\sum_{t=1}^{15} t}}{\frac{\sum_{i=1}^{240} \left(\sum_{t=1}^{15} I_{i,t} \right)}{\sum_{t=1}^{15} t * \sum_{i=1}^{240} i}} \right) \to 0 \text{ , than } P_{r_{i,t}} = 2 \qquad (2)$$

$$\text{If } \lim_{t \to \infty} \left(\frac{\frac{\sum_{t=1}^{15} I_{i,t}}{\sum_{t=1}^{15} t}}{\frac{\sum_{i=1}^{240} \left(\sum_{t=1}^{15} I_{i,t} \right)}{\sum_{t=1}^{15} t * \sum_{i=1}^{240} i}} \right) = 0 \text{ , than } P_{r_{i,t}} = 3 \qquad (3)$$

If $\lim_{t \to \infty} \left(\frac{\frac{(\sum_{t=1}^{15} I_{i,t})}{\sum_{t=1}^{15} t}}{\frac{\sum_{i=1}^{240} (\sum_{t=1}^{15} I_{i,t})}{\sum_{t=1}^{15} t * \sum_{i=1}^{240} i}} \right) \to 1$, than $Pr_{i,t} = 4$ (4)

If $\lim_{t \to \infty} \left(\frac{\frac{(\sum_{t=1}^{15} I_{i,t})}{\sum_{t=1}^{15} t}}{\frac{\sum_{i=1}^{240} (\sum_{t=1}^{15} I_{i,t})}{\sum_{t=1}^{15} t * \sum_{i=1}^{240} i}} \right) \to max$, than $Pr_{i,t} = 5$ (5)

where: $Pr_{i,t}$—regional performance in basic terms, without the effects of the COVID-19 pandemic; $I_{i,t}$—the value of the 14 aforementioned indicators for the 240 regions over the 15-year horizon (data collected from Eurostat 2006–2020); i—number of EU regions (240); t—the time horizon for which the analysis was performed; and coefficients 1, 2, 3, 4, 5—the scalar values shown in Figure 3.

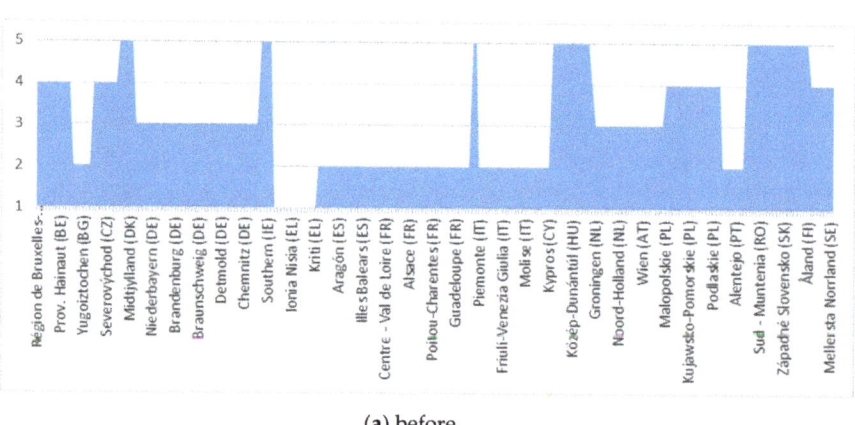

(a) before

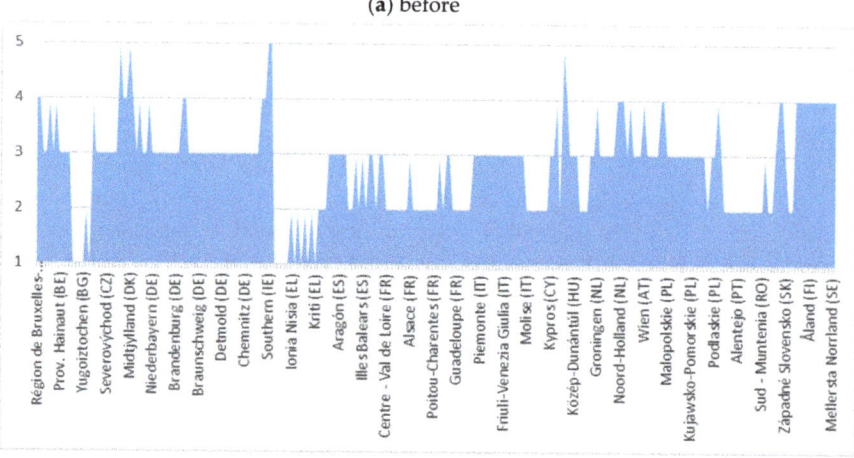

(b) after adjustment

Figure 3. Refugee migration.

For the scalar evaluation of the European population and of the refugees' migration phenomenon, we analysed data from the specialized literature and the official figures presented by Eurostat. Finally, we made our own dimension based on the reality in each Member State regarding the migration and its impact on the destination state, as well as on the migration of the European population from states with less developed economies to those with developed economies. The empirically and statistically evaluated data are presented in Figures 3 and 4.

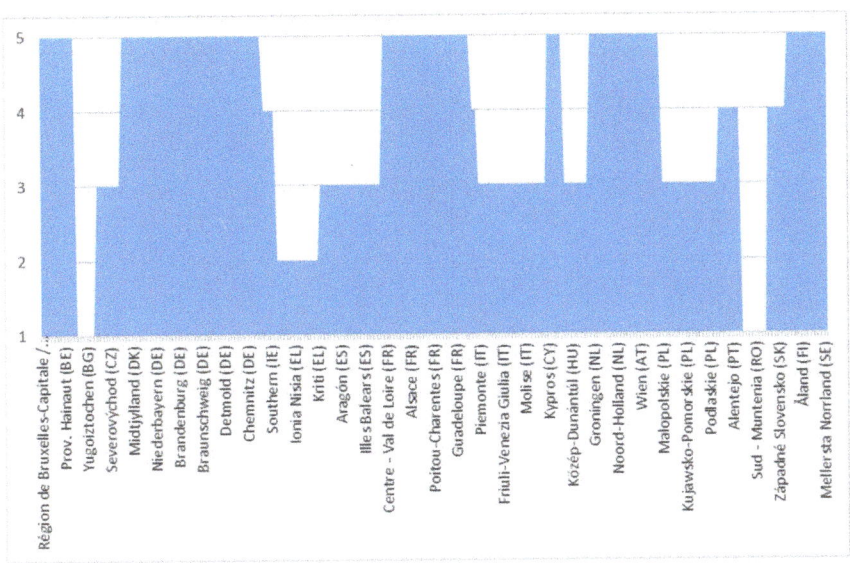

(a) before

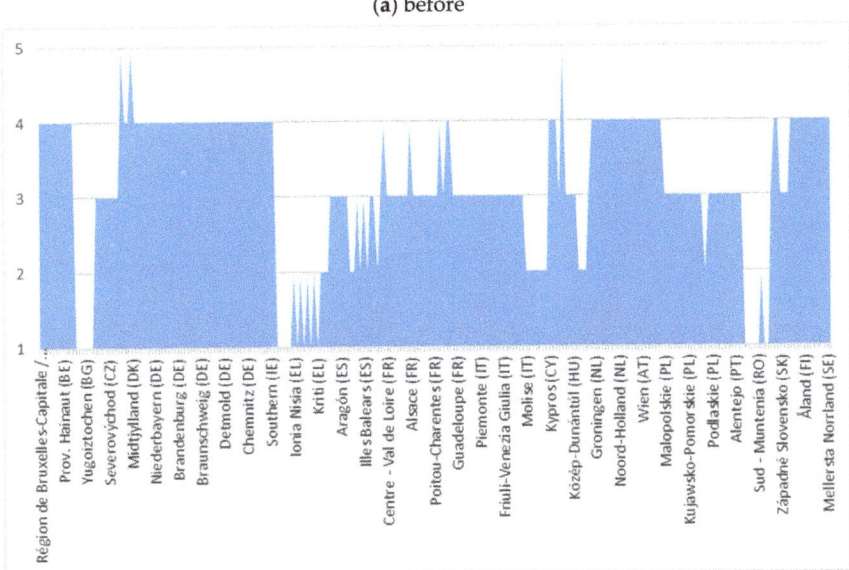

(b) after adjustment

Figure 4. EU population's migration.

Following the analysis of the migration phenomenon through the lens of the proposed model, there is an increase in the impact of the phenomenon on European regions, especially on those with a low level of influence of the indicators in the initial (unadjusted) version. According to the figure, the trend is one of evenness/reduction in disparities, but towards the high impact area.

In Figure 4, we have analysed the migration of the European population within the Union, showing a more pronounced trend compared to the baseline period, but less pronounced than in the case of refugee migration. Under the impact of the refugee crisis, we estimate that some of the restrictive measures will also have an effect on the migration of the European population, which can be seen by comparing the fitted diagrams in Figures 3 and 4.

For the homogeneity of the analysis process, we used the same scale in Figure 3, so that our new model allows data parity. After estimating the data series (point "a" in Figures 5 and 6), their adjustment was made regarding the impact on the versatility of regional administrative capacity through the analysed disturbance factor (internal migration + refugees).

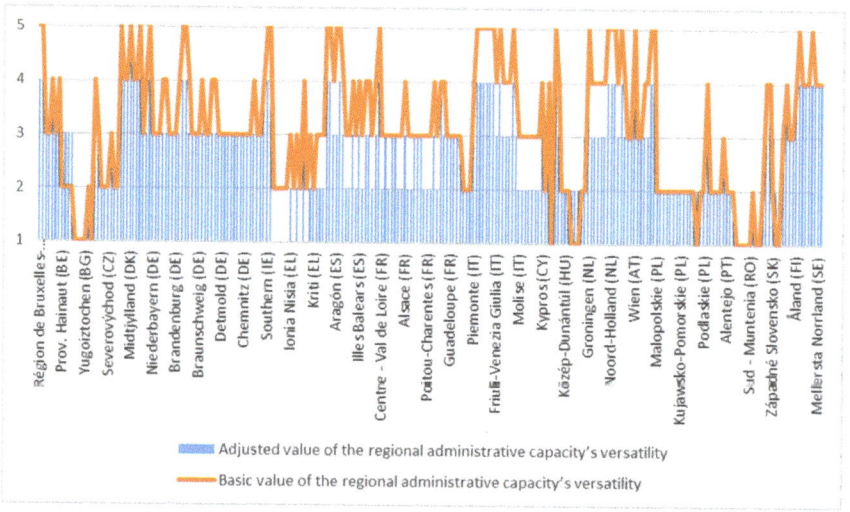

Figure 5. Regional administrative capacity under the conditions of the analysed disturbed factors.

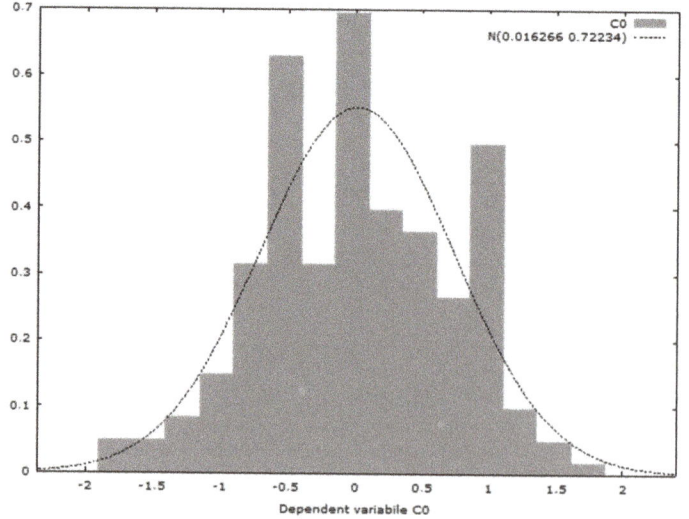

Figure 6. Distribution of the dependent variable.

The adjustment model started from the results obtained by calculating the basic administrative capacity at the regional level, on which the consecutive impact of the two phenomena was evaluated according to the formula:

$$\text{If } \lim_{i \to \infty} \left(\frac{M_i}{\frac{\sum_{i=1}^{240}(M_i)}{\sum_{i=1}^{240} i}} \right) \to \min, \text{ than } M_i = 1 \tag{6}$$

$$\text{If } \lim_{i \to \infty} \left(\frac{M_i}{\frac{\sum_{i=1}^{240}(M_i)}{\sum_{i=1}^{240} i}} \right) \to 0, \text{ than } M_i = 2 \tag{7}$$

$$\text{If } \lim_{i \to \infty} \left(\frac{M_i}{\frac{\sum_{i=1}^{240}(M_i)}{\sum_{i=1}^{240} i}} \right) = 0, \text{ than } M_i = 3 \tag{8}$$

$$\text{If } \lim_{i \to \infty} \left(\frac{M_i}{\frac{\sum_{i=1}^{240}(M_i)}{\sum_{i=1}^{240} i}} \right) \to 1, \text{ than } M_i = 4 \tag{9}$$

$$\text{If } \lim_{i \to \infty} \left(\frac{M_i}{\frac{\sum_{i=1}^{240}(M_i)}{\sum_{i=1}^{240} i}} \right) \to \max, \text{ than } M_i = 5 \tag{10}$$

$$P_{r_{i,t}}{}^1 = \sqrt{P_{r_{i,t}} \times M_i} \tag{11}$$

where: M_i—the intensity of the migration phenomenon in region i, $i \in [1, 240]$, $P_{r_{i,t}}{}^1$—adjusting the basic model with the scalar afferent to the migration phenomenon calculated based on the above formula.

$$\text{If } \lim_{i \to \infty} \left(\frac{R_i}{\frac{\sum_{i=1}^{240}(R_i)}{\sum_{i=1}^{240} i}} \right) \to \min, \text{ than } R_i = 1 \tag{12}$$

$$\text{If } \lim_{i \to \infty} \left(\frac{R_i}{\frac{\sum_{i=1}^{240}(R_i)}{\sum_{i=1}^{240} i}} \right) \to 0, \text{ than } R_i = 2 \tag{13}$$

$$\text{If } \lim_{i \to \infty} \left(\frac{R_i}{\frac{\sum_{i=1}^{240}(R_i)}{\sum_{i=1}^{240} i}} \right) = 0, \text{ than } R_i = 3 \tag{14}$$

$$\text{If } \lim_{i \to \infty} \left(\frac{R_i}{\frac{\sum_{i=1}^{240}(R_i)}{\sum_{i=1}^{240} i}} \right) \to 1, \text{ than } R_i = 4 \tag{15}$$

$$\text{If } \lim_{i \to \infty} \left(\frac{R_i}{\frac{\sum_{i=1}^{240}(R_i)}{\sum_{i=1}^{240} i}} \right) \to \max, \text{ than } R_i = 5 \tag{16}$$

$$P_{r_{i,t}}{}^2 = \sqrt{P_{r_{i,t}} \times R_i} \tag{17}$$

where: R_i—the intensity of the refugee migration phenomenon in region i, $i \in [1, 240]$, $P_{r_{i,t}}{}^2$—adjusting the basic model with the scalar of the refugee migration phenomenon calculated based on the above formula.

Regarding the impairment of regional administrative capacity with the scalar values of the impact due to the COVID-19 pandemic in EU regions, we used the data communicated on the statista.com website, which presents in detail the distribution of the regional spread of the diseases with COVID-19 in each Member State. These data were centralized by the authors, compared with the demographic values reported by Eurostat through the population on 1 January by NUTS 2 region persons indicator at the level of 2019, calculating the regional disease rate defined as COVID-19's rate, according to Appendix B (Table A1).

The scaling procedure was similar to those presented above, namely:

$$\text{If } \lim_{i \to \infty} \left(\frac{COVID-19_i}{\frac{\sum_{i=1}^{240}(COVID-19_i)}{\sum_{i=1}^{240} i}} \right) \to min \text{, than } COVID-19_i = 1 \quad (18)$$

$$\text{If } \lim_{i \to \infty} \left(\frac{COVID-19_i}{\frac{\sum_{i=1}^{240}(COVID-19_i)}{\sum_{i=1}^{240} i}} \right) \to 0 \text{, than } COVID-19_i = 2 \quad (19)$$

$$\text{If } \lim_{i \to \infty} \left(\frac{COVID-19_i}{\frac{\sum_{i=1}^{240}(COVID-19_i)}{\sum_{i=1}^{240} i}} \right) = 0 \text{, than } COVID-19_i = 3 \quad (20)$$

$$\text{If } \lim_{i \to \infty} \left(\frac{COVID-19_i}{\frac{\sum_{i=1}^{240}(COVID-19_i)}{\sum_{i=1}^{240} i}} \right) > 1 \text{, than } COVID-19_i = 4 \quad (21)$$

$$\text{If } \lim_{i \to \infty} \left(\frac{COVID-19_i}{\frac{\sum_{i=1}^{240}(COVID-19_i)}{\sum_{i=1}^{240} i}} \right) \to max \text{, than } COVID-19_i = 5 \quad (22)$$

$$P_{r_{i,t}}{}^3 = \sqrt{P_{r_{i,t}} \times COVID-19_i} \quad (23)$$

where: $COVID-19$—the intensity of the population infection phenomenon following the outbreak of the pandemic in region i, $i \in [1, 240]$, $P_{r_{i,t}}{}^3$—adjusting the basic model with the scalar afferent to the phenomenon of population infection following the outbreak of the pandemic, calculated based on the above formula.

In order to evaluate the impact of the economic crisis, a two-step formula was applied. In the first step, the scalar indicators I7, I9 and I13 were used: I7, people living in households with very low work intensity, predicted as the percentage of the total population aged less than 60, Eurostat code: 0sdg_01_40; I9, real GDP per capita, predicted as chain-linked volumes (2010), EUR per capita, Eurostat code: 0sdg_08_10 GDP; and I13, employment rates of the recent graduates by sex, predicted as % of population aged 20 to 34 with at least upper secondary education, Eurostat code: 0sdg_04_50.

In the second stage, the scalar indicator calculated for COVID-19 was used, according to the formula:

$$\text{If } \lim_{t \to \infty} \left(\frac{\frac{(\sum_{n=1}^{3} I_{i,n})}{\sum_{n=1}^{3} n} + COVID-19_i}{2} \right) \to min \text{, than } C_i = 1 \quad (24)$$

$$\text{If } \lim_{t \to \infty} \left(\frac{\frac{\left(\sum_{n=1}^{3} I_{i,n}\right)}{\sum_{n=1}^{3} n} + COVID-19_i}{2} \right) \to 0 \text{, than } C_i = 2 \qquad (25)$$

$$\text{If } \lim_{t \to \infty} \left(\frac{\frac{\left(\sum_{n=1}^{3} I_{i,n}\right)}{\sum_{n=1}^{3} n} + COVID-19_i}{2} \right) = 0 \text{, than } C_i = 3 \qquad (26)$$

$$\text{If } \lim_{t \to \infty} \left(\frac{\frac{\left(\sum_{n=1}^{3} I_{i,n}\right)}{\sum_{n=1}^{3} n} + COVID-19_i}{2} \right) \to 1 \text{, than } C_i = 4 \qquad (27)$$

$$\text{If } \lim_{t \to \infty} \left(\frac{\frac{\left(\sum_{n=1}^{3} I_{i,n}\right)}{\sum_{n=1}^{3} n} + COVID-19_i}{2} \right) \to \max \text{, than } C_i = 5 \qquad (28)$$

$$P_{r_{i,t}}{}^3 = \sqrt{P_{r_{i,t}} \times C_i} \qquad (29)$$

where: C_i—the scalar coefficient of the economic crisis impact on the regional administrative capacity calculated according to the above formula; $I_{i,n}$—scalar indicators I7, I9 and I13; $P_{r_{i,t}}{}^4$—adjusting the basic model with the scalar afferent to the phenomenon after the outbreak of the pandemic, calculated based on the above formula.

The composite value of the versatility indicator of regional administrative capacity in relation to the 3 disturbing phenomena (economic crisis, COVID-19 pandemic and migration) was calculated based on the 4 intermediate values, adjusted by rounded arithmetic mean to the value of the scalars defined in Figure 1, according to the formula:

$$P_{r_{i,t}}{}^* = \frac{P_{r_{i,t}}{}^1 + P_{r_{i,t}}{}^2 + P_{r_{i,t}}{}^3 + P_{r_{i,t}}{}^4}{4} \qquad (30)$$

The graphical representation of the predicted final values for the analysed indicator, namely the versatility of the regional administrative capacity under the conditions of the analysed disturbed factors, is shown in Figure 5:

From Figure 5, it emerges that the final predictive values for regional administrative capacity versatility under the disturbing factors denote an evolving amplitude for most regions. There are cases where the versatility of regional administrative capacity is reduced by at least one point of influence from the base level. This means that disturbing factors constitute monitoring elements for the regional administrations on the basis of which the regional policies can be rebuilt in the short and medium term, with the advantage of maintaining the stability of the regional capacity by mitigating or eliminating the influence of these disturbing factors.

4. Results

We designed an econometric model in order to test the correlation between the previously presented variables, with the title of global phenomena with negative impact, namely the economic crisis, the refugees and the migration, and not lastly, the impact of the COVID-19 pandemic. These variables allowed the calculation of the scalar coefficients of regional administrative capacity in the absence of the disturbing factors (C0) and in the presence of each individual (C1–C4) in order to finally allow the calculation of the regional administrative capacity versatility under the current crisis conditions. The definitions of the aforementioned terms are:

F1—Economic crisis' impact;
F2—Refugees' impact;
F3—Migration's impact;
F4—COVID-19's impact;

C0—Basic regional administrative capacity;
C1—Refugees' impact on regional administrative capacity;
C2—Migration's impact on regional administrative capacity;
C3—COVID-19's impact on regional administrative capacity;
C4—Economic crisis' impact on regional administrative capacity;
R—Regional administrative capacity.

The new proposed model is based on the following hypotheses H1–H3:

Hypothesis 1 (H1). *There is a direct and quantifiable dependence between the regional administrative capacity and the regional economic power quantified in real GDP/capita. In the absence of the disturbing factors, it is estimated that the growth trend of the regional economies is directly related to the regional administrative capacity and in terms of economic growth in the EU as a whole.*

Hypothesis 2 (H2). *In the presence of the disturbing factors, it is estimated that the greatest impact quantified by the correlation between the scalar of the phenomenon and the impact on the regional administrative capacity is generated by F4 (COVID-19 pandemic) and F1 (Economic crisis' impact).*

Hypothesis 3 (H3). *There is a demonstrable econometric correlation through the same dependent variable between the scalar value of the disturbing factors with regional manifestation and the scalar value of the regional administrative capacity through a high statistical confidence regarding the test of bivalent correlation between C0, R and the factors Fi.*

In the above context of the hypotheses and the methodological concepts presented in Section 3, we define the correlational econometric model based on the two-stage least squares regression. The model used Gretl software version 2019, according to the regression equation as follows:

$$\begin{cases} C0 = +2.19 \times F1 + 0.105 \times F2 + 0.0501 \times F3 - 1.34 \times F4 \\ \langle n = 240. R - \text{squared} = 0.729 \rangle \\ \\ C0 = +1.13 \times R \\ \langle n = 240. R - \text{squared} = 0.968 \rangle \end{cases} \qquad (31)$$

According to this regression equation, we find highly significant statistical values of the model for the dependent variable C0, the regressors Fi and the instrumented variables Ci. In this case, the statistical significance test indicates the value of 72.9%, while the C0-R correlation indicates a 96.8% value of the statistical significance test, which leads to a first conclusion of the model's validity. In order to consolidate this conclusion, the statistical tests were performed for the TSLS model applied to the EU 240 NUTS 2 regions, obtaining significant values of the p-value indicator for the variable regression scales F1, F4 and F2 (see Table 2). The p-value is medium significant for F2, while it is highly significant for F1 and F4.

The heteroscedasticity test reveals that, in the case of the null hypothesis, the heteroscedascity is not present, and the test for the residual normality reflects that the error is normally distributed, according to the distribution diagram of the Gaussian curve.

Hausman test—null hypothesis: OLS estimates are consistent; asymptotic statistical test: Hi square (4) = 728.81 with p-value = $2.01207e^{-156}$; Pesaran–Taylor test for heteroskedasticity—null hypothesis: heteroscedasticity is not present; asymptotic statistical test: z = 0.329671 with p-value = 0.741648; test for residual normality—null hypothesis: the error is normally distributed; statistical test: Hi square (2) = 2.79135 with p-value = 0.247665; weak instrument test—Cragg–Donald minimum eigenvalue = 50.9864 (see Figure 6).

Table 2. Model TSLS using observations 1–240. Dependent variable: C0; Instrumented: F1 F2 F3 F4; Instruments: C1 C2 C3 C4.

	Coefficient	Std. Error	t-Ratio	p-Value	
F1	2.18552	0.100009	21.85	<0.0001	***
F2	0.105132	0.0479492	2.193	0.0293	**
F3	0.0501419	0.0431048	1.163	0.2459	
F4	−1.33810	0.0780583	−17.14	<0.0001	***
Mean dependent var	3.150000	S.D. dependent var		1.150950	
The sum of the squares residuals	123.2029	Standard error of regression		0.722528	
Uncentred R-squared	0.728780	Centred R-squared		0.901506	
F (4.236)	1277.098	p-value(F)		$1.5e^{-158}$	
Log-likelihood	−2566.499	Akaike criterion		5140.998	
Schwarz criterion	5154.920	Hannan–Quinn		5146.608	

***—high significance; **—medium significance.

The predicted analysis of the amplitude of the dependent variable variation achieves over the 95% confidence interval and shows a significant impairment of the values of the basic regional capacity (C0) in the presence of the disturbing factors. This forecast is shown in the diagram (Figure 7):

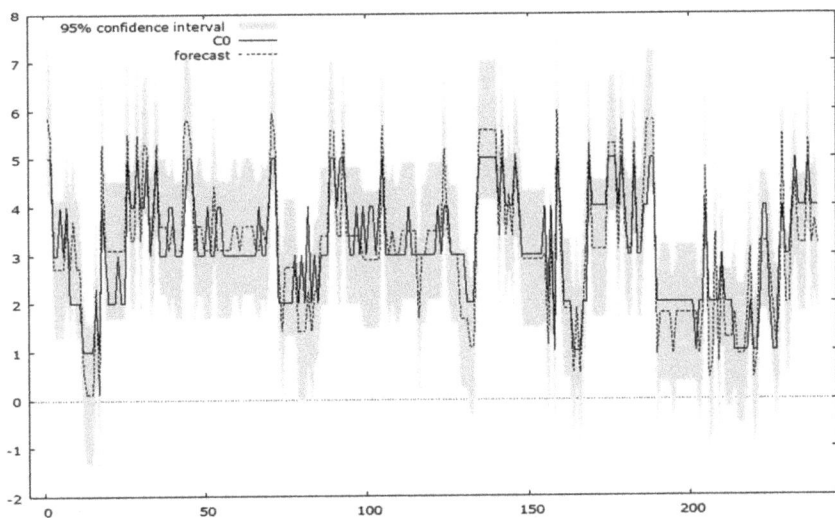

Figure 7. Predicted distribution diagram of the dependent variable for the 95% confidence interval.

The model proposed in this paper objectively evaluated the versatility of the regional administrative capacity in relation to the disturbing factors, finding a high influence of F1 and F4 and an average influence of F2 on the dependent variable. Variable F3 represents a residual regressor in the proposed model because it is concerned with the measures adopted during the pandemic and economic crisis to limit the movement of people and to control the social distance.

5. Discussion

Through the analysis performed during the present research, the working hypotheses were demonstrated as follows:

H1 demonstration: *There is a direct and quantifiable dependence between the regional administrative capacity and the regional economic power quantified in real GDP/capita, so that, in the absence of disturbing factors, it is estimated that the growth trend of the regional economies is directly related to the regional administrative capacity and in terms of economic growth in the EU as a whole. This aspect was also highlighted by Asahi K, Undurraga EA, Valdés R and Wagner R. (2021) [15], who pointed out that, during the crisis period, there is an impairment of the regional economy compared to the development experienced by these regions before the crisis (see Table 1).*

This aspect was demonstrated because for the calculation of the regional administrative capacity, 14 regional statistical indicators were integrated: I1. investment share of GDP by institutional sectors, I2. early leavers from education and training by sex, I3. gross domestic expenditure on R&D by sector, predicted as % of GDP, I4. employment in high- and medium-high-technology manufacturing and knowledge-intensive services, I5. people at risk of poverty or social exclusion, I6. people at risk of income poverty after social transfers, I7. people living in households with very low work intensity, I8. share of renewable energy in gross final energy consumption by sector, I9. real GDP per capita, I10. long-term unemployment rate by sex, I11. R&D personnel by sector, I12. patent applications to the European Patent Office, I13. employment rates of recent graduates by sex and I14. energy import dependency by products.

$$(\text{I9. real GDP per capita}) = +0.936 \times (\text{C0. basic regional administrative capacity}) \quad (32)$$

n = 240, R-squared = 0.956.

The correlation diagram is shown in Figure 8.

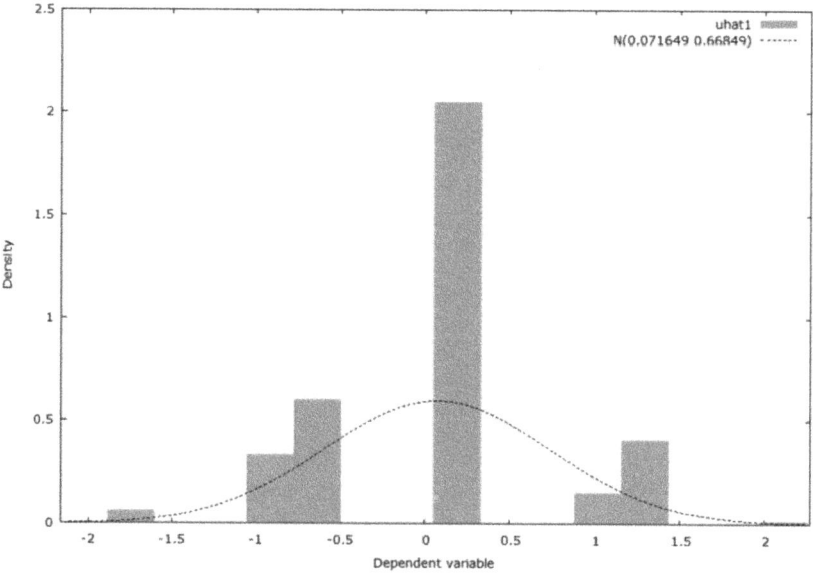

Figure 8. The correlation diagram.

H2 demonstration: *In the presence of disturbing factors, it is estimated that the greatest impact quantified by the correlation between the phenomenon scalar and the impact on the regional administrative capacity is generated by F4 (COVID-19 pandemic) and F1 (Economic crisis' impact). In the paper "Economic interventions to ameliorate the impact of COVID-19 on the economy and health: an international comparison," [13] the authors show that the immediate measures taken by the authorities in the developed countries have a high fiscal impact in terms of combating the* effects of the pandemic. Moreover, the authors show that there are common elements in the strategies adopted, namely reducing taxes and adopting measures to support the population. (see Table 1).

As we demonstrated in Section 4, the *p*-values of the two scalar factors are less than 0.0001 and are smaller than the other 2 scalar factors (F2, F3), contributing to the homogeneity of the proposed model.

H3 demonstration: *There is a demonstrable econometric correlation through the same dependent variable between the scalar value of the disturbing factors with regional manifestation and the scalar value of the regional administrative capacity through a high statistical confidence regarding the test of bivalent correlation between C0, R and the factors Fi.* Some authors [6] show that the effect of population health on economic growth can be assessed by a directional model of valuation which, we believe, would be adjusted by the impact value of the disturbing factors. Additionally, other authors [7] consider that the impact of the pandemic on the health status of the population can be measured directly and on the pandemic indirectly based on a Markov chain model, demonstrating the need for a review of public health policies and measures to be implemented to reduce uncertainty. Some researchers [8] presented an analysis of the impact of the disruptive factors on the global economy during the economic crises. They show that these factors act as markers of the flattening of the growth curve. As shown in Table 1, their proposed model can be improved by adding social protection variables with an impact on the economic recovery.

The correlation is demonstrated for a high level of statistical representativeness, 96.8% for the C0-R correlation and 72.9% for the C0-Fi correlation. These values were presented together with the model equation in Section 4, demonstrating the correlations presented in the Methodology and indicating, together with the statistical tests, that the proposed model is reasonable, homogeneous, well determined and representative in relation to the analysed disturbing phenomena.

The objectives of the study are aimed primarily at the structured assessment of regional administrative capacity in the initial version, based on statistical indicators, and in the current version, after the outbreak of the pandemic, based on quantifying the impact of the disturbing factors.

The first objective defined according to the above was achieved by the authors carrying out a structured analysis of regional administrative capacity, based on the disturbing factors, obtaining the following results:

The regional administrative capacity is affected for the F1 scale in the critical value range 1–2, on the segment of the regional economies whose basic variable of the administrative capacity registers values towards the minimum interval (the lower values of the pre-crisis administrative capacity, assessed on the basis of the 14 Eurostat statistical indicators, lead to a higher impact of the economic crisis that disturbs the administrative capacity in the period after this phenomenon occurs). In the same sense, impairments are also found for the strengthened administrative capacities, in the sense of reducing or declassifying those to the average area of the range of scalar values (see Figure 9).

In the case of factor F2 (the impact of refugees), there is a major impairment of administrative capacity for those regional units whose basic administrative capacity C0 registers scalar values in the critical interval (1–2). It can be seen from the figure below (Figure 10) that the administrative capacities that had higher positions in the scalar ranking preceded by the crisis will not be significantly affected by the phenomenon, except the declassification from the maximum category to category.

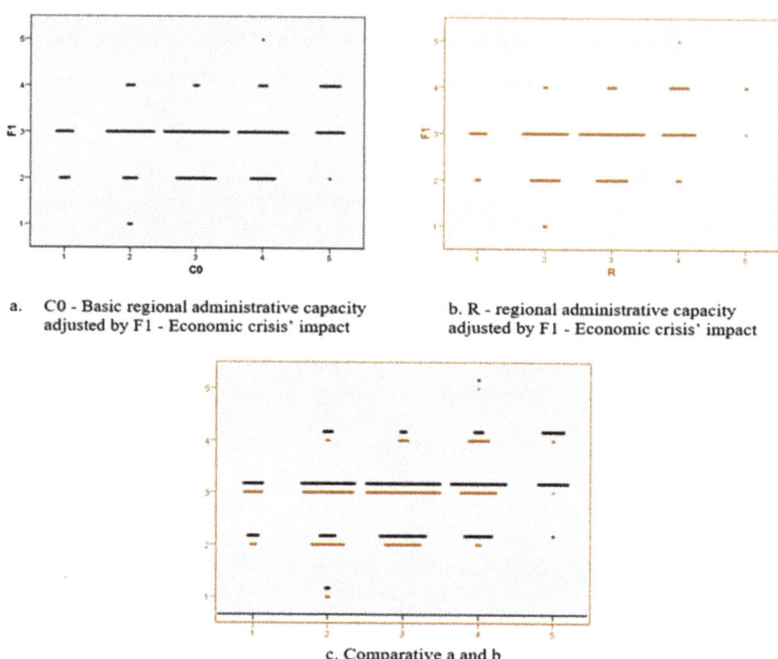

Figure 9. Two-dimensional plot diagram for analysing the C0-R variables in relation to F_1.

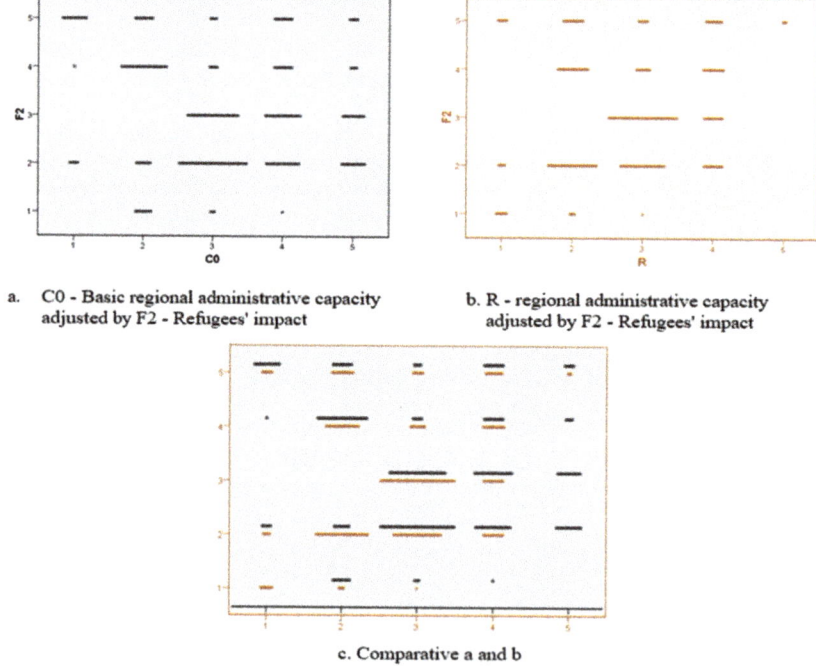

Figure 10. Two-dimensional plot diagram for analysing the C0-R variables in relation to F_2.

124

A situation similar to the F2 phenomenon, but with a high impact in the area of the average declassification of the regional administrative capacities, is the phenomenon of the migration of European citizens inside the community space. On the upper segment, the analysis does not involve significant disturbances (see Figure 11).

The F4 and F1 factors are the real challenges for the current European context. In the case of F4, there is an increase in the vulnerabilities of the regional administrative capacity both for the regions in the upper echelon and for those in administrative difficulty, because the COVID-19 pandemic socially affects the regions in which it is triggered and requires economic support measures for liquidation of its propagation. According to Figure 12, a translation of the adjusted scalar value F4 of the administrative capacity against the background of the pandemic in the upper echelon is observed, and a maximization of the reduced values for the administrative capacities already in difficulty, according to C0.

The second objective of the study aims to evaluate the reaction of the administrative units according to their capacity in the economic problems in the region, in the sense of improving the performance of the regional economies.

The aspects discussed in the case of the F1 impact (economic crisis) are likely to recommend for the crisis period the implementation of specific measures to increase the regional administrative capacity through proactive methods of supporting the economy, including the improvement of the administrative apparatus relationship with the business environment, creating some databases for connecting small producers with communities that can generate demand for goods and services, setting up e-commerce platforms managed by economic levers to help SMEs, creating a mechanism of decision-making transparency through online portals to help the economic entities affected by the crisis and the improvement and intensification of the activity of the unemployment offices in order to redistribute the surplus of labour on the market affected by the crisis.

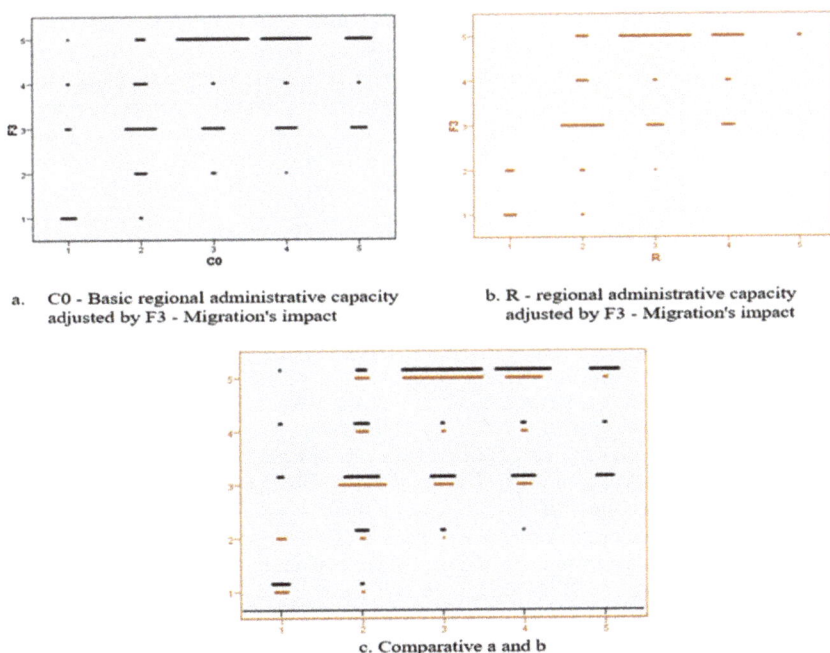

Figure 11. Two-dimensional plot diagram for analysing the C0-R variables in relation to F_3.

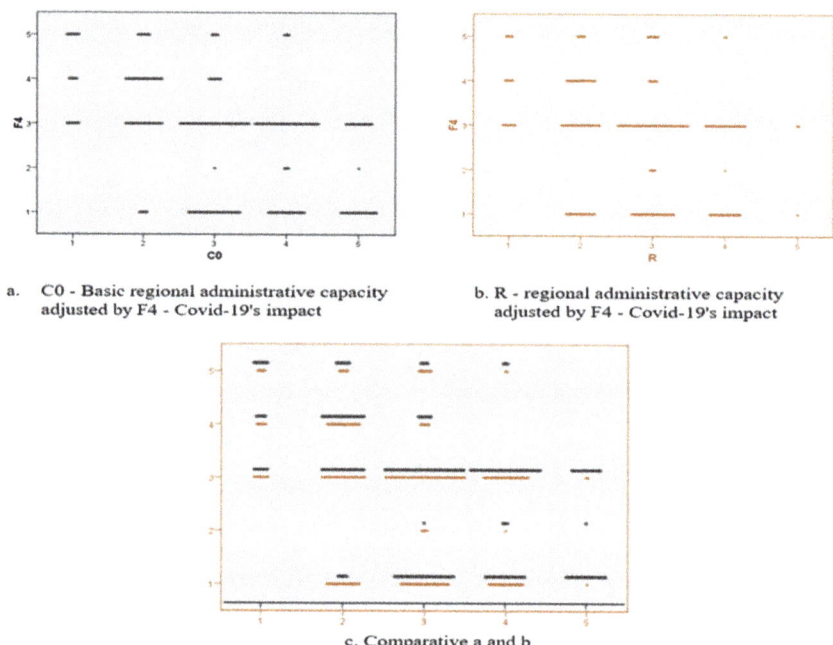

Figure 12. Two-dimensional plot diagram for analysing the C0-R variables in relation to F_4.

Following the regression of correlation analysis of the administrative capacity variable in relation to the impact factor F2, the need to adopt at the EU level some measures to help the affected regions by primary migration was identified, in order to provide technical and financial assistance for weighting the migration phenomenon in the affected areas and to provide superior management of the situation. In this regard, some projects of social insertion and the elimination of any kind of discrimination can be primarily directed to the areas identified as having difficulties, these areas being represented graphically and in the Figure A1 in the Appendix A.

From the analysis of the community migration impact, we found that there is an impairment of the administrative capacity of the reduced impact model (as shown by the model presented in Section 4), on which it was determined that F3 has a low impact in relation to the other factors (p-value having the highest coefficient according to the statistical tests performed by modelling). In practice, there is a latent labour demand in the developed regional economies for the primary and secondary sectors; however, community migration is not represented only by the active labour, and there is a population that, due to conjugate factors, fails to reach the developed region and to integrate into the labour market, becoming a social burden for the new region. This population segment represents a real challenge for the regional economies, which will have to identify, in times of economic crisis, real possibilities of engaging them in economic activity, based on the fact that this segment of population that is uninsured and unable to contribute to the regional economy will be at the forefront of potential social conflicts.

The COVID-19 pandemic represents an unprecedented global challenge that has led to a major rate of disease and death among the population, especially the aging population. The cumulative administrative burden cannot be managed in this regional context, with many Member States adopting national strategies and declaring a state of national emergency to prevent the spread of the disease.

The first major effect of the pandemic is the short-circuiting of the health system, given that it was not designed to cope with such a pandemic. At the same time, a food and disinfectant crisis can be induced successively, which raises challenges for the big regional units in order to ensure the optimal conditions of hygiene and health for the regional population in public areas, public transport and in spaces destined for commercial activities.

Some of the regions with low C0 values (the NE region of Romania, for example) encountered, at the outbreak of the pandemic, major problems in the management of the three disruptive factors, which required the institutionalized intervention of the armed forces, and of the ministry of internal affairs to manage the situation, which had escaped control in the region and was resolved with a far greater number of victims than the national average.

6. Conclusions

The study carried out in this paper constitutes, by the amplitude of the analysed phenomenon and by the proposed model, a step forward for forecasting the need to strengthen the regional administrative capacity in European space, and it is intended to be a useful tool for competent bodies in the management of the territorial level.

The authors intend to use the results of this research to conduct a further regional impact study, which offers concrete solutions to regional decision makers, in order to efficiently manage the current crisis and its consequences in the short and medium term.

Following the study, it was found that it is necessary to implement immediate economic recovery measures according to the ones presented in the Discussion section, measures that should be integrated into regional plans with economic–administrative specificity.

The results of the present study can be implemented in order to increase the effectiveness of public policies at the regional and local level in the fight against the negative impact of the pandemic on society.

From our point of view, the local and regional public administrations should establish best-practice models in the fight against the effects of COVID-19, and should increase administrative capacity. A starting point in this approach can be the monitoring of the indicators proposed in this paper, and the adoption of an adaptive policy such as the one we have formulated.

The limitations of the study include the introduction of a restricted number of disturbing factors, but the proposed model allows us to remedy this disadvantage by introducing other variables into the analysis.

Author Contributions: Conceptualization, R.-V.I. and V.M.A.; methodology, R.-V.I. and M.L.Z.; validation, R.-V.I., M.L.Z. and V.M.A.; formal analysis, V.M.A.; investigation, R.-V.I. and M.L.Z.; resources, V.M.A.; data curation, M.L.Z.; writing—original draft preparation, R.-V.I. and M.L.Z.; writing—review and editing, M.L.Z. and V.M.A.; visualization, V.M.A.; supervision, R.-V.I. All authors have read and agreed to the published version of the manuscript.

Funding: This research received no external funding.

Institutional Review Board Statement: Not applicable.

Informed Consent Statement: Not applicable.

Data Availability Statement: We used public data from Eurostat and the World Health Organization.

Conflicts of Interest: The authors declare no conflict of interest.

Appendix A

Distribution of the scalar values of the disturbing factors across the Member States, and their impact on regional administrative capacity.

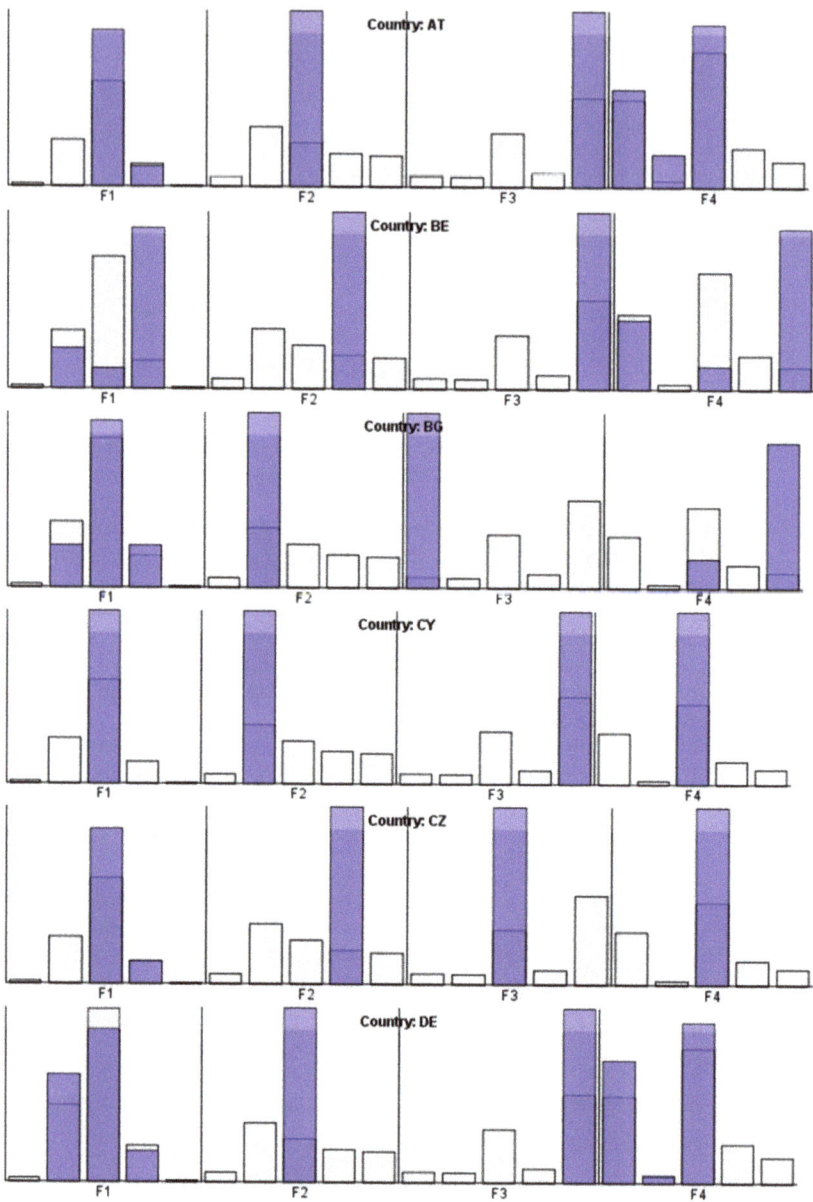

Figure A1. Cont.

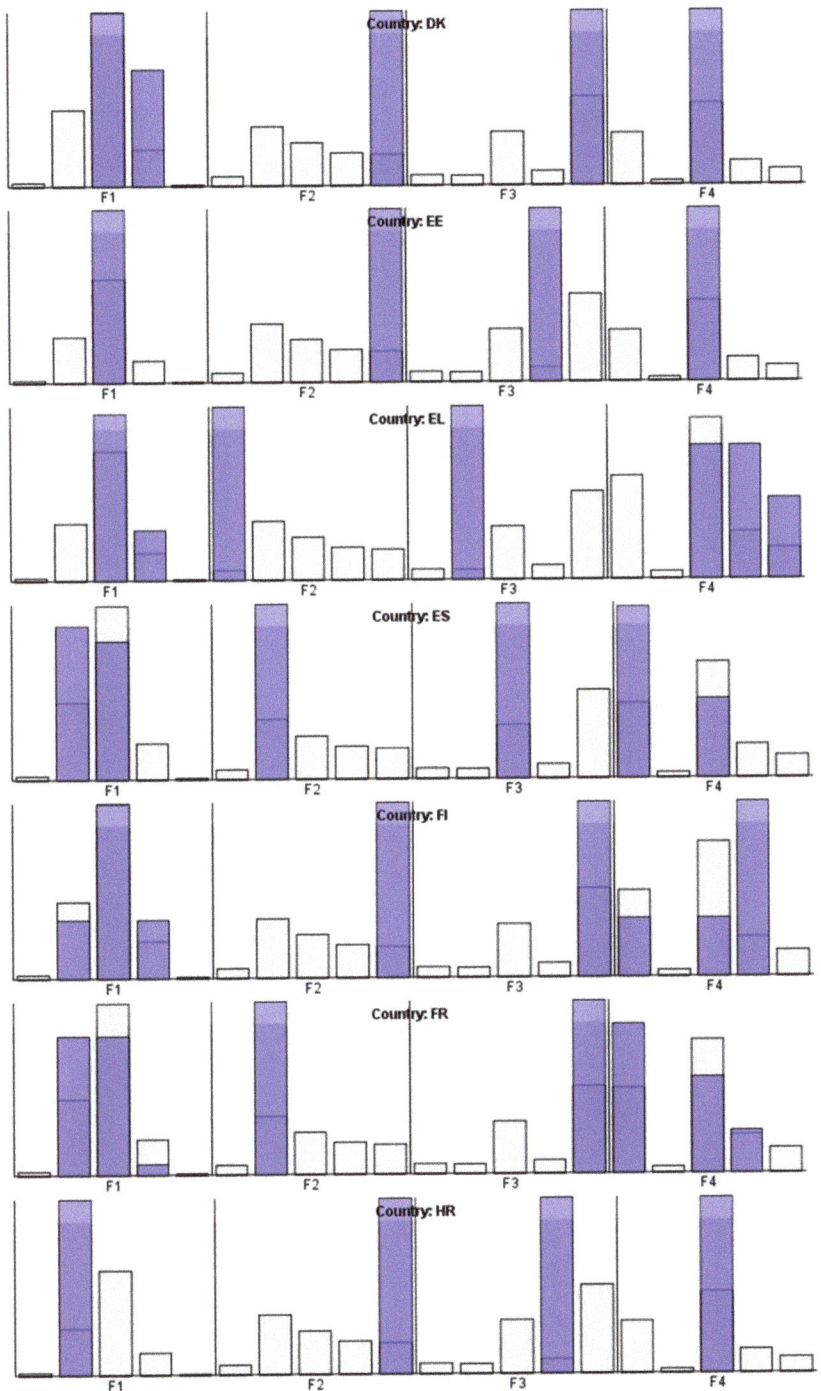

Figure A1. *Cont.*

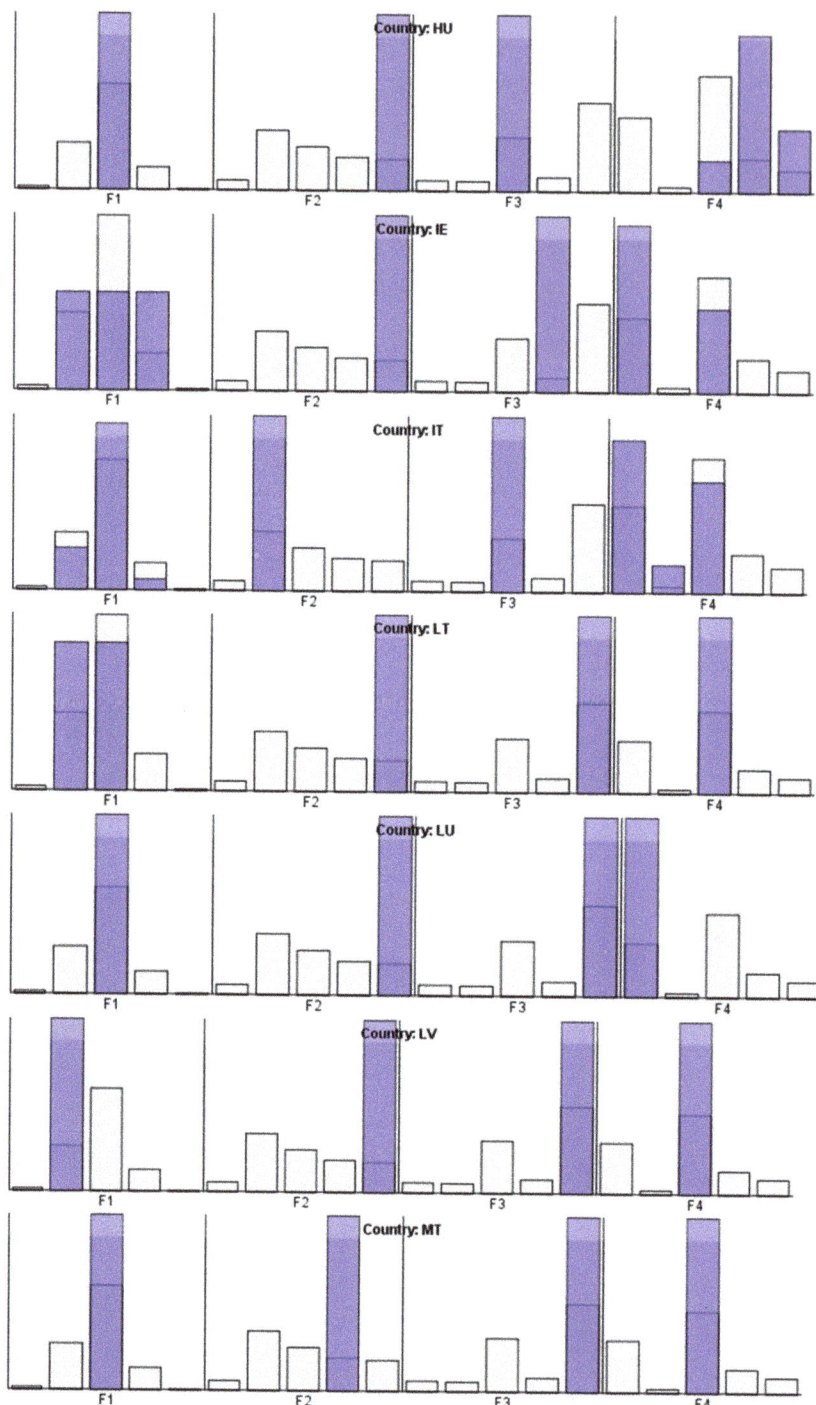

Figure A1. *Cont.*

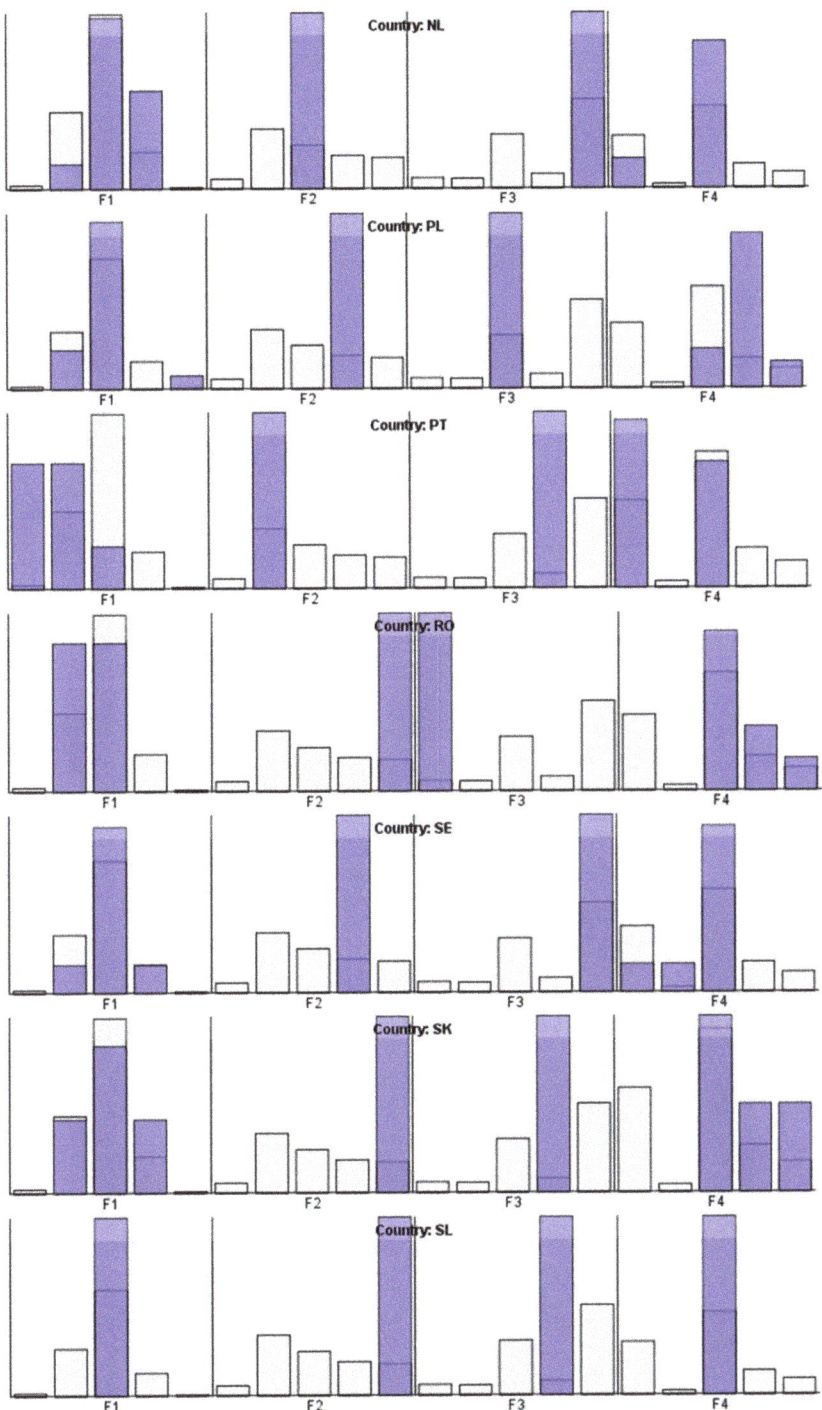

Figure A1. F1—Economic crisis' impact; F2—Refugees' impact; F3—Migration's impact; F4—COVID-19's impact.

Appendix B

Table A1. COVID-19's impact on NUTS 2 regions.

Regions	COVID-19 Region Cases	Population on 1 January 2019 by NUTS 2 Region	COVID-19 Rate	COVID-19 Scalar	Regions	COVID-19 Region Cases	Population on 1 January 2019 by NUTS 2 Region	COVID-19 Rate	COVID-19 Scalar
Région de Bruxelles/Brussels	2352	1,215,290	0.19%	1	Languedoc-Roussillon	4150	2,838,966	0.15%	1
Antwerpen	363	1,860,470	0.02%	3	Midi-Pyrénées	4480	3,060,243	0.15%	1
Limburg	0	875,842	0.00%	5	Auvergne	1990	1,362,576	0.15%	1
Oost-Vlaanderen	0	1,516,283	0.00%	5	Rhône-Alpes	5720	6,643,306	0.09%	3
Vlaams-Brabant	0	1,146,643	0.00%	5	Provence-Alpes-Côte d'Azur	7380	5,048,405	0.15%	1
West-Vlaanderen	0	1,196,995	0.00%	5	Corse	225	341,554	0.07%	3
Brabant wallon	5809	404,270	1.44%	1	Guadeloupe	76	416,474	0.02%	3
Hainaut	0	1,346,082	0.00%	5	Martinique	66	363,484	0.02%	3
Liège	12,289	1,110,083	1.11%	1	Guyane	28	283,539	0.01%	4
Luxembourg	0	286,685	0.00%	5	La Réunion	94	857,961	0.01%	4
Namur	0	496,891	0.00%	5	Mayotte	35	269,471	0.01%	4
Severozapaden	588	742,304	0.08%	3	Jadranska Hrvatska	611	1,374,071	0.04%	3
Severen tsentralen	0	784,168	0.00%	5	Kontinentalna Hrvatska	671	2,702,175	0.02%	3
Severoiztochen	0	929,035	0.00%	5	Piemonte	13,343	4,356,406	0.31%	1
Yugoiztochen	0	1,032,079	0.00%	5	Valle d'Aosta	835	125,666	0.66%	1
Yugozapaden	0	2,102,205	0.00%	5	Liguria	4757	1,550,640	0.31%	1
Yuzhen tsentralen	0	1,410,248	0.00%	5	Lombardia	52,325	10,060,574	0.52%	1
Praha	1234	1,308,632	0.09%	3	Provincia Autonoma di Bolzano	1811	531,178	0.34%	1
Střední Čechy	606	1,369,332	0.04%	3	Provincia Autonoma di Trento	2476	541,098	0.46%	1
Jihozápad	298	1,226,805	0.02%	3	Veneto	11,925	4,905,854	0.24%	1
Severozápad	278	1,115,005	0.02%	3	Friuli-Venezia Giulia	2153	1,215,220	0.18%	1
Severovýchod	1300	1,513,693	0.09%	3	Emilia-Romagna	17,825	4,459,477	0.40%	1
Jihovýchod	334	1,696,941	0.02%	3	Toscana	6173	3,729,641	0.17%	1
Střední Morava	450	1,215,413	0.04%	3	Umbria	1263	882,015	0.14%	2
Moravskoslezsko	506	1,203,299	0.04%	3	Marche	4710	1,525,271	0.31%	1
Hovedstaden	1901	1,835,562	0.10%	3	Lazio	4149	5,879,082	0.07%	3
Sjælland	203	836,738	0.02%	3	Abruzzo	1799	1,311,580	0.14%	2
Syddanmark	472	1,223,348	0.04%	3	Molise	224	305,617	0.07%	3
Midtjylland	584	1,320,678	0.04%	3	Campania	3148	5,801,692	0.05%	3
Nordjylland	501	589,755	0.08%	3	Puglia	2514	4,029,053	0.06%	3
Stuttgart	3189	4,113,418	0.08%	3	Basilicata	291	562,869	0.05%	3
Karlsruhe	2234	2,805,129	0.08%	3	Calabria	833	1,947,131	0.04%	3
Freiburg	2084	2,264,469	0.09%	3	Sicilia	2097	4,999,891	0.04%	3
Tübingen	7432	1,856,517	0.40%	1	Sardegna	935	1,639,591	0.06%	3
Oberbayern	2123	4,686,163	0.05%	3	Kypros	494	875,899	0.06%	3
Niederbayern	3112	1,238,528	0.25%	1	Latvija	548	1,919,968	0.03%	3
Oberpfalz	4311	1,109,269	0.39%	1	Sostinės regionas	412	810,538	0.05%	3
Oberfranken	2120	1,067,482	0.20%	1	Vidurio ir vakarų Lietuvos regionas	468	1,983,646	0.02%	3
Mittelfranken	1234	1,770,401	0.07%	3	Luxembourg	2970	613,894	0.48%	1
Unterfranken	3214	1,317,124	0.24%	1	Budapest	345	1,752,286	0.02%	3
Schwaben	1245	1,887,754	0.07%	3	Pest	153	1,278,874	0.01%	4
Berlin	3670	3,644,826	0.10%	3	Közép-Dunántúl	139	1,058,236	0.01%	4
Brandenburg	2345	2,511,917	0.09%	3	Nyugat-Dunántúl	86	989,343	0.01%	4
Bremen	2811	682,986	0.41%	1	Dél-Dunántúl	4	879,596	0.00%	5
Hamburg	2993	1,841,179	0.16%	1	Észak-Magyarország	82	1,126,360	0.01%	4
Darmstadt	1121	3,998,724	0.03%	3	Észak-Alföld	33	1,450,960	0.00%	5
Gießen	1125	1,047,262	0.11%	3	Dél-Alföld	70	1,237,101	0.01%	4
Kassel	1889	1,219,823	0.15%	1	Malta	293	493,559	0.06%	3
Mecklenburg-Vorpommern	2346	1,609,675	0.15%	1	Groningen	207	583,990	0.04%	3
Braunschweig	1256	1,596,396	0.08%	3	Friesland	215	647,672	0.03%	3
Hannover	1084	2,149,805	0.05%	3	Drenthe	222	492,167	0.05%	3
Lüneburg	1111	1,710,914	0.06%	3	Overijssel	1211	1,156,431	0.10%	3
Weser-Ems	3456	2,525,333	0.14%	2	Gelderland	2210	2,071,972	0.11%	3
Düsseldorf	2412	5,202,321	0.05%	3	Flevoland	264	416,546	0.06%	3
Köln	1525	4,468,904	0.03%	3	Utrecht	1476	1,306,912	0.11%	3
Münster	3500	2,623,619	0.13%	3	Noord-Holland	2891	2,853,359	0.10%	3
Detmold	2235	2,055,310	0.11%	3	Zuid-Holland	3361	3,709,139	0.09%	3
Arnsberg	2768	3,582,497	0.08%	3	Zeeland	279	383,032	0.07%	3
Koblenz	2987	1,495,885	0.20%	1	Noord-Brabant	4456	2,544,806	0.18%	1

132

Table A1. Cont.

Regions	COVID-19 Region Cases	Population on 1 January 2019 by NUTS 2 Region	COVID-19 Rate	COVID-19 Scalar	Regions	COVID-19 Region Cases	Population on 1 January 2019 by NUTS 2 Region	COVID-19 Rate	COVID-19 Scalar
Trier	3456	531,007	0.65%	1	Limburg	2011	1,116,137	0.18%	1
Rheinhessen-Pfalz	1567	2,057,952	0.08%	3	Burgenland	234	293,433	0.08%	3
Saarland	4321	990,509	0.44%	1	Niederösterreich	1978	1,677,542	0.12%	3
Dresden	3189	1,598,199	0.20%	1	Wien	1777	1,897,491	0.09%	3
Chemnitz	4567	1,436,445	0.32%	1	Kärnten	333	560,939	0.06%	3
Leipzig	3111	1,043,293	0.30%	1	Steiermark	1354	1,243,052	0.11%	3
Sachsen-Anhalt	2345	2,208,321	0.11%	3	Oberösterreich	2061	1,482,095	0.14%	2
Schleswig-Holstein	2723	2,896,712	0.09%	3	Salzburg	1085	555,221	0.20%	1
Thüringen	3456	2,143,145	0.16%	1	Tirol	2804	754,705	0.37%	1
Eesti	1149	1,324,820	0.09%	3	Vorarlberg	764	394,297	0.19%	1
Northern and Western	1389	867,947	0.16%	1	Malopolskie	1247	3,360,545	0.04%	3
Southern	2510	1,624,381	0.15%	1	Slaskie	601	4,488,998	0.01%	4
Eastern and Midland	1810	2,411,912	0.08%	3	Wielkopolskie	349	3,473,172	0.01%	4
Anatoliki Makedonia, Thraki	367	599,723	0.06%	3	Zachodniopomors	133	1,675,502	0.01%	4
Kentriki Makedonia	215	1,873,777	0.01%	4	Lubuskie	127	1,003,310	0.01%	4
Dytiki Makedonia	314	267,008	0.12%	3	Dolnoslaskie	527	2,865,072	0.02%	3
Ipeiros	98	333,696	0.03%	3	Opolskie	107	946,038	0.01%	4
Thessalia	412	718,640	0.06%	3	Kujawsko-Pomorskie	264	2,055,433	0.01%	4
Ionia Nisia	190	203,869	0.09%	3	Warminsko-Mazurskie	87	1,404,441	0.01%	4
Dytiki Ellada	78	655,189	0.01%	4	Pomorskie	135	2,305,077	0.01%	4
Sterea Ellada	58	555,960	0.01%	4	Lódzkie	358	2,453,167	0.01%	4
Peloponnisos	70	574,447	0.01%	4	Swietokrzyskie	120	1,226,243	0.01%	4
Attiki	12	3,742,235	0.00%	5	Lubelskie	192	2,097,294	0.01%	4
Voreio Aigaio	15	221,098	0.01%	4	Podkarpackie	371	2,086,135	0.02%	3
Notio Aigaio	0	344,027	0.00%	5	Podlaskie	168	1,152,074	0.01%	4
Kriti	3	634,930	0.00%	5	Warszawski stoleczny	62	3,053,104	0.00%	5
Galicia	6331	2,700,441	0.23%	1	Mazowiecki regionalny	0	2,327,207	0.00%	5
Principado de Asturias	1679	1,022,205	0.16%	1	Norte	1777	3,572,583	0.05%	3
Cantabria	1501	581,641	0.26%	1	Algarve	1561	438,864	0.36%	1
País Vasco	9021	2,177,880	0.41%	1	Centro	1823	2,216,569	0.08%	3
Navarra	3355	649,946	0.52%	1	Lisboa	1789	2,846,332	0.06%	3
La Rioja	2846	313,571	0.91%	1	Alentejo	1813	705,478	0.26%	1
Aragón	3449	1,320,586	0.26%	1	Região Autónoma dos Açores	1800	242,846	0.74%	1
Madrid	40,469	6,641,649	0.61%	1	Madeira	1879	253,945	0.74%	1
Castilla y León	9581	2,407,733	0.40%	1	Nord-Vest	276	2,552,112	0.01%	4
Castilla-la Mancha	11,077	2,034,877	0.54%	1	Centru	425	2,318,272	0.02%	3
Extremadura	2116	1,065,424	0.20%	1	Nord-Est	1743	3,198,564	0.05%	3
Cataluña	28,323	7,566,431	0.37%	1	Sud-Est	362	2,396,171	0.02%	3
Comunidad Valenciana	7443	4,974,969	0.15%	1	Sud-Muntenia	282	2,929,832	0.01%	4
Illes Balears	1369	1,188,220	0.12%	3	Bucuresti-Ilfov	697	2,315,173	0.03%	3
Andalucía	8767	8,427,405	0.10%	3	Sud-Vest Oltenia	72	1,926,860	0.00%	5
Región de Murcia	1283	1,487,663	0.09%	3	Vest	565	1,777,474	0.03%	3
Ciudad Autónoma de Ceuta	83	84,829	0.10%	3	Vzhodna Slovenija	501	1,094,435	0.05%	3
Ciudad Autónoma de Melilla	92	84,689	0.11%	3	Zahodna Slovenija	558	986,473	0.06%	3
Canarias	1725	2,206,901	0.08%	3	Bratislavský kraj	147	659,598	0.02%	3
Île de France	17,910	12,244,807	0.15%	1	Západné Slovensko	76	1,826,145	0.00%	5
Centre-Val de Loire	3750	2,565,258	0.15%	1	Stredné Slovensko	72	1,339,242	0.01%	4
Bourgogne	1569	1,619,728	0.10%	3	Východné Slovensko	286	1,625,436	0.02%	3
Franche-Comté	24,920	1,173,605	2.12%	1	Länsi-Suomi	90	1,379,749	0.01%	4
Basse-Normandie	688	1,464,500	0.05%	3	Helsinki	1438	1,671,024	0.09%	3
Haute-Normandie	1753	1,848,840	0.09%	3	Etelä-Suomi	154	1,152,719	0.01%	4
Nord-Pas-de-Calais	5930	4,052,299	0.15%	1	Pohjois- ja Itä-Suomi	118	1,284,638	0.01%	4
Picardie	2820	1,925,138	0.15%	1	Åland	508	29,789	1.71%	1

Table A1. Cont.

Regions	COVID-19 Region Cases	Population on 1 January 2019 by NUTS 2 Region	COVID-19 Rate	COVID-19 Scalar	Regions	COVID-19 Region Cases	Population on 1 January 2019 by NUTS 2 Region	COVID-19 Rate	COVID-19 Scalar
Alsace	2770	1,894,144	0.15%	1	Stockholm	3279	2,344,124	0.14%	2
Champagne-Ardenne	1920	1,314,964	0.15%	1	Östra Mellansverige	1133	1,708,813	0.07%	3
Lorraine	3390	2,316,183	0.15%	1	Småland med öarna	632	864,630	0.07%	3
Pays-de-la-Loire	368	3,787,400	0.01%	4	Sydsverige	366	1,521,848	0.02%	3
Bretagne	603	3,333,720	0.02%	3	Västsverige	674	2,039,166	0.03%	3
Aquitaine	1082	3,450,045	0.03%	3	Norra Mellansverige	554	855,220	0.06%	3
Limousin	1070	729,981	0.15%	1	Mellersta Norrland	576	375,733	0.15%	1
Poitou-Charentes	2640	1,806,292	0.15%	1	Övre Norrland	478	520,651	0.09%	3

References

1. Eurostat. SDG INDICATORS: GOAL BY GOAL. Eurostat Datbase. 2021. Available online: https://ec.europa.eu/eurostat/web/sdi/indicators (accessed on 2 March 2021).
2. World Health Organization. WHO Health Emergency Dashboard. WHO (COVID-19) Homepage. 2021. Available online: https://covid19.who.int/ (accessed on 15 March 2021).
3. Iamsiraroj, S. The Foreign direct investment–economic growth nexus. *Int. Rev. Econ. Financ.* **2016**, *42*, 116–133. [CrossRef]
4. Meyer, D.; Shera, A. The impact of remittances on economic growth: An econometric model. *EconomiA* **2017**, *18*, 147–155. [CrossRef]
5. Pradhan, R.P.; Arvin, M.B.; Hall, J.H.; Nair, M. Innovation, financial development and economic growth in Eurozone countries. *Appl. Econ. Lett.* **2016**, *23*, 1141–1144. [CrossRef]
6. Bloom, J.J.; Canning, D.E.; Kotschy, D.; Prettner, R.; Schunemann, K. Health and Economic Growth. *Handb. Econ. Growth* **2014**, *2*, 623–682.
7. Atkeson, A. What Will Be the Economic Impact of COVID-19 in the US? Rough Estimates of Disease Scenarios. *Natl. Bur. Econ. Res. Work. Pap. Ser.* **2020**, *26867*, 1–27.
8. Gilchrist, S.; Schoenle, R.; Sim, J.; Zakrajšek, E. Inflation Dynamics during the Financial Crisis. *Am. Econ. Rev.* **2017**, *107*, 785–823. [CrossRef]
9. Adrian, T.; Fleming, M.; Shachar, O.; Vogt, E. Market Liquidity After the Financial Crisis. *Annu. Rev. Financ. Econ.* **2017**, *9*, 43–83. [CrossRef]
10. Kreichauf, R. From forced migration to forced arrival: The campization of refugee accommodation in European cities. *Comp. Migr. Stud.* **2018**, *6*, 7. [CrossRef] [PubMed]
11. Hangartner, D.; Dinas, E.; Marbach, M.; Matakos, K.; Xefteris, D. Does Exposure to the Refugee Crisis Make Natives More Hostile? *Am. Polit. Sci. Rev.* **2019**, *113*, 442–455. [CrossRef]
12. Harteveld, E.; Schaper, J.; De Lange, S.L.; Van Der Brug, W. Blaming Brussels? The Impact of (News about) the Refugee Crisis on Attitudes towards the EU and National Politics. *JCMS J. Common Mark. Stud.* **2018**, *56*, 157–177. [CrossRef]
13. Danielli, S.; Patria, R.; Donnelly, P.; Ashrafian, H.; Darzi, A. Economic interventions to ameliorate the impact of COVID-19 on the economy and health: An international comparison. *J. Public Health* **2020**, *43*, 42–46. [CrossRef] [PubMed]
14. Umar, M.; Xu, Y.; Mirza, S.S. The impact of COVID-19 on Gig economy. *Econ. Res. Istraživanja* **2021**, *34*, 2284–2296. [CrossRef]
15. Asahi, K.; Undurraga, E.A.; Valdés, R.; Wagner, R. The effect of COVID-19 on the economy: Evidence from an early adopter of localized lockdowns. *J. Glob. Health* **2021**, *11*, 5002. [CrossRef] [PubMed]
16. Vitenu-Sackey, P.; Barfi, R. The Impact of COVID-19 Pandemic on the Global Economy: Emphasis on Poverty Alleviation and Economic Growth. *Financ. Res. Lett.* **2021**, *8*, 32–43. [CrossRef]
17. Khurshid, A.; Khan, K. How COVID-19 shock will drive the economy and climate? A data-driven approach to model and forecast. *Environ. Sci. Pollut. Res.* **2021**, *28*, 2948–2958. [CrossRef] [PubMed]

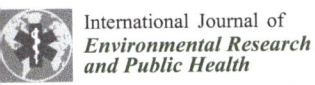

Article

Feeling Uncertainty during the Lockdown That Commenced in March 2020 in Greece

Dimitris Zavras

Department of Public Health Policy, School of Public Health, University of West Attica, 11521 Athens, Greece; dzavras@uniwa.gr

Abstract: The coronavirus disease 2019 (COVID-19) pandemic has resulted in significant uncertainty for the global population. However, since not all population groups experience the impacts of the pandemic in the same way, the objective of this study was to identify the individual characteristics associated with the feeling of uncertainty during the lockdown that commenced in March 2020 in Greece. The study used data from the "Public Opinion in the European Union (EU) in Time of Coronavirus Crisis" survey. The sample consisted of 1050 individuals aged between 16 and 54 years. According to the analysis, which was based on a logistic regression model, the emotional status of older individuals, those who experienced income and job losses since the beginning of the pandemic, and middle-class and high-class individuals, is more likely to be described as a feeling of uncertainty. In addition, the emotional status of individuals with less concern for their own health and that of family and friends is less likely to be described as a feeling of uncertainty. Although the results related to age, income, and job losses, as regards concern for health, agree with the international literature, the limited health literacy of lower-class individuals may explain the reduced likelihood of their experiencing feelings of uncertainty. The results confirm the international literature describing several aspects of uncertainty due to the COVID-19 crisis.

Keywords: coronavirus disease 2019 pandemic; lockdown; uncertainty; age; income loss; job loss; social class; health literacy; concern for health

1. Introduction

Because public health emergencies adversely affect the health, safety, and well-being of individuals and communities, they may provoke a range of emotional reactions [1]. Thus, it is not surprising that during the coronavirus disease 2019 (COVID-19) pandemic, a substantial proportion of society has felt uncertainty [2].

Uncertainty exists when details of situations are ambiguous, complex, unpredictable, or probabilistic, when information is unavailable or inconsistent, and when people feel insecure about their own state of knowledge or the state of knowledge in general [3].

Uncertainty in events is considered to be a consequence of a gap between knowledge of the actual occurrence of events in the real world and the availability of knowledge regarding these events [4], that is, uncertainty refers to a state characterized by a lack of information about whether, where, when, how, or why an event has occurred or will occur [5].

Since it is impossible to assign probabilities to the likelihood of future events, it is difficult to judge the future impact of uncertainty due to unpredictable or uncontrollable external events such as economic fluctuations [6] and pandemics [7].

Unpredictable events are complex and one of the main sources of uncertainty [8]; other sources of uncertainty include situations that are unfamiliar or not easily resolved and situations that are novel or insoluble. The period of anticipation prior to the confrontation with a potentially harmful event and the notion that negative events may occur without a definitive means of predicting them can also cause uncertainty [9].

During the period of the COVID-19 pandemic, most of these sources have contributed to the high degree of global uncertainty in the context of the pandemic's physical, psychological, financial, and social impacts [10]. Uncertainty is therefore related not only to the seriousness of the threats to people's physical health and lives, the lack of early knowledge about quarantine duration, the real risk of exposure, and the unpredictability of symptomatology, but also to the impacts on personal, economic, and societal levels [11]. Thus, uncertainty arises from various aspects of the COVID-19 crisis.

That is, in parallel with the uncertainties related to infectiousness, viral lethality [12], mutations [13], and prevention and treatment [14], the COVID-19 pandemic has created a pervasive atmosphere of general uncertainty, concerning both personal finances and the overall state of the economy and finance [15,16], as well as uncertainty concerning the costs and benefits of lockdown-lifting strategies [17].

Indeed, due to the pandemic, the global community has been facing not only a public health crisis, but also an economic crisis [18]. According to Kose and Sugawara, the current recession is the first, since 1870, to be driven solely by a pandemic [19].

Economic recessions cause individuals to have feelings of uncertainty that are associated with their finances, reduced income, or fear of losing their jobs [20], which have also been experienced during the current pandemic [21–23]; however, even though a person may not experience income or job losses, feelings of uncertainty may arouse as a result of working under pressure or being exposed to so many deaths [24].

In addition, feelings of uncertainty may be triggered by the risk of contracting the COVID-19 virus, which causes a potentially life-threatening infection [25,26].

Moreover, the stringent measures implemented to control the spread of the virus, as well as the resulting social disruption and physical distancing due to the pandemic, have had the same effect [27–29].

The previous points justify the feelings of uncertainty during the COVID-19 pandemic [30].

In Greece, the first COVID-19 case was diagnosed on 26 February 2020, and the first death was reported on 12 March 2020. As of 29 April 2021, 337,723 confirmed cases and 10,179 deaths have been reported in Greece [31]. A few weeks after the first cases of COVID-19, strict containment measures were introduced, including the closure of schools, universities, non-essential shops, cafes and restaurants, public spaces, as well as movement restrictions including a ban on gatherings and travel [32].

Because uncertainty is considered one of the more obvious consequences of lockdowns [33], based on the previous points, the objective of this study was to identify the individual characteristics associated with a feeling of uncertainty during the lockdown that commenced in March 2020 in Greece.

2. Materials and Methods

For the purpose of this study, data from the "Public Opinion in the EU in Time of Coronavirus Crisis" [34] survey were used. The survey was conducted using Kantar's online access panel between 23 April and 1 May 2020, among 21,804 respondents in 21 EU Member States. The survey was limited to respondents aged between 16 and 64 years. In some countries, including Greece, the sample was limited to respondents aged between 16 and 54 years. Representativeness at the national level was ensured by quotas concerning gender, age, and region. The sample size was $n = 1050$ in Greece. The data collection took place between 23 April and 27 April 2020.

The business and workplace suspensions implemented in Greece between 10 March and 18 March 2020 included the following: (a) closure of schools and universities on 10 March; (b) closure of movie theaters, courtrooms, and gyms on 12 March; (c) closure of malls, cafés, restaurants, bars, museums, archaeological sites, and beauty parlors on 13 March; (d) closure of all organized beaches and ski resorts on 14 March; (e) closure of all stores with the exception of supermarkets and pharmacies on 18 March. In addition, a nationwide restriction of movement was imposed on 23 March (3 May was the last day of the lockdown). Business restrictions were gradually relaxed up to the end of May [35].

The variable under study was whether or not uncertainty is among the feelings that best describe respondents' current emotional status. The respondents were asked the question "What feelings best describe your current emotional status?" One of the response options was "uncertainty", and the remaining response options were (a) frustration, (b) hope, (c) fear, (d) anger, (e) helpfulness, (f) confidence, (g) helplessness, and (h) other. Respondents could choose a maximum of three different response options. From the above-mentioned variable, a dichotomous variable, i.e., the response, was derived as follows: (a) uncertainty was among the feelings that best described respondents' current emotional status (1), i.e., in this case, respondents chose uncertainty either alone or in combination with other feelings (one or two); and (b) uncertainty was not among the feelings that best described respondents' current emotional status (0), i.e., in this case, respondents chose exclusively other feelings.

Thus, as in Powell et al.'s article (2007) [36], in this study, uncertainty is defined as an individual's perception. Because a person who believes himself or herself to be uncertain is uncertain [3], the responses in this study reflect the self-perceived event of uncertainty.

Because the response was binary, a logistic regression model was used. The potential predictors used in the analysis are presented in Table 1.

Table 1. Potential predictors.

Variable	Category	Code (Range)
Geographic Region	Attica	1
	Macedonia and Thrace	2
	Epirus and Western Macedonia	3
	Thessaly and Central Greece	4
	Peloponnese, Western Greece and Ionian Islands	5
	Aegean Islands and Crete	6
Gender	Female	0
	Male	1
Age		16–54
Marital Status	Married/Living with Partner	1
	Never Married (Single)	2
	Divorced/Widowed	3
	Living with Parents	4
	Domestic Partner/Living with Other Adults	5
Presence of Children	No	0
	Yes	1
Social Class	Low	1
	Middle	2
	High	3
Experiencing Loss of Income since the Beginning of the COVID-19 Pandemic	No	0
	Yes	1
Experiencing Unemployment or Partial Unemployment since the Beginning of the COVID-19 Pandemic	No	0
	Yes	1
Current Employment Status	Employed (Full-Time)	1
	Employed (Part-Time)	2
	Self-Employed	3
	Retired/Unable to Work/Disabled	4
	Still at School	5
	In Full-Time Higher Education	6
	Unemployed and Seeking Work	7
	Not Working and Not Seeking Work	8

Table 1. Cont.

Variable	Category	Code (Range)
COVID-19-Related Concern for Own Health	Very Concerned	1
	Fairly Concerned	2
	Not Very Concerned	3
	Not at All Concerned	4
COVID-19-Related Concern for Family and Friends' Health	Very Concerned	1
	Fairly Concerned	2
	Not Very Concerned	3
	Not at All Concerned	4

Social class was based on the occupation of the main earner of the household: (a) 1: low–semi-skilled or unskilled manual workers, students, retired and living on state pension only, unemployed (for over six months), or not working due to long-term sickness; (b) 2: middle–skilled manual workers, supervisory or clerical/junior managerial/professional/ administrator; (c) 3: high–intermediate managerial/professional/administrative, higher managerial/professional/administrative.

Helmert coding was applied to the ordinal variables (a) social class, (b) COVID-19-related concern for one's own health, and (c) COVID-related concern for one's family and friends' health. The Helmert contrast compares each category of an ordinal variable (except the last) with the mean of the subsequent levels. Indicator coding was applied to the following nominal variables: (a) region, (b) marital status, and (c) current employment status. Indicator contrast was used to compare the reference category of a nominal variable with the remaining categories. The binary variables "experiencing loss of income since the beginning to the COVID-19 pandemic", "experiencing unemployment or partial unemployment since the beginning of the COVID-19 pandemic", "gender", and "presence of children" were treated as such.

The model's goodness of fit was tested using the Hosmer and Lemeshow test. The calibration of the model was tested using the calibration belt test. In addition, the model was tested for specification error using the link test.

The STATA 14 statistical software package was used for the analysis. Specifically, the commands desmat [37], logistic, linktest, and calibrationbelt [38] were used.

3. Results

Regarding gender, 50% of the respondents were female, and 50% were male. The mean age of the respondents was 37.14 years (± 10.47), while 17.05% of the respondents were aged between 16 and 24 years, 22.29% between 25 and 34 years, 29.90% between 35 and 44 years, and 30.76% between 45 and 54 years. The respondents' characteristics are presented in Table 2.

Table 2. Respondents' Characteristics.

Age	Gender % (n)	
	Male	Female
16–24	8.57 (90)	8.48 (89)
25–34	11.05 (116)	11.24 (118)
35–44	14.95 (157)	14.95 (157)
45–54	15.43 (162)	15.33 (161)

According to the descriptive analysis, 69.13% of the respondents of the survey declared that uncertainty was among the feelings that best described their current emotional status. Uncertainty was ranked first among the nine feelings.

In addition, 41.33% of the respondents had experienced loss of income since the beginning of the COVID-19 pandemic, and 28.29% of the respondents had experienced unemployment or partial unemployment.

Furthermore, it is worth noting that only 11.35% of the respondents were very concerned for their own health, and 23.29% of the respondents were very concerned for the health of their family and friends (Table 3).

Table 3. Concern for Health.

Category	Concern for Own Health % (n)	Concern for Family and Friends' Healtth % (n)
Very Concerned	11.35 (118)	23.29 (241)
Fairly Concerned	35.29 (367)	47.44 (491)
Not Very Concerned	37.98 (395)	21.74 (225)
Not at All Concerned	15.38 (160)	7.54 (78)

According to the results shown in Table 4, uncertainty was among the feelings that best described the current emotional status of older individuals (OR = 1.015 (>1), 95% Confidence Interval (CI): 1.001–1.030), as well as of those experiencing income loss (OR = 1.386 (>1), 95% CI: 1.031–1.865), those experiencing unemployment or partial unemployment (OR = 1.903 (>1), 95% CI: 1.348–2.686), those who were not very concerned for their own health as compared with those who were not at all concerned for their own health (OR = 1.621 (>1), 95% CI: 1.033–2.544), those who were not very concerned for family and friends' health as compared with those who were not at all concerned for family and friends' health (OR = 2.030 (>1), 95% CI: 1.124–3.667), those who were fairly concerned for family and friends' health as compared with those who were not very concerned for family and friends' health and those who were not at all concerned for family and friends' health (OR = 2.257 (>1), 95% CI: 1.495–3.407), and those who were very concerned for family and friends' health as compared with those who were fairly concerned for family and friends' health, those who were not very concerned for family and friends' health, and those who were not at all concerned for family and friends' health (OR = 2.725 (>1), 95% CI: 1.713–4.333). However, it is less likely that uncertainty was among the feelings that best described the current emotional status of lower-social-class individuals (OR = 0.604 (<1), 95% CI: 0.437–0.833) as compared with middle- and higher-social-class individuals.

Table 4. Logistic regression model.

Variable	OR	p	95% CI	
Age	1.015	0.030	1.001	1.030
Income Loss	1.386	0.031	1.031	1.865
Job Loss	1.903	<0.001	1.348	2.686
Social Class		0.007		
Low vs. Middle and High	0.604	0.002	0.437	0.833
Middle vs. High	1.059	0.739	0.757	1.481
COVID-19-Related Concern for own Health		0.038		
Very Concerned vs. Subsequent Levels	0.637	0.097	0.374	1.084
Fairly Concerned vs. Subsequent Levels	1.106	0.603	0.757	1.616
Not Very Concerned vs. Not at all Concerned	1.621	0.036	1.033	2.544
COVID-19-Related Concern for Health of Family and Friends		<0.001		
Very Concerned vs. Subsequent Levels	2.725	<0.001	1.713	4.333
Fairly Concerned vs. Subsequent Levels	2.257	<0.001	1.495	3.407
Not Very Concerned vs. Not at all Concerned	2.030	0.019	1.124	3.667
Constant	0.695	0.198	0.400	1.210

According to the link test (Table 5), the model did not suffer from specification error.

Table 5. Link Test.

Variable	Coefficient	p	95% Confidence Interval	
h	0.879	<0.001	0.540	1.218
h^2	0.104	0.376	−0.127	0.336
Constant	−0.012	0.911	−0.230	0.205

In addition, both the Hosmer and Lemeshow tests ($p = 0.102$) and the calibration belt test ($p = 0.375$) indicated a good fit.

Based on the logistic regression model, income and job losses since the beginning of the pandemic were linked to increased odds of feeling uncertainty during the lockdown.

4. Conclusions

The COVID-19 pandemic has resulted in significant uncertainty for the global population [39].

According to the results of this study, the probability that uncertainty is among the feelings that best describe individuals' emotional status depends on age, income and job losses, social class, concern for own health and concern for family and friends' health. The influence of both economic factors (income and job losses) and health-related factors (concern for health) indicates that uncertainty arises from various aspects of the COVID-19 crisis, i.e., economic impacts, health impacts, and social impacts.

In regard to age, the explanation for the positive association (OR = 1.015 > 1) with feelings of uncertainty may be that for this particular COVID-19 viral infection, age increases vulnerability, even prior to the age of 65 [40]. The epidemiologic data and daily information in Greece are consistent with this evidence. As of 27 April 2020, the mean age of COVID-19 confirmed cases was 49 years, and the mean age of COVID-19-related deaths was 74 years [41].

Furthermore, there is a positive association between income loss and the probability that uncertainty is one of the feelings that best describes individuals' current emotional status, since OR = 1.386 (>1). Similarly, job loss was positively associated with the probability that uncertainty is among the feelings that best describe individuals' current emotional status, since OR = 1.903 (>1). The plausible explanation is that during the COVID-19 pandemic, individuals have been exposed to increasing job and financial insecurities [42,43] due to job and income losses [44], which have been associated with the deterioration of security and stability of individuals' personal finances, all of which could be linked to strong feelings of uncertainty [45].

Because income and job losses are directly associated with financial uncertainty, as mentioned above, the results of this study are consistent with the literature. Furthermore, in combination with the unpredictability of illness, which may expose individuals to unexpected financial expenses [46], the potential but realistic threat of future income and job losses generate additional financial uncertainty.

In addition, because health emergencies lead to economic impacts through (a) unanticipated healthcare costs, (b) forced limitation of other essential expenditure to meet healthcare costs, and (c) income losses through inability to work, individual illness, or caring for another person [47], it is not surprising that income and job losses are positively associated with the probability of feeling uncertain.

The literature indicates that an individual's vulnerability to uncertainty depends largely on that individual's place in society [48]. As such, one would expect that uncertainty would be among the feelings that best describe the emotional status of lower-class individuals. According to the results, this was not confirmed, since the OR of lower-social-class individuals as compared with middle- and higher-social-class individuals was lower than one (OR = 0.604). Thus, although limited resources and uncertainty characterize the social context of lower-class individuals in general [49], it seems that in the case of COVID-19, the feelings of uncertainty that restrictions and lockdowns generate [50] may have another predictor. One explanation may be health literacy.

Health literacy is defined as "the degree to which individuals have the capacity to obtain, process, and understand basic health information and services needed to make appropriate health decisions" [51]. It is evident that limited health literacy exists among those whose social status is very low or low [52].

Due to the high degree of multidimensional uncertainty, interpreting COVID-19-related news and official recommendations is of particular difficulty. Integrating this large volume of information into behavioral actions is a task that requires critical health literacy and becomes a significant challenge for individuals [53]. In other words, in this uncertain era, health literacy is a key factor for survival [54]. Because it is evident that the health literacy of those who believe they are less likely to be infected with COVID-19 is lower [55], we may argue that individuals with limited health literacy, including lower-class individuals, may have a limited capacity to conceive the uncertainties surrounding the COVID-19 pandemic.

Finally, the emotional status of individuals with higher levels of concern for their own health and higher levels of concern for family and friends' health is more likely to be described as a feeling of uncertainty. Specifically, in regard to the concern for one's own health, it is more likely that uncertainty is one of the feelings that best describe the current emotional status of those who are not very concerned for their own health as compared with those who are not at all concerned for their own health, since OR was equal to 1.621 (>1). This same trend of a higher likelihood of feeling uncertain is evident for the concern that individuals have about their family and friend's health (OR = 2.030 > 1, OR = 2.257 > 1, OR = 2.725 > 1).

Because it is evident that one's fears and concerns affect his/her emotions, i.e., he/she may feel uncertain, depressed, anxious, etc. [56], the results regarding the influence of concern for health agree with the international literature. That is, feelings of uncertainty are also generated by the unpredictability of who will get infected or become sick, the duration of the pandemic, and its short-term or long-term effects [57]. Therefore, the pandemic period represents a long-lasting highly stressful event involving constant and prolonged feelings of uncertainty and worry related to the risk of infection [58].

The aim of this study was to confirm the complexity of the feelings of uncertainty experienced by individuals during a lockdown and that such feelings result from the direct effects of the pandemic, i.e., changes in individuals' personal finances and concerns for one's own health and for that of family and friends. Since uncertainty arises from various aspects of the COVID-19 pandemic, namely, economic, health-related, and social, this study integrates the way that several sources of uncertainty related to the COVID-19 pandemic translate to feelings of uncertainty.

The uncertainty generated by the COVID-19 pandemic over the short and long term is likely to have different effects on different sociodemographic groups. Furthermore, these effects are also likely to be modified by a country's welfare system and the emergency interventions of its institutions [59]. Although uncertainty cannot be eliminated, better management would help to minimize its damage [60].

The previous discussion indicates that it is clear that policy is vital for coping with the COVID-19 pandemic. However, the formation of COVID-19 policy must address the uncertainties surrounding the nature of the disease, the dynamics of transmission, and behavioral responses. That is, to make useful predictions of policy impacts and reasonable policy decisions, a credible means of measuring COVID-19 uncertainty is needed [61]. Because policies should compromise between preventing an outbreak that would overwhelm domestic resources and mitigating economic loss [62], this evaluation is a difficult task.

Funding: This research received no external funding.

Institutional Review Board Statement: The survey was conducted for the European Parliament by Kantar.

Informed Consent Statement: Informed consent was obtained from all subjects involved in the study.

Data Availability Statement: The data are available by the Public Opinion Monitoring Unit. Directorate General for Communication. European Parliament.

Conflicts of Interest: The author declares no conflict of interest.

References

1. Pfefferbaum, B.; North, C.S. Mental Health and the Covid-19 Pandemic. *N. Engl. J. Med.* **2020**, *383*, 510–512. [CrossRef] [PubMed]
2. Sardar, S.; Abdul-Khaliq, I.; Ingar, A.; Amaidia, H.; Mansour, N. 'COVID-19 Lockdown: A Protective Measure or Exacerbator of Health Inequalities? A Comparison between the United Kingdom and India.' a Commentary on "the Socio-Economic Implications of the Coronavirus and COVID-19 Pandemic: A Review.". *Int. J. Surg.* **2020**, *83*, 189–191. [CrossRef] [PubMed]
3. Brashers, D.E. Communication and Uncertainty Management. *J. Commun.* **2001**, *51*, 477–497. [CrossRef]
4. Wasserkrug, S. Uncertainty in Events. In *Encyclopedia of Database Systems*; Liu, L., Özsu, M.T., Eds.; Springer: Boston, MA, USA, 2009; pp. 3221–3225, ISBN 978-0-387-35544-3.
5. Bar-Anan, Y.; Wilson, T.D.; Gilbert, D.T. The feeling of uncertainty intensifies affective reactions. *Emotion* **2009**, *9*, 123–127. [CrossRef]
6. van Horen, F.; Mussweiler, T. Experimental Research Examining How People Can Cope with Uncertainty Through Soft Haptic Sensations. *J. Vis. Exp.* **2015**, e53155. [CrossRef] [PubMed]
7. Vescovi, G.; Riter, H.S.; Azevedo, E.C.; Pedrotti, B.G.; Frizzo, G.B. Parenting, mental health and Covid-19: A rapid systematic review. *Psicol. Teoria e Prática* **2021**, *23*, 1–28. [CrossRef]
8. van der Wal, A.J.; van Horen, F.; Grinstein, A. Temporal Myopia in Sustainable Behavior under Uncertainty. *Int. J. Res. Mark.* **2018**, *35*, 378–393. [CrossRef]
9. Hillen, M.A.; Gutheil, C.M.; Strout, T.D.; Smets, E.M.; Han, P.K. Tolerance of uncertainty: Conceptual analysis, integrative model, and implications for healthcare. *Soc. Sci. Med.* **2017**, *180*, 62–75. [CrossRef]
10. Ma, C.S.; Bs, K.M.; Gorrell, S.; Reilly, E.E.; Ma, J.M.D.; Anderson, D.A. Eating disorder pathology and compulsive exercise during the COVID-19 public health emergency: Examining risk associated with COVID-19 anxiety and intolerance of uncertainty. *Int. J. Eat. Disord.* **2020**, *53*, 2049–2054. [CrossRef]
11. Glowacz, F.; Schmits, E. Psychological distress during the COVID-19 lockdown: The young adults most at risk. *Psychiatry Res.* **2020**, *293*, 113486. [CrossRef]
12. Altig, D.; Baker, S.; Barrero, J.M.; Bloom, N.; Bunn, P.; Chen, S.; Davis, S.J.; Leather, J.; Meyer, B.; Mihaylov, E.; et al. Economic uncertainty before and during the COVID-19 pandemic. *J. Public Econ.* **2020**, *191*, 104274. [CrossRef]
13. Santos-Pinto, L.; Mata, J. Strategies for COVID-19: The Option Value of Waiting. VoxEU CERP. 2020. Available online: https://voxeu.org (accessed on 24 January 2021).
14. Sun, N. Applying Siracusa: A Call for a General Comment on Public Health Emergencies. *Health Hum. Rights J* **2020**, *22*, 387–390.
15. Hansel, T.C.; Saltzman, L.Y.; Bordnick, P.S. Behavioral Health and Response for COVID-19. *Disaster Med. Public Health Prep.* **2020**, *14*, 670–676. [CrossRef]
16. Godinić, D.; Obrenovic, B.; Khudaykulov, A. Effects of Economic Uncertainty on Mental Health in the COVID-19 Pandemic Context: Social Identity Disturbance, Job Uncertainty and Psychological Well-Being Model. *Int. J. Innov. Econ. Dev.* **2020**, *6*, 61–74. [CrossRef]
17. Raboisson, D.; Lhermie, G. Living with COVID-19: A Systemic and Multi-Criteria Approach to Enact Evidence-Based Health Policy. *Front. Public Health* **2020**, *8*, 294. [CrossRef] [PubMed]
18. Susskind, D.; Vines, D. The economics of the COVID-19 pandemic: An assessment. *Oxf. Rev. Econ. Policy* **2020**, *36*, S1–S13. [CrossRef]
19. World Bank. *Global Economic Prospects, June 2020*; World Bank: Washington, DC, USA, 2020; p. 15.
20. Greenglass, E.; Marjanovic, Z.; Fiksenbaum, L.; Antoniou, A.-S.; Cooper, C. The impact of the recession and its af-termath on individual health and well-being. In *The Psychology of the Recession on the Workplace*; Edward Elgar Publishing: Cheltenham, UK, 2013; pp. 42–58.
21. Simone, M.; Emery, R.L.; Hazzard, V.M.; Eisenberg, M.E.; Larson, N.; Neumark-Sztainer, D. Disordered Eating in a Population-based Sample of Young Adults during the COVID-19 Outbreak. *Int. J. Eat. Disord.* **2021**. [CrossRef]
22. Brock, R.L.; Laifer, L.M. Family Science in the Context of the COVID-19 Pandemic: Solutions and New Directions. *Fam. Proc.* **2020**, *59*, 1007–1017. [CrossRef] [PubMed]
23. Brown, J.D.; Vouri, S.M.; Manini, T.M. Survey-Reported Medication Changes among Older Adults during the SARS-CoV-2 (COVID-19) Pandemic. *Res. Soc. Adm. Pharm.* **2020**. [CrossRef] [PubMed]
24. Di Giusto, M.; Grover, P.; Castillo, C.; Jimenez, I.; García, J.; Tijerina, R.; Ramos-Usuga, D.; Arango-Lasprilla, J. The State of Pulmonary Rehabilitation in Latin America during the COVID-19 Pandemic. *J. Int. Soc. Phys. Rehabil. Med.* **2021**, *4*, 40. [CrossRef]
25. Marko, C.; Košec, A.; Brecic, P. Stay Home While Going out—Possible Impacts of Earthquake Co-Occurring with COVID-19 Pandemic on Mental Health and Vice Versa. *Brain Behav. Immun.* **2020**, *87*, 82–83. [CrossRef]
26. Benke, C.; Autenrieth, L.K.; Asselmann, E.; Pané-Farré, C.A. Lockdown, Quarantine Measures, and Social Distancing: Associations with Depression, Anxiety and Distress at the Beginning of the COVID-19 Pandemic among Adults from Germany. *Psychiatry Res.* **2020**, *293*, 113462. [CrossRef] [PubMed]

27. Sinha, M.; Kumar, M.; Zeitz, L.; Collins, P.Y.; Kumar, S.; Fisher, S.; Foote, N.; Sartorius, N.; Herrman, H.; Atwoli, L. Towards Mental Health Friendly Cities during and after COVID-19. *Cities Health* **2020**. [CrossRef]
28. Faulkner, G.; Rhodes, R.E.; Vanderloo, L.M.; Chulak-Bozer, T.; O'Reilly, N.; Ferguson, L.; Spence, J.C. Physical Activity as a Coping Strategy for Mental Health Due to the COVID-19 Virus: A Potential Disconnect Among Canadian Adults? *Front. Commun.* **2020**, *5*, 571833. [CrossRef]
29. Nitschke, J.P.; Forbes, P.A.G.; Ali, N.; Cutler, J.; Apps, M.A.J.; Lockwood, P.L.; Lamm, C. Resilience during Uncertainty? Greater Social Connectedness during COVID-19 Lockdown Is Associated with Reduced Distress and Fatigue. *Br. J. Health Psychol.* **2021**, *26*, 553–569. [CrossRef] [PubMed]
30. van Maurik, I.S.; Bakker, E.D.; van den Buuse, S.; Gillissen, F.; van de Beek, M.; Lemstra, E.; Mank, A.; van den Bosch, K.A.; van Leeuwenstijn, M.; Bouwman, F.H.; et al. Psychosocial Effects of Corona Measures on Patients With Dementia, Mild Cognitive Impairment and Subjective Cognitive Decline. *Front. Psychiatry* **2020**, *11*, 585686. [CrossRef]
31. World Health Organization. WHO Coronavirus Disease (COVID-19) Dashboard. 2020. Available online: https://covid19.who.int/ (accessed on 29 April 2021).
32. Organization for Economic Co-operation and Development. Policy Responses to the COVID-19 Crisis. 2020. Available online: http://www.oecd.org/social/Covid-19-Employment-and-Social-Policy-Responses-by-Country.xlsx (accessed on 19 April 2021).
33. Ballivian, J.; Alcaide, M.L.; Cecchini, D.; Jones, D.L.; Abbamonte, J.M.; Cassetti, I. Impact of COVID–19-Related Stress and Lockdown on Mental Health Among People Living with HIV in Argentina. *JAIDS J. Acquir. Immune Defic. Syndr.* **2020**, *85*, 475–482. [CrossRef] [PubMed]
34. European Parliament. Public Opinion in the EU in Time of Coronavirus Crisis. 2020. Available online: https://www.europarl.europa.eu/at-your-service/en/be-heard/eurobarometer/public-opinion-in-the-eu-in-time-of-coronavirus-crisis (accessed on 18 September 2020).
35. National Public Health Organization. Current State of Covid-19 Outbreak in Greece and Timeline of Key Containment Events. 2020. Available online: https://eody.gov.gr/en/current-state-of-covid-19-outbreak-in-greece-and-timeline-of-key-containment-events/ (accessed on 19 April 2021).
36. Powell, M.; Dunwoody, S.; Griffin, R.; Neuwirth, K. Exploring lay uncertainty about an environmental health risk. *Public Underst. Sci.* **2007**, *16*, 323–343. [CrossRef]
37. Hendrickx, J. Using Categorical Variables in Stata. *Stata Tech. Bull.* **1999**, *STB-52*, 2–8.
38. Nattino, G.; Lemeshow, S.; Phillips, G.; Finazzi, S.; Bertolini, G. Assessing the calibration of dichotomous outcome models with the calibration belt. *Stata J.* **2017**, *17*, 1003–1014. [CrossRef]
39. Rettie, H.; Daniels, J. Coping and tolerance of uncertainty: Predictors and mediators of mental health during the COVID-19 pandemic. *Am. Psychol.* **2020**. [CrossRef] [PubMed]
40. Wiemers, E.E.; Abrahams, S.; AlFakhri, M.; Hotz, V.J.; Schoeni, R.F.; Seltzer, J.A. Disparities in vulnerability to complications from COVID-19 arising from disparities in preexisting conditions in the United States. *Res. Soc. Stratif. Mobil.* **2020**, *69*, 100553. [CrossRef]
41. National Public Health Organization. Daily Reports on COVID-19. 2020. Available online: https://eody.gov.gr/ (accessed on 15 December 2020). (In Greek)
42. Armitage, R.; Nellums, L.B. COVID-19: Compounding the Health-Related Harms of Human Trafficking. *EClinicalMedicine* **2020**, *24*, 100409. [CrossRef] [PubMed]
43. Brener, A.; Mazor-Aronovitch, K.; Rachmiel, M.; Levek, N.; Barash, G.; Pinhas-Hamiel, O.; Lebenthal, Y.; Landau, Z. Lessons learned from the continuous glucose monitoring metrics in pediatric patients with type 1 diabetes under COVID-19 lockdown. *Acta Diabetol.* **2020**, *57*, 1511–1517. [CrossRef]
44. Witteveen, D. Sociodemographic Inequality in Exposure to COVID-19-Induced Economic Hardship in the United Kingdom. *Res. Soc. Stratif. Mobil.* **2020**, *69*, 100551. [CrossRef]
45. Marjanovic, Z.; Greenglass, E.R.; Fiksenbaum, L.; Bell, C.M. Psychometric evaluation of the Financial Threat Scale (FTS) in the context of the great recession. *J. Econ. Psychol.* **2013**, *36*, 1–10. [CrossRef]
46. Maruotti, A. Fairness of the national health service in Italy: A bivariate correlated random effects model. *J. Appl. Stat.* **2009**, *36*, 709–722. [CrossRef]
47. Clarke, L. An introduction to economic studies, health emergencies, and COVID-19. *J. Evid. Based Med.* **2020**, *13*, 161–167. [CrossRef]
48. Marris, P. The social construction of uncertainty. In *Attachment across the Life Cycle*; Parkes, C.M., Stevenson-Hinde, J., Marris, P., Eds.; Routledge: New York, NY, USA, 2004; pp. 77–90.
49. Kraus, M.W.; Piff, P.K.; Mendoza-Denton, R.; Rheinschmidt, M.L.; Keltner, D. Social class, solipsism, and contextualism: How the rich are different from the poor. *Psychol. Rev.* **2012**, *119*, 546–572. [CrossRef]
50. Serafini, G.; Parmigiani, B.; Amerio, A.; Aguglia, A.; Sher, L.; Amore, M. The psychological impact of COVID-19 on the mental health in the general population. *QJM Int. J. Med.* **2020**, *113*, 531–537. [CrossRef]
51. Selden, C.R.; Zorn, M.; Ratzan, S.; Parker, R.M. *Health Literacy*; National Library of Medicine: Bethesda, MD, USA, 2000. Available online: http://www.nlm.nih.gov/pubs/cbm/hliteracy.html (accessed on 11 November 2020).

52. Sørensen, K.; Pelikan, J.M.; Röthlin, F.; Ganahl, K.; Slonska, Z.; Doyle, G.; Fullam, J.; Kondilis, B.; Agrafiotis, D.; Uiters, E.; et al. Health literacy in Europe: Comparative results of the European health literacy survey (HLS-EU). *Eur. J. Public Health* **2015**, *25*, 1053–1058. [CrossRef]
53. Abel, T.; McQueen, D. Critical health literacy and the COVID-19 crisis. *Health Promot. Int.* **2020**, *35*, 1612–1613. [CrossRef]
54. Spring, H. Health Literacy and COVID-19. *Health Inf. Librar. J.* **2020**, *37*, 171–172. [CrossRef] [PubMed]
55. Bailey, S.C.; Serper, M.; Opsasnick, L.; Persell, S.D.; O'Conor, R.; Curtis, L.M.; Benavente, J.Y.; Wismer, G.; Batio, S.; Eifler, M.; et al. Changes in COVID-19 Knowledge, Beliefs, Behaviors, and Preparedness Among High-Risk Adults from the Onset to the Acceleration Phase of the US Outbreak. *J. Gen. Intern. Med.* **2020**, *35*, 3285–3292. [CrossRef]
56. Levkovich, I.; Shinan-Altman, S. Impact of the COVID-19 pandemic on stress and emotional reactions in Israel: A mixed-methods study. *Int. Health* **2020**. [CrossRef] [PubMed]
57. Whitehead, B.R.; Torossian, E. Older Adults' Experience of the COVID-19 Pandemic: A Mixed-Methods Analysis of Stresses and Joys. *Gerontologist* **2021**, *61*, 36–47. [CrossRef] [PubMed]
58. Diolaiuti, F.; Marazziti, D.; Beatino, M.F.; Mucci, F.; Pozza, A. Impact and Consequences of COVID-19 Pandemic on Complicated Grief and Persistent Complex Bereavement Disorder. *Psychiatry Res.* **2021**, *300*, 113916. [CrossRef] [PubMed]
59. Settersten, R.A.; Bernardi, L.; Härkönen, J.; Antonucci, T.C.; Dykstra, P.A.; Heckhausen, J.; Kuh, D.; Mayer, K.U.; Moen, P.; Mortimer, J.T.; et al. Understanding the effects of Covid-19 through a life course lens. *Adv. Life Course Res.* **2020**, *45*, 100360. [CrossRef]
60. Koffman, J.; Gross, J.; Etkind, S.N.; Selman, L. Uncertainty and COVID-19: How are we to respond? *J. R. Soc. Med.* **2020**, *113*, 211–216. [CrossRef]
61. Manski, C.F. Forming COVID-19 Policy under Uncertainty. *J. Benefit-Cost Anal.* **2020**, *11*, 341–356. [CrossRef]
62. Al Zobbi, M.; Alsinglawi, B.; Mubin, O.; Alnajjar, F. Measurement Method for Evaluating the Lockdown Policies during the COVID-19 Pandemic. *Int. J. Environ. Res. Public Health* **2020**, *17*, 5574. [CrossRef] [PubMed]

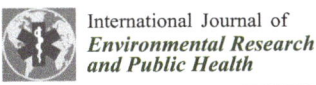

Article

Amid the COVID-19 Pandemic, Unethical Behavior in the Name of the Company: The Role of Job Insecurity, Job Embeddedness, and Turnover Intention

Ibrahim A. Elshaer [1,2,*] and Alaa M. S. Azazz [3,4,*]

1. Management Department, College of Business Administration, King Faisal University, Al-Hassa 31982, Saudi Arabia
2. Hotel Studies Department, Faculty of Tourism and Hotels, Suez Canal University, Ismailia 41522, Egypt
3. Department of Tourism and Hospitality, Arts College, King Faisal University, Al-Ahsa 380, Saudi Arabia
4. Tourism Studies Department, Faculty of Tourism and Hotels, Suez Canal University, Ismailia 41522, Egypt
* Correspondence: ielshaer@kfu.edu.sa (I.A.E.); aazazz@kfu.edu.sa (A.M.S.A.)

Abstract: The worldwide economic crisis initiated by the COVID-19 pandemic certainly altered the perception of regular job insecurity dimensions and brought these to the ultimate level. When employees feel insecure, they may decide to participate in unethical behavior in the name of the company to avoid layoff and become retained employees. This study investigated the relationship between job insecurity and unethical organizational behavior through the mediating role of job embeddedness and turnover intention. A total of 685 employees working in five- and four-star hotels and category A travel agents participated in this study. Data were analyzed using structural equation modeling. Job embeddedness and turnover intention were found to be partially mediated by the impact of job insecurity on unethical organizational behavior. Theoretical and practical implications were identified and discussed.

Keywords: job insecurity; unethical organizational behavior; job embeddedness; turnover intention; COVID-19; tourism industry

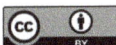

1. Introduction

Until the recent outbreak of the COVID-19 virus, which has spread throughout the globe, organizational life in the twenty-first century had never been more challenging. This pandemic, which spread across numerous countries at the same time, has harmed billions of people worldwide [1]. As a response to this pandemic, more than 30 million employees are expected to lose their jobs in the United States [2]. The leisure and hospitality industry was the most impacted, with 7.7 million jobs lost, or 47% of the total positions worldwide [3]. Prior to the current epidemic, the travel and tourist industry had remarkable resilience, contributing more than 10% of global GDP and a similar percentage of jobs [4]. However, due to the lockdowns and bans on internal and international travel executed by a large number of countries, this sector is currently the most affected [5]. Many countries' hospitality businesses have begun laying off employees to cope with the massive losses. Marriott International hotel chains® have begun to lay off tens of thousands of employees around the world [6]. Similarly, Airbnb® laid off almost a quarter of its workforce [7]. Even employees who survive the layoffs are apprehensive about their future careers and have a high level of job insecurity under these conditions. According to previous research, job insecurity is one of the most significant hindrance-related stressors [8–10] that has negative impacts on the hospitality industry's desirable work outcomes [11,12]—and causes absenteeism, nervousness [13], and higher turnover intentions [14].

Though job insecurity has been thoroughly researched, further research can explore the specific employee's reactions to adapt and deal with job insecurity [8,15]. According to [16], job insecurity can be combined with high achievement to eliminate work withdrawal.

Additionally, employees with a higher feeling of job embeddedness can use their capabilities to avoid layoff and become retained employees [17]. They may wish to show their managers that they can make a positive contribution to the company, especially in a time when job instability is on the rise [18]. As a result, they may not see any moral boundaries to engaging in unethical behavior actions that are beneficial to the organization [19].

The issue of employees engaging in unethical behavior to contend with the feeling of job insecurity has been previously highlighted in the literature [20]. However, impacted employees could decide to participate in unethical behavior in the name of the organization but contradict the international ethical standards. A salesperson, for example, could exaggerate the characteristics of a product they were selling to a consumer in order to meet their sales target and assist their company to earn more money. Alternatively, an accountant may falsify figures in order to decrease a company's tax liability [21]. By executing these unethical practices in the name of the company, the employee may be perceived as a successful employee by their managers [21].

The current study first explores the relationship between job insecurity and unethical organizational behavior. This relationship is examined in the context of increasing the fear of job loss with the tendency for employees to engage in unethical behavior that provides short-term advantages to the organization. Second, this study tests the mediating role of job embeddedness in the relationship between job insecurity and unethical organizational behavior, and finally, the study also highlights the mediating effects of turnover intention in the relationship between job insecurity and unethical organizational behavior. Though job insecurity has been extensively investigated, further research can explore the specific employee's reactions to adapt and deal with job insecurity [8,15]. Thus, this study proposed a model that may contribute to enhancing academics' understanding in which job insecurity affects employees' unethical organizational behavior through the mediating role of job embeddedness and turnover intention.

Testing these relationships has implications for practitioners as well. Employees who participated in unethical organizational behavior in the name of the company can be for personal gains and such behaviors can reduce the reputation of the organization. Therefore, managers amid such a pandemic should avoid sending signals that can promote employees' perceptions of job insecurity.

2. Literature Review and Hypotheses Development

2.1. Job Insecurity and Unethical Organizational Behavior

Job insecurity is a 'perceptual phenomenon' that focuses on the threat to an individual's current job stability [22]. The authors of [23] propose two dimensions of job insecurity: quantitative 'threats to the job as such' and qualitative 'threats to valued job features'. Quantitative job insecurity emphasizes the predicted job loss caused by intended/unintended organizational signals, or employees' appraisal reports [22]. Qualitative job insecurity explains an employee's perceived future job loss based on their presumed threat [22]. Given the substantial negative impact of the COVID-19 pandemic on the economy, which affects both demand and supply, organizational restructuring through downsizing has become a popular approach. Downsizing is a strategy for cutting and controlling labor expenses (typically by reducing the number of employees or lowering compensation), streamlining operations, and boosting organizational competitiveness [24]. According to researchers [25,26], downsizing could threaten employees and their jobs. Organizational restructure, according to [27], increases employees' job insecurity. Employees may experience employment insecurity as a result of COVID-19. In the same vein, employees often experience stress because of perceived job insecurity. An employees' stress response frequently stimulates employees to participate in unethical behaviors that help to cope with the perceived threat [28]. Employees can participate in unethical organizational behavior by acting in their self-interest or the best interests of the organization.

Organizational unethical behavior is an unethical practice that is intended to benefit the organization rather than the person [21]. For example, supplying incorrect information to a customer in order to accomplish the organization's quarterly predetermined goals could be one of these practices.

As proposed by the self-regulation theory [29,30], exercising self-control necessitates the application of a limited number of self-regulatory resources. The application of these self-regulatory systems depletes these resources, reducing a person's ability to demonstrate the self-control required to make ethical decisions. Additionally, when employees' moral resources have been diminished, their cognitive capabilities are drained, and their successive skill to self-regulate is impeded. When employees' self-regulatory resources are depleted, employees may decide to participate in unethical behavior that benefits the organization or themselves. Therefore, the following hypothesis is proposed as shown in Figure 1:

Hypothesis 1 (H1). *Job insecurity has a positive significant impact on unethical organizational behavior.*

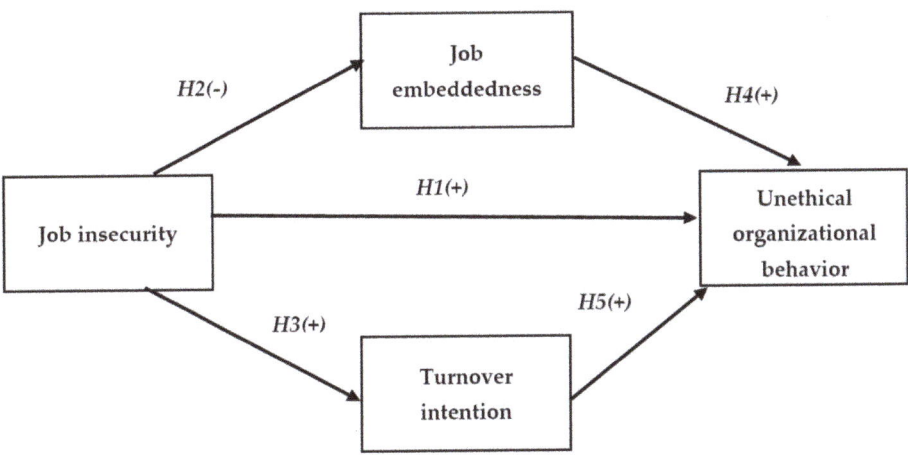

Figure 1. A research framework (developed by authors).

2.2. Job Insecurity, Job Embeddedness, and Turnover Intention

When the organization members face and feel job insecurity, threats to financial resources can be devastating. The high risk of losing a job threatens the employees' feelings of embeddedness and fit with the organization. Job embeddedness has been explained as a solid net through which employees at the workplace are attached [31]. The more connections at the workplace that employees have, the more embedded the employee is. The previous literature provides evidence that job insecurity stimulates a lower level of job embeddedness [32].

Employees' feelings of job insecurity will stimulate a search for new job opportunities and increase the possibilities of turnover. The tourism and hospitality industry is one of the industries with the highest employee turnover rates [33], which may be caused by an unstable environment [34]. The worldwide economic crisis initiated by the COVID-19 pandemic certainly altered the perception of regular job insecurity dimensions and brought these to the ultimate level due to the failure to expect the strength and duration of the pandemic [35]. The meta-analytical research conducted by [36] endorses the claim that job insecurity is a major stressor that is directly related to low job satisfaction and high levels of job withdrawal. Notwithstanding, and based on Adams' [37,38] equity theory, employees regularly compare their ratio of inputs and outputs as compared to their peers in the organization, and if an imbalance exists an inequity exists. The authors of [36] argue that employees' feelings of job insecurity could stimulate an imbalanced feeling between their input efforts and output gains. More specifically, employees, compare their organizational loyalty with their perceived job security. On the other hand, as employees' feelings of job insecurity increase, their intention to leave the organization will increase [39]. Accordingly, the following hypotheses are proposed.

Hypothesis 2 (H2). *Job insecurity has a negative significant impact on job embeddedness.*

Hypothesis 3 (H3). *Job insecurity has a positive significant impact on turnover intention.*

2.3. Job Embeddedness and Unethical Organizational Behavior

Job embeddedness defines the affective and cognitive connection with the organization, concerned with the organization–employee fit, and builds the internal and external links in the organization and the sacrifices resulting from the breaking of these links [40]. Therefore, it is defined as a set of 'combined forces' that bind an employee to the job [41,42]. Job embeddedness refers to a person's social involvement within their company [43]. As a result, people who are emotionally attached to their jobs are unlikely to leave the company [40].

Embedded workers are aware of the advantages of being attached to their job. Employees with a high level of job embeddedness feel comfortable and compatible with their coworkers, which leads to heightened levels of attachment to the company [44]. While work embeddedness provides heightened degrees of commitment to the company, it also creates an inherent amount of dependence on the organization in terms of job insecurity [44]. According to self-regulation theory, employees make a conscious effort to match their practices and behaviors with accepted norms [45,46]. Employees with higher levels of embeddedness will demonstrate behaviors that are aligned with the organization as a result of increasing levels of fit and connection. Individuals with low levels of embeddedness, on the other hand, have not developed a strong attachment or fondness for the organization [40]. While work embeddedness increases degrees of attachment to the organization, it also produces an inherent level of dependence on the organization, which contributes to job insecurity [44]. Self-regulation theory argued that employees exert a conscious effort to associate their behaviors with established standards [45,46]. Employees who have higher levels of embeddedness will exhibit ethical and/or unethical behaviors in the name of the organization [40]. Therefore, the following hypothesis is proposed:

Hypothesis 4 (H4). *Job embeddedness has a positive significant impact on unethical organizational behavior.*

2.4. Turnover Intention and Unethical Organization Behavior

Employees who are facing turnover intention may participate in unethical organizational behaviors in the hopes that their sacrifices will be rewarded with ongoing employment. However, these unethical behaviors can generate succeeding harms to the organization. On the other hand, employees also may choose to participate in unethical behavior such as padding work hours in an attempt to release some of the disappointment they are suffering regarding the possible job loss [45] and, hence, the following hypothesis is proposed:

Hypothesis 5 (H5). *Turnover intention has a positive and significant impact on unethical organizational behavior.*

3. Methodological Approach

3.1. Instrument Development and Research Measures

The current study scales were developed based on a survey of existing theoretical items and a review of the literature. This survey yields four factors, each with its own set of items, which have been customized to fit the tourism sector. The operationalization of the study concepts was derided from previous literature. The study scale was developed using a five-point Likert-type scale anchored by '1 = strongly disagree and 5 = strongly agree', as suggested by [47,48]. Similarly, turnover intention (TrnOvr) was measured by three items developed by [34,49,50]. Job insecurity (JobInsc) was measured by six quantitative and qualitative items adopted from [51] (e.g., 'I am worried that I will have to leave my job before I would like to'). Job embeddedness (JobEmb) was operationalized by six items developed by [31] (i.e., 'I like the authority and responsibility I have at this company'). Finally, from Umphress et al. [21], seven items to measure unethical organizational behavior were employed (i.e., 'If my organization needed me to, I would give a good recommendation on the behalf of an incompetent employee in the hope that the person will become another organization's problem instead of my own').

The instrument was created in English at first. Back-translation was then conducted [52]. The research instrument was translated from English to Arabic by three academics. In addition, the back translation from Arabic to English was done by a group of two more distinct academics. Both versions were identical. There were no discernible discrepancies between the original and translated instruments. Five academics in the tourism industry, thirty employees, eleven experts, and managers from twenty different hotels were used to validate the research instrument. The pilot respondents provided positive feedback on the consistency, content, and face validity of the scale. The final form of the scale was directed to 700 employees working in five- and four-star hotels in Egypt.

3.2. Data Collections

The drop and collect method of distributing and collecting the study questionnaires was employed to ensure a high response rate [53]. Survived employees, who may have an intention to leave the hotel amid the COVID-19 pandemic, were targeted to answer the study instrument. Twenty-five enumerators (faculty students) were instructed to collect data from the respondents in greater Cairo, Hurghada, and Sharm Elsheikh (the biggest tourist cities in Egypt). This method was employed to avert the usual low response rate of mail and/or online approach of data collection and to avert the reluctance to answer the anonymous questionnaires. Enumerators were taught to follow hygiene protocols to minimize the risk of infection for themselves and respondents amid the data collection process during July and August 2021. Respondents were asked to sign a consent form before starting the survey.

With a usable response rate of 97%, 685 employees working in the Egyptian five- and four-star hotels and travel agent category A participated in the study survey. A total of 65 four-star hotels, 60 five-star hotels, and 60 category A travel agents were represented in the survey. Four/five questionnaires were sent to each hotel/ travel agent to deal with over-or under-representation. The majority (51%) of the respondents were aged between 31 to 40 and were married (66%). The distribution of the respondents according to gender is nearly equivalent, with 55% male and 45% female. The majority of respondents were normal employees (85%), while only 15% were supervisors. The full-time employees comprised the highest percentage, at 86%, as did employees who had obtained a university degree (85%). A high percentage (43%) of respondents have an annual salary below 4000$, as shown in Table 1.

Table 1. The Demographic characteristics (developed by authors).

N = 685		%	Groups		Number of Responses
Age			Five-star Hotels	65	235
21–30	185	27	Five-star Hotels	60	210
31–40	350	51	Travel agents	60	240
>41	150	22	Total		685
Gender					
Male	380	55			
Female	305	45			
Marital status					
Married	450	66			
Unmarried	235	34			
	200	20			
Occupation					
Supervisors	105	15			
Normal employees	580	85			
Type of employment					
Full time	590	86			
Part time	95	14			
Education level					
Less than high school degree	185	27			
	200	20			
High school degree	100	15			
University graduate	400	58			
Annual Salary ($)					
Under 4000	300	43			
4001–6000	150	22			
6001–8000	150	22			
Over 8000	85	13			

3.3. Non-Response and Common Bias Tests

Two different methods were employed to deal with the potential non-response bias: univariate analysis 'independent samples *t*-test, analysis of the variance (ANOVA) and multivariate analysis 'multivariate analysis of the variance (MANOVA). The findings of the two tests did not statistically generate any significant discrepancies at a 95% confidence level for early and late respondents [54]. To test the potential common method variance, Harmon's one-factor test method, as suggested by [55], was conducted. The one factor extracted solution accounts for 25% of the variance, which gives evidence that no one factor accounted for the majority of the variance, implying that common method variance is not fully responsible for our findings.

Questionnaire items had a maximum and minimum value of 5 and 1, respectively. The mean scores for all answers ranged from 3.31 to 4.08, with standard deviation values ranging from 1.230 to 0.603 (see Table 2), indicating that the study data is more dispersed and less condensed around the mean value [56]. Furthermore, the skewness and kurtosis values in Table 2 indicated that the data did not violate the normality rules [57].

Table 2. Descriptive statistics (developed by authors based on previous literature).

Abbr.	Items	Min	Max	M	S.D	Skewness	Kurtosis
Job Insecurity							
JobInsc_1	"I am worried that I will have to leave my job before I would like to".	1	5	3.33	1.086	−0.353	−0.422
JobInsc_2	"I worry about being able to keep my job".	1	5	3.33	1.101	−0.328	−0.489
JobInsc_3	"I am afraid I may lose my job shortly".	1	5	3.36	1.060	−0.343	−0.385
JobInsc_4	"I worry about getting less stimulating work tasks in the future".	1	5	3.31	1.127	−0.399	−0.364
JobInsc_5	"I worry about my future wage development".	1	5	3.31	1.123	−0.404	−0.344
JobInsc_6	"I feel worried about my career development in the organization".	1	5	3.31	1.140	−0.432	−0.328
Job Embeddedness							
JobEmb_1	"I like the members of my workgroup".	1	5	3.57	1.220	−0.394	−0.953
JobEmb_2	"My coworkers are similar to me".	1	5	3.54	1.169	−0.334	−0.918
JobEmb_3	"My job utilizes my skills and talents well".	1	5	3.59	1.162	−0.328	−0.957
JobEmb_4	"I feel like I am a good match for this company".	1	5	3.47	1.191	−0.324	−0.938
JobEmb_5	"I fit with the company's culture".	1	5	3.51	1.184	−0.346	−0.904
JobEmb_6	"I like the authority and responsibility I have at this company".	1	5	3.62	1.184	−0.396	−0.953
Turnover Intention							
trnOvr_1	"I often think about leaving that career".	1	5	4.08	.618	−1.439	1.485
trnOvr_2	"It would not take much to make me leave this career".	1	5	4.07	.629	−1.463	1.198
trnOvr_3	"I will probably be looking for another career soon".	1	5	4.08	.603	−1.439	1.993
Unethical Organizational Behavior							
Unethic_1	"If it would help my organization, I would misrepresent the truth to make my organization look good".	1	5	3.85	1.203	−1.073	0.275
Unethic_2	"If it would help my organization, I would exaggerate the truth about my "company's products or services to customers and clients"."	1	5	3.76	1.230	−0.974	−0.020
Unethic_3	"If it would benefit my organization, I would withhold negative information about my company or its products from customers and clients".	1	5	3.80	1.208	−1.016	0.171
Unethic_4	"If my organization needed me to, I would give a good recommendation on the behalf of an incompetent employee in the hope that the person will become another organization's problem instead of my own".	1	5	3.79	1.224	−1.031	0.140
Unethic_5	"If my organization needed me to, I would withhold issuing a refund to a customer or client accidentally overcharged".	1	5	3.76	1.222	−0.963	0.031
Unethic_6	"If needed, I would conceal information from the public that could be damaging to my organization".	1	5	3.75	1.250	−0.981	−0.013
Unethic_7	"I would do whatever it takes to help my organization".	1	5	3.74	1.245	−0.945	−0.085

4. Results

4.1. Confirmatory Factor Analysis

Confirmatory factor analysis (CFA) was employed to evaluate the overall model fit with the data and to determine the unidimensionality of the study constructs. Several researchers recommended that (χ^2/df) should be less than 3 and that all fit indices, such as Comparative Fit Index (CFI) and Tucker-Lewis Index (TLI), should be greater than 0.9, while root-mean-square error of approximation (RMSEA) and root-mean-square residual (RMR) should be less than 0.08 [57–59]. To assess the factors' reliability and validity, Analysis of Moment Structures (AMOS) v25 was employed to test a first-order confirmatory factor analysis with all of the study's dependent and independent variables. The result of our CFA model in Table 3 revealed that the overall fit statistics indicate a satisfactory model fit, as all obtained fit statistics met the recommended cut-off values.

Convergent and discriminant validity for each construct were evaluated to determine the construct validity. Table 3 showed that factor loadings for all study constructs' items are all significant at the 0.001 level, exceeding the minimum criteria of 0.5. Furthermore, all of the research constructs had AVEs greater than 0.5, and the construct reliability values for all four constructs exceed the 0.70 criterion. Overall, the previous results showed good convergent validity, as recommended by [60,61]

Table 3. Convergent and discriminant validity (developed by authors).

Dimensions and Items	Loading	CR	AVE	MSV	1	2	3	4
1-Job Insecurity (a = 0.965)		0.9590	0.7970	0.0210	0.8930			
JobInsc_1	0.934							
JobInsc_2	0.965							
JobInsc_3	0.962							
JobInsc_4	0.836							
JobInsc_5	0.829							
JobInsc_6	0.818							
-2-Job Embeddedness (a = 0.981)		0.9820	0.8990	0.003	−0.055	0.9480		
JobEmb_1	0.948							
JobEmb_2	0.974							
JobEmb_3	0.958							
JobEmb_4	0.913							
JobEmb_5	0.952							
JobEmb_6	0.943							
3-Turnover Intention (a = 0.918)		0.9180	0.7890	0.0210	0.1440	0.0230	0.888	
trnOvr_1	0.887							
trnOvr_2	0.916							
trnOvr_3	0.861							
4-Unethical Organizational Behavior (a = 0.978)		0.9770	0.8590	0.0130	−0.116	−0.040	0.0370	0.927
Unethic_1	0.916							
Unethic_2	0.885							
Unethic_3	0.936							
Unethic_4	0.916							
Unethic_5	0.975							
Unethic_6	0.968							
Unethic_7	0.886							

Model fit: (χ^2 (203, N = 685) = 585.046, $p < 0.001$, normed χ^2 = 2.882, RMSEA = 0.049, SRMR = 0.050, CFI = 0.937, TLI = 0.924, NFI = 0.938, PCFI = 0.797 and PNFI = 0.816). CR: composite reliability; AVE: average variance extracted; MSV: maximum shared value; Diagonal values: the square root of AVE for each dimension; Below diagonal values: intercorrelation between dimensions.

Cronbach alpha values, correlation matrix, and the square root of AVEs were utilized to test the discriminant validity [62]. Table 3 shows the average variance extracted (AVE), correlation matrix, and composite Cronbach alphas for the research variables. As shown in Table 3, the square root of AVEs was higher than the off-diagonal values, which represent the correlations among those constructs, confirming discriminant validity for research factors as suggested by [62]. Moreover, the average variance extracted (AVE) scores for job insecurity (0.797), job embeddedness (0.899), turnover intention (0.789), and unethical organizational behavior (0.859) exceeded the maximum shared variance (MSV) (ranging from 0.021 to 003), further confirmed that the discriminant validity is supported, as suggested by [59,62]. Additionally, for discriminant validity, the inter-correlations scores for each factor (below diagonal value) should not surpass the square root values of the AVE for each factor (bold diagonal) as shown in Table 3, which further support the discriminant validity of the research variables.

4.2. Structural Equations Modeling (SEM) Results

After ensuring that the validity and reliability of the measures were adequate, structural equation modeling was employed to test the impact of job insecurity on unethical organizational behavior via job embeddedness and turnover intention. Two criteria are employed to assess the proposed model: overall goodness of model fit "χ^2/df, CFI, TLI. RMSEA, and RMR" and the statistical significance of the hypothesized relationships. The overall model fit values for the structural model demonstrated satisfactory values, as displayed in Table 4. Moreover, Figure 2 and Table 4 explain the proposed model output.

The relationships in the proposed model involving the five hypotheses investigate the impact of job insecurity on unethical organizational behavior via job embeddedness and turnover intention. The results show that the four paths (H1, H3, H4, and H5) are positive and significant with $p < 0.05$, whereas one path was negative but significant (H2). The significant positive effect of job insecurity on unethical organizational behavior had been supported ($\beta 1 = +0.29$ with t-value = 6.320, $p < 0.001$). Nevertheless, job insecurity has a significant but negative link with job embeddedness that supports H2 ($\beta 2 = -0.36$ with t-value = -9.448, $p < 0.001$). The model findings also demonstrate that job insecurity significantly and positively impacts turnover intention ($\beta 3 = +0.41$ with t-value = 10.221, $p < 0.001$) that proves H3. As assumed in H4, job embeddedness has a positive and significant effect on unethical organizational behavior ($\beta 4 = +0.47$ with t-value = 11.116, $p < 0.001$) that endorses H4. Similarly, turnover intention was found to have a positive significant impact on unethical organizational behavior, which supports H5 ($\beta 5 = +0.32$ with t-value = 7.252, $p > 0.001$).

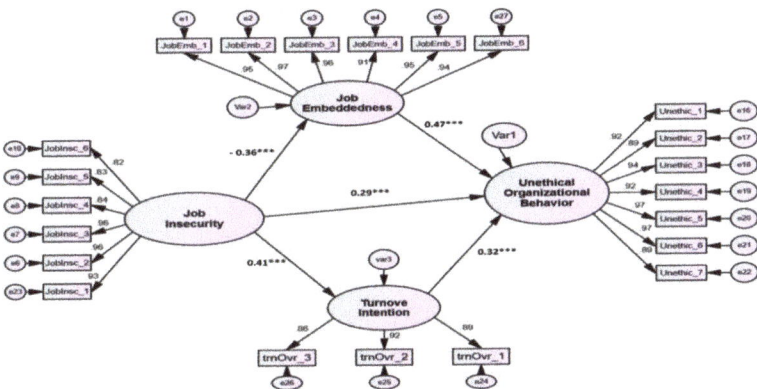

Figure 2. Research model (developed by authors). *** Significant level is less than 0.001.

Table 4. Result of the structural model (developed by authors).

		Hypotheses	Beta (β)	C-R (T-Value)	R^2	Hypotheses Results
H1	Job Insecurity	Unethical organizational behavior	0.29 ***	6.320		Supported
H2	Job Insecurity	Job embeddedness	−0.36 ***	−9.448		Supported
H3	Job Insecurity	Turnover intention	0.41 ***	10.221		Supported
H4	Job embeddedness	Unethical organizational behavior	0.47 ***	11.116		Supported
H5	Turnover intention	Unethical organizational behavior	0.32 ***	7.252		Supported
	Unethical organizational behavior				0.42	

Model fit: (χ^2 (204, N = 685) = 612.204, $p < 0.001$, normed χ^2 = 3.001, RMSEA = 0.050, SRMR = 0.051, CFI = 0.924, TLI = 0.927, NFI = 0.929, PCFI = 0.719 and PNFI = 0.706). *** $p < 0.00$, n/s = not significant.

The power of the tested structural model is further proven by the significant coefficient of determination (R^2) value of 0.42 percent of the variance in unethical organizational behavior can be explained through job insecurity, job embeddedness, and turnover intention.

Additionally, besides the previous direct relationships, the Amos output can provide further information about the indirect effects that can be employed to test the mediation effects in the tested model. To investigate the mediation of job embeddedness and turnover intention in the relationship between job insecurity and unethical organizational behavior, the recommendations of [63,64] were adopted. According to Zhao et al. [64], for a direct-only non-mediation impact, only a direct relationship must exist and be significant; for complementary mediation, both direct and indirect effects must exist and be significant with the same signs. Finally, if both direct and indirect effects are significant with opposite signs, competitive mediation is obtained.

Accordingly, as pictured in Figure 2 and displayed in Table 4, the direct path from job insecurity to turnover intention is positive and significant (β = +0.29, $p < 0.001$); and turnover intention positively and significantly affects unethical organizational behavior (β = +0.32, $p > 0.001$), hence complementary mediation is supported for the mediation effect of turnover intention in the relationship between job insecurity and unethical organizational behavior. On the other hand, the direct path from job insecurity to job embeddedness is negative but significant (β = −0.36, $p < 0.001$); and job embeddedness positively and significantly affects unethical organizational behavior (β = +0.47, $p > 0.001$); hence, competitive mediation is supported for the mediation effect of job embeddedness in the relationship between job insecurity and unethical organizational behavior.

5. Discussion and Contributions

The COVID-19 pandemic has spread across multiple countries at the same time and has harmed numerous industries, including the hospitality industry. Multiple approaches have been used to flatten the COVID-19 curve, including lockdowns, social distancing measures, quarantine at home, and travel restrictions, resulting in the temporary closure of many hospitality organizations [65]. Accordingly, hospitality businesses have reacted to the massive losses experienced amid the pandemic by laying off most of their employees. Because employees in developing countries (i.e., Egypt) may be more exposed to job insecurity as a result of inadequate employment protection laws or poor economic environments [66,67], the current study has an exceptional context by testing the impacts of job insecurity on unethical organization behavior among hospitality employees (hotels and travel agents) in a developing country (i.e., Egypt) amid the COVID-19 pandemic.

This paper has attempted to explore and understand the psychological process through which unethical behaviors and decisions are conducted by employees who encountered job insecurity. A total of 650 employees working in the hotel industry and travel agent companies were surveyed to better explain and predict in what way and under what circumstances employees faced with potential job loss amid the COVID-19 pandemic are prone to participate in unethical behaviors. Job embeddedness and turnover intention were employed as mediating variables.

Consistent with the expectations and previous studies' results [68–74], job insecurity was found to reduce job embeddedness, reinforce the turnover intention, and promote employees' unethical organizational behavior. However, there are scarce studies conducted in non-Western countries on these relationships [75]. Consequently, this research contributed to the literature by studying these relationships in the Egyptian context. Scholars have found that employees overcome the perception of job insecurity by working hard, seeking help from others [34,76], and engaging in impression management [77]. However, there is scarce research that examines employees' reactions to job insecurity by practicing behaviors that are unethical but are in the name of the company.

Job insecurity was found to directly increase employees' unethical behavior in the name of the company. Employees may practice unethical organizational behavior that may, in turn, assist them to be perceived as valuable to the organization and, accordingly, retain employment or employment benefits. This result is consistent with [21], in which it was found that job insecurity promotes employees' unethical behavior.

Following [74,78], job insecurity was found to have a negative impact on employee embeddedness to the organizations, especially amid the COVID-19 pandemic. When employees feel the risk of future job loss and insecurity, they begin to reconsider their job and their future career path in the company [32]. This causes them to lose association with their supervisors and destruction in the match and alignment between their beliefs and values and those of the organization. Due to a lack of empirical study on the factors that influence job embeddedness [79], this result can enhance our understanding of such a relationship. Job embeddedness, in turn, was found to promote employees' unethical behavior in the name of the company. This result is consistent with [31], who argued that, as a result of increased levels of alignment and attachment between the employees and the company, employees with higher levels of embeddedness will exhibit unethical behaviors in the name of the organization.

Additionally, the current study gives evidence that when employees feel insecure, their turnover intention is increased. This result is consistent with the study by [80]. Furthermore, several previous studies have shown that job insecurity impacts job dissatisfaction and intention to quit the job [81,82]. Turnover intention, in turn, can increase the employees' unethical behaviors in the name of the company in the hopes that their sacrifices will be rewarded with ongoing employment.

This study provides two contributions to practitioners and academics. First, job insecurity should be a high priority for top-level management and human resource managers in hospitality organizations because it leads to a variety of negative consequences not only for employees but for the organization as well. These consequences can include reduced job embeddedness, low job satisfaction, reduced trust in management, poor organizational performance, increases in unethical organizational behavior, and high turnover intention. The study, as well, highlighted the mediating role of job embeddedness and turnover intention in increasing the effect of job insecurity on unethical organizational behavior, as the direct impact of job insecurity on unethical organizational behavior was further strengthened through these two mediators. Testing these relationships may enhance academic's understanding of the nature of the relationships between job insecurity and unethical behavior.

Second, the study has further implications for managers in the hospitality industry. In the context of a developing country (e.g., Egypt), where unemployment levels are substantially high [8], job insecurity amid the pandemic may have destructive outcomes for hospitality businesses. Perceived job insecurity may threaten the reputation and goodwill of the hospitality industry due to employee's practicing unethical behavior in the name of the company to retain employment or employment benefits. Consequently, amid such a severe pandemic, managers in the hospitality industry should avoid sending out signals that may cause their employees to believe that they are in danger of losing their jobs. Any uncertainty or miscommunication on the side of management can lead to workers' feelings of insecurity, resulting in low job embeddedness and high turnover intention, and can promote unethical behavior in the name of the company.

6. Study Limitations and Directions for Future Research

This study has four limitations. First, job embeddedness and turnover intention were found to be partially mediated by the impact of job insecurity on unethical organizational behavior. However, other variables (e.g., justice, job satisfaction, and trust in supervisor,) may also intervene in this relationship. As a result, future studies should look at whether the impacts are direct or are mediated by factors other than job embeddedness and turnover intention. Second, due to the cross-sectional nature of the data obtained, causal correlations among the variables cannot be deduced. Third, although we attempted to avoid common technique bias [36], future researchers could employ longitudinal data or a variety of data sources. Fourth, a different model can be employed to test these relationships in different contexts using a multi-group analysis technique [83].

Author Contributions: Conceptualization, I.A.E. and A.M.S.A.; methodology, I.A.E. and A.M.S.A.; software, I.A.E.; validation, I.A.E. and A.M.S.A.; formal analysis, I.A.E. and A.M.S.A.; investigation, I.A.E. and A.M.S.A.; resources, I.A.E.; data curation, I.A.E.; writing—original draft preparation, I.A.E. and A.M.S.A.; writing—review and editing, I.A.E. and A.M.S.A.; visualization, I.A.E.; supervision, I.A.E.; project administration, I.A.E. and A.M.S.A.; funding acquisition, I.A.E. and A.M.S.A. All authors have read and agreed to the published version of the manuscript.

Funding: The authors acknowledge the Deanship of Scientific Research at King Faisal University for the financial support under Nasher Track (Grant No. NA000163).

Institutional Review Board Statement: The study was conducted according to the guidelines of the Declaration of Helsinki and approved by the deanship of scientific research ethical committee, King Faisal University (project number: NA000163, date of approval: 1 October 2021).

Informed Consent Statement: Informed consent was obtained from all subjects involved in the study.

Data Availability Statement: Data is available upon request from researchers who meet the eligibility criteria. Kindly contact the first author privately through e-mail.

Conflicts of Interest: The authors declare no conflict of interest.

References

1. International Labor Organization. *ILO: As job losses escalate, nearly half of global workforce at risk of losing livelihoods*; International Labour Organization, 2020. Available online: https://www.ilo.org/global/about-the-ilo/newsroom/news/WCMS_743036/lang--en/index.htm (accessed on 30 April 2019).
2. Jones, L.; Palumbo, D.; Brown, D. Coronavirus: A Visual Guide to the Economic Impact. *BBC News*. 2020. Available online: https://www.unic.ac.cy/da/2020/05/08/coronavirus-a-visual-guide-to-the-economic-impact-bbc-news/ (accessed on 3 December 2020).
3. Frank, T. *Hardest-Hit Industries: Nearly Half the Leisure and Hospitality Jobs were Lost in April*; CNBC, 2020. Available online: https://www.cnbc.com/2020/05/08/l (accessed on 30 April 2019).
4. Calderwood, L.U.; Soshkin, M. *The Travel & Tourism Competitiveness Report 2019. Travel and Tourism at a Tipping Point*; World Economic Forum: Geneva, Switzerland, 2019. Available online: https://apo.org.au/node/257631 (accessed on 30 April 2019).
5. Rivera, M. Hitting the reset button for hospitality research in times of crisis: COVID-19 and beyond. *Int. J. Hosp. Manag.* **2020**, *87*, 102528. [CrossRef] [PubMed]
6. Karmin, C. Marriott begins furloughing tens of thousands of employees. *Wall Str. J.* **2020**. Available online: https://www.wsj.com/articles/marriott-starting-to-furlough-tens-of-thousands-of-employees-11584459417 (accessed on 30 April 2019).
7. Kelly, J. Airbnb lays off 25% of its employees: CEO brian chesky gives a master class in empathy and compassion. *Forbes* **2020**. Available online: https://www.forbes.com/sites/jackkelly/2020/05/06/airbnb-lays-off-25-of-its-employees-ceo-brian-chesky-gives-a-master-class-in-empathy-and-compassion/ (accessed on 30 April 2019).
8. Saad, S.K.; Elshaer, I.A. Justice and trust's role in employees "resilience and business" continuity: Evidence from Egypt. *Tour. Manag. Perspect.* **2020**, *35*, 100712. [CrossRef]
9. Cheng, G.H.L.; Chan, D.K.S. Who suffers more from job insecurity? A meta-analytic review. *Appl. Psychol.* **2008**, *57*, 272–303. [CrossRef]
10. Jung, H.S.; Jung, Y.S.; Yoon, H.H. COVID-19: The effects of job insecurity on the job engagement and turnover intent of deluxe hotel employees and the moderating role of generational characteristics. *Int. J. Hosp. Manag.* **2021**, *92*, 102703. [CrossRef] [PubMed]
11. Darvishmotevali, M.; Arasli, H.; Kilic, H. Effect of job insecurity on frontline employee's performance. *Int. J. Contemp. Hosp. Manag.* **2017**, *29*, 1724–1744. [CrossRef]

12. Etehadi, B.; Karatepe, O.M. The impact of job insecurity on critical hotel employee outcomes: The mediating role of self-efficacy. *J. Hosp. Mark. Manag.* **2019**, *28*, 665–689. [CrossRef]
13. Shin, Y.; Hur, W.M. When do service employees suffer more from job insecurity? The moderating role of coworker and customer incivility. *Int. J. Environ. Res. Public Health* **2019**, *16*, 1298. [CrossRef]
14. Akgunduz, Y.; Eryilmaz, G. Does turnover intention mediate the effects of job insecurity and co-worker support on social loafing? *Int. J. Hosp. Manag.* **2018**, *68*, 41–49. [CrossRef]
15. Boswell, W.R.; Olson-Buchanan, J.B.; Harris, T.B. I cannot afford to have a life: Employee adaptation to feeling of job insecurity. *Pers. Psychol.* **2014**, *67*, 887–915. [CrossRef]
16. Yi, X.; Wang, S. Revisiting the curvilinear relation between job insecurity and work withdrawal: The moderating role of achievement orientation and risk aversion. *Hum. Resour. Manag.* **2015**, *54*, 499–515. [CrossRef]
17. Hirsch, P.M.; De Soucey, M. Organizational restructuring and its consequences: Rhetorical and structural. *Annu. Rev. Sociol.* **2006**, *32*, 171–189. [CrossRef]
18. Burchell, B. The prevalence and redistribution of job insecurity and work intensification. In *Job Insecurity and Work Intensification*; Burchell, B., Ladipo, D., Wilkinson, F., Eds.; Routledge: London, UK, 2002; pp. 61–76.
19. Debus, M.E.; Probst, T.M.; Konig, C.J.; Kleinmann, M. Catch me if I fall! Enacted uncertainty avoidance and the social safety net as country-level moderators in the job insecurity-job attitudes link. *J. Appl. Psychol.* **2012**, *97*, 690–698. [CrossRef]
20. Keim, A.C.; Landis, R.S.; Pierce, C.A.; Earnest, D.R. Why do employees worry about their job? A meta-analytical review of predictors of job insecurity. *J. Occup. Health Psychol.* **2014**, *19*, 269–290.
21. Umphress, E.E.; Bingham, J.B.; Mitchell, M.S. Unethical behavior in the name of the company: The moderating effect of organizational identification and positive reciprocity beliefs on unethical pro-organizational behavior. *J. Appl. Psychol.* **2010**, *95*, 769. [CrossRef]
22. Greenhalgh, L.; Rosenblatt, Z. Evolution of research on job insecurity. *Int. Stud. Manag. Organ.* **2010**, *40*, 6–19. [CrossRef]
23. Tu, Y.; Long, L.; Wang, H.J.; Jiang, L. To prevent or to promote: How regulatory focus moderates the differentiated effects of quantitative versus qualitative job insecurity on employee stress and motivation. *Int. J. Stress Manag.* **2020**, *27*, 1–135. [CrossRef]
24. Martin, K.D.; Cullen, J. Continuities and extensions of ethical climate theory: A meta-analytic review. *J. Bus. Ethics* **2006**, *69*, 175–194. [CrossRef]
25. Frone, M.R. What happened to the employed during the Great Recession? A US population study of net change in employee insecurity, health, and organizational commitment. *J. Vocat. Behav.* **2018**, *107*, 246–260. [CrossRef]
26. Meyer, J.P.; Allen, N.J. Testing the 'side-bet theory' of organizational commitment: Some methodological considerations. *J. Appl. Psychol.* **1984**, *69*, 372–378. [CrossRef]
27. Niesen, W.; Hootegem, A.V.; Handaja, Y.; Battistelli, A.; De Witte, H. Quantitative and qualitative job insecurity and idea generation: The mediating role of psychological contract breach. *Scan. J. Work. Organ. Psychol.* **2018**, *3*, 1–14. [CrossRef]
28. Vohs, K.D.; Schmeichel, B.J. Self-regulation and extended now: Controlling the self-alters the subjective experience of time. *J. Pers. Soc. Psychol.* **2003**, *85*, 217. [CrossRef] [PubMed]
29. Baumeister, R.F. Esteem threat, self-regulatory breakdown, and emotional distress. *Rev. Gen. Psychol.* **1997**, *2*, 145–174. [CrossRef]
30. Baumeister, R.F. Ego depletion, the executive function, and self-control: An energy model of the self in personality. In *Personality Psychology in the Workplace: Decade of Behavior: 299–316*; Roberts, B.W., Hogan, R., Eds.; American Psychological Association: Washington, DC, USA, 2001.
31. Mitchell, T.R.; Holtom, B.C.; Lee, T.W.; Sablynski, C.J.; Erez, M. Why people stay: Using job embeddedness to predict voluntary turnover. *Acad. Manage. J.* **2001**, *44*, 1102–1121.
32. Murphy, W.M.; Burton, J.P.; Henagan, S.C.; Briscoe, J.P. Employee reactions to job insecurity in a declining economy: A longitudinal study of the mediating role of job embeddedness. *Group. Organ. Manag.* **2013**, *38*, 512–537. [CrossRef]
33. Gok, O.A.; Akgunduz, Y.; Alkan, C. The effects of job stress and perceived organizational support on turnover intentions of hotel employees *Ozge. J. Tour.* **2012**, *3*, 23–32.
34. Elshaer, I.A.; Saad, S.K. Political instability and tourism in Egypt: Exploring survivors' attitudes after downsizing. *J. Policy Res. Tour. Leis. Events* **2017**, *9*, 3–22.
35. Bajrami, D.D.; Terzić, A.; Petrović, M.D.; Radovanović, M.; Tretiakova, T.N.; Hadoud, A. Will we have the same employees in hospitality after all? The impact of COVID-19 on employees' work attitudes and turnover intentions. *Int. J. Hosp. Manag.* **2021**, *94*, 102754.
36. Podsakoff, N.P.; LePine, J.A.; LePine, M.A. Differential challenge stressor-hindrance stressor relationships with job attitudes, turnover intentions, turnover, and withdrawal behavior: A meta-analysis. *J. Appl. Psychol.* **2007**, *92*, 438–454. [CrossRef]
37. Adams, J.S. Toward an understanding of inequity. *J. Abnorm. Soc. Psychol.* **1963**, *67*, 422–436. [CrossRef]
38. Adams, J.S. Inequity in social exchange. In *Advances in Experimental Social Psychology*; Berkowitz, L., Ed.; Academic Press: Cambridge, MA, USA, 1965; Volume 2, pp. 267–299.
39. Hanafiah, M. Pengaruh kepuasan kerja dan ketidakamanan kerja (job insecurity) dengan intensi pindah kerja (turnover) pada karyawan PT. *J. Psikol.* **2014**, *1*, 303–312.
40. Yaqub, R.M.S.; Mahmood, S.; Hussain, N.; Sohail, H.A. Ethical leadership and turnover intention: A moderated mediation model of job embeddedness and organizational commitment. *Bull. Bus. Econ.* **2021**, *10*, 16–34.

41. Crossley, C.D.; Bennett, R.J.; Jex, S.M.; Burnfield, J.L. Development of a global measure of job embeddedness and integration io a traditional model of voluntary turnover. *J. Appl. Psychol.* **2007**, *92*, 1031–1042. [CrossRef] [PubMed]
42. Yao, T.; Qiu, Q.; Wei, Y. Retaining hotel employees as internal customers: Effect of organizational commitment on attitudinal and behavioral loyalty of employees. *Int. J. Hosp. Manag.* **2019**, *76*, 1–8. [CrossRef]
43. Holtom, B.C.; Inderrieden, E.J. Integrating the unfolding model and job embeddedness model to better understand voluntary turnover. *J. Manag.* **2006**, *18*, 435–452.
44. Eberly, M.; Holtmon, B.; Lee, T.; Mitchell, T. Control voluntary turnover by understanding its causes. In *Handbook of Principles of Organizational Behavior*; Locke, E.A., Ed.; John Wiley & Sons: New York, NY, USA, 2009.
45. Baumeister, R.F. The self. In *Handbook of Social Psychology*, 4th ed.; Gilbert, D.T., Fiske, S.T., Lindzey, G., Eds.; McGraw-Hill: New York, NY, USA, 1998; pp. 680–740.
46. Baumeister, R.F.; Bushman, B.J. *Social Psychology and Human Nature*, 2nd ed.; Wadsworth: Belmont, CA, USA, 2010.
47. Maddox, R.N. Measuring satisfaction with tourism. *J. Travel. Res.* **1985**, *23*, 2–5. [CrossRef]
48. Churchill, G.A., Jr. A paradigm for developing better measures of marketing constructs. *J. Mark. Res.* **1979**, *16*, 64–73. [CrossRef]
49. Karatepe, O. An investigation of the joint effects of organizational tenure and supervisor support on work-family conflict and turnover intentions. *J. Hosp. Tour. Manag.* **2009**, *16*, 73–81. [CrossRef]
50. Singh, J.; Verbeke, W.; Rhoads, G.K. Do Organizational Practices Matter in Role Stress Processes? A Study of Direct and Moderating Effects for Marketing-Oriented Boundary Spanners. *J. Mark.* **1996**, *60*, 69–86. [CrossRef]
51. Hellgren, J.; Sverke, M.; Isaksson, K. A two-dimensional approach to job insecurity: Consequences for employee attitudes and well-being. *Eur. J. Work. Organ. Psychol.* **1999**, *8*, 179–195. [CrossRef]
52. Douglas, S.P.; Craig, C.S. Collaborative and iterative translation: An alternative approach to back translation. *J. Int. Mark.* **2007**, *15*, 30–43. [CrossRef]
53. Ibeh, K.; Brock, J.K.U.; Zhou, Y.J. The drop and collect survey among industrial populations: Theory and empirical evidence. *Ind. Mark. Manag.* **2004**, *33*, 155–165. [CrossRef]
54. Armstrong, J.S.; Overton, T. Estimating nonresponse bias in mail surveys. *J. Mark. Res.* **1977**, *14*, 396–402. [CrossRef]
55. Podsakoff, P.M.; Organ, D.W. Self-reports in organizational research: Problems and prospects. *J. Manag.* **1986**, *12*, 531–544. [CrossRef]
56. Bryman, A.; Cramer, D. *Quantitative Data Analysis with IBM SPSS 17, 18 & 19: A Guide for Social Scientists*; Routledge: London, UK, 2012.
57. Kline, R.B. *Principles and Practice of Structural Equation Modeling*; Guilford Publications: New York, NY, USA, 2015.
58. Guo, L.; Xiao, J.J.; Tang, C. Understanding the psychological process underlying customer satisfaction and retention in a relational service. *J. Bus. Res.* **2009**, *62*, 1152–1159. [CrossRef]
59. Hair, J.; Anderson, R.; Tatham, R.; Black, W. *Multivariate Data Analysis*; Prentice Hall: Saddle River, NJ, USA, 2014.
60. Anderson, J.C.; Gerbing, D.W. Structural equation modeling in practice: A review and recommended two-step approach. *Psychol. Bull.* **1988**, *103*, 411. [CrossRef]
61. Joreskog, K.G. Analysis of covariance structures. In *The Handbook of Multivariate Experimental Psychology*; Cattell, R.B., Nessclroade, J.R., Eds.; Plenum Press: New York, NY, USA, 1988; pp. 207–230.
62. Fornell, C.; Larcker, D. Evaluating structural equation models with unobservable variables and measurement error. *J. Mark. Res.* **1981**, *18*, 39–50. [CrossRef]
63. Kelloway, E.K. Structural equation modelling in perspective. *J. Organ. Behav.* **1995**, *16*, 215–224. [CrossRef]
64. Zhao, X.; Lynch, J.G., Jr.; Chen, Q. Reconsidering Baron and Kenny: Myths and truths about mediation analysis. *J. Consum. Res.* **2010**, *37*, 197–206. [CrossRef]
65. Bartik, A.W.; Bertrand, M.; Cullen, Z.B.; Glaeser, E.L.; Luca, M.; Stanton, C.T. *How are Small Businesses Adjusting to Covid-19? Early Evidence from a Survey (No. w26989)*; National Bureau of Economic Research: Chicago, IL, USA, 2020.
66. Raja, U.; Sheikh, R.A.; Abbas, M.; Bouckenooghe, D. Do procedures really matter when rewards are more important? A Pakistani perspective on the effects of distributive and procedural justice on employee behaviors. *Eur. Rev. Appl. Psychol.* **2018**, *68*, 79–88. [CrossRef]
67. Sulemana, I.; Bofah, R.O.; Nketiah-Amponsah, E. Job insecurity and life satisfaction in Ghana. *J. Fam. Econ. Issues* **2020**, *41*, 172–184.
68. Abbas, M.; Malik, M.; Sarwat, N. Consequences of job insecurity for hospitality workers amid COVID-19 pandemic: Does social support help? *J. Hosp. Mark. Manag.* **2021**, *30*, 957–981. [CrossRef]
69. Chirumbolo, A.; Hellgren, J. Individual and organizational consequences of job insecurity: A European study. *Econ. Ind. Democr.* **2003**, *24*, 217–240. [CrossRef]
70. Emberland, J.S.; Rundmo, T. Implications of job insecurity perceptions and job insecurity responses for psychological well-being, turnover intentions and reported risk behavior. *Saf. Sci.* **2010**, *48*, 452–459. [CrossRef]
71. Ghosh, S.K. The direct and interactive effects of job insecurity and job embeddedness on unethical pro-organizational behavior: An empirical examination. *Pers. Rev.* **2017**, *46*, 1–17. [CrossRef]
72. Lawrence, E.R.; Kacmar, K.M. Exploring the impact of job insecurity on employees' unethical behavior. *Bus. Ethics Q.* **2017**, *27*, 39–70. [CrossRef]
73. Obeng, A.F.; Quansah, P.E.; Boakye, E. The Relationship between Job Insecurity and Turnover Intention: The Mediating Role of Employee Morale and Psychological Strain. *Management* **2020**, *10*, 35–45.

74. Safavi, H.P.; Karatepe, O.M. The effect of job insecurity on employees' job outcomes: The mediating role of job embeddedness. *J. Manag. Dev.* **2019**, *38*, 288–297. [CrossRef]
75. Hur, H.; Perry, J.L. The relationship between job security and work attitudes: A meta-analysis examining competing theoretical models. In Proceedings of the APSA 2014 Annual Meeting Paper, Indiana University, Bloomington, CA, USA, 21 August 2014. Bloomington School of Public & Environmental Affairs Research Paper (No. 2452082).
76. Armstrong-Stassen, M. Determinants of how managers cope with organisational downsizing. *Appl. Psychol.* **2006**, *55*, 1–26. [CrossRef]
77. Huang, G.H.; Zhao, H.H.; Niu, X.Y.; Ashford, S.J.; Lee, C. Reducing job insecurity and increasing performance ratings: Does impression management matter? *J. Appl. Psychol.* **2013**, *98*, 852. [CrossRef]
78. King, J.E. White Collar Reactions to Job Insecurity and the Role of the Psychological Contract: Implications of Human Resource Management. *Hum. Resour. Manag.* **2000**, *39*, 79–92. [CrossRef]
79. Singh, R. Developing organisational embeddedness: Employee personality and social networking. *Int. J. Hum. Resour. Manag.* **2019**, *30*, 2445–2464. [CrossRef]
80. Brougham, D. and Haar, J. Technological disruption and employment: The influence on job insecurity and turnover intentions: A multi-country study. *Technol. Forecast. Soc. Change* **2020**, *161*, 120276. [CrossRef]
81. Ashford, S.J.; Lee, C.; Bobko, P. Content, cause, and consequences of job insecurity: A theory-based measure and substantive test. *Acad. Manag. J.* **1989**, *32*, 803–829.
82. Davy, J.A.; Kinicki, A.J.; Scheck, C.L. Developing and testing a model of survivor responses to layoffs. *J. Vocat. Behav.* **1991**, *38*, 302–317. [CrossRef]
83. Elshaer, I.A.; Augustyn, M.M. Testing the dimensionality of the quality management construct. *Total. Qual. Manag. Bus. Excell.* **2016**, *27*, 353–367. [CrossRef]

Article

An Unethical Organizational Behavior for the Sake of the Family: Perceived Risk of Job Insecurity, Family Motivation and Financial Pressures

Ibrahim A. Elshaer [1,2,*], Marwa Ghanem [3] and Alaa M. S. Azazz [3,4,*]

1. Department of Management, College of Business Administration, King Faisal University, Al-Ahsaa 31982, Saudi Arabia
2. Hotel Studies Department, Faculty of Tourism and Hotels, Suez Canal University, Ismailia 41522, Egypt
3. Tourism Studies Department, Faculty of Tourism and Hotels, Suez Canal University, Ismailia 41522, Egypt; marwamagdy00@gmail.com or M_ghanem@tourism.suez.edu.eg
4. Department of Tourism and Hospitality, Arts College, King Faisal University, Al-Ahsaa 31982, Saudi Arabia
* Correspondence: ielshaer@kfu.edu.sa (I.A.E.); aazazz@kfu.edu.sa (A.M.S.A.)

Abstract: In organizations, unethical behaviors are pervasive and costly, and considerable recent research attention has been paid to various types of workplace unethical behavior. This study examines employees' behaviors that are carried out for the benefit of one's family but violate societal and organizational moral standards. Drawing upon the self-maintenance and bounded ethicality theories, this study examines the engagement of unethical organization behaviors (UOB) in the name of the family during the COVID-19 pandemic. It examines the influence of job instability and the mediating role of family financial pressure and family motivation. A total of 770 employees in hotels and travel agents in Egypt were targeted, and the data were analyzed using structural equation modeling. The results posit that perceived risk of job insecurity predicts engagement in unethical organizational behaviors, while intentions of UOB increase by high family motivation and financial pressures. Toward the end of this paper, a discussion on the theoretical and practical implications and are presented.

Keywords: unethical organizational behaviors; job insecurity; family financial pressure; family motivation; COVID-19 pandemic; tourism

1. Introduction

Job loss and job insecurity were among the topics that were of most concern as consequences of the worldwide spread of the coronavirus. Export-dependent economies and economies that rely on tourism have struggled adjusting to fluctuating and shifting demand. The World Travel and Tourism Council (WTTC) suggested that the global job market was at risk for 75 million people in 2020 [1], while the World Economic Forum reported that the lockdown and layoff practices during the COVID-19 pandemic resulted in 114 million job losses in 2020 [2]. Even employees who survive the layoffs become anxious about their career and suffer high levels of job insecurity [3,4]. According to prior studies, job insecurity is a significant hindrance-related stress that negatively influence tourism business's ability to achieve its desired work [4–6] and can lead to absenteeism and anxiety [7].

As a result of the COVID-19 pandemic and according to social cognitive theory, employees who face job insecurity in addition to increased family financial strain are more likely to use moral disengagement practices to disable moral self-regulation, resulting in increased levels of unethical behavior. Moreover, researchers asserted that the heavy losses suffered by business organizations created significant unethical organizational practice [3,8,9]. Approximately 90% of companies indicate that COVID-19 is a risk to ethical behavior at work, according to a report from Ernst and Young [10]. Similarly, in a survey conducted in India by Bhattacharyya [11] during the COVID-19 outbreak, many employees were found to be willing to engage in unethical behavior, such as falsifying records of customers (32%) and disclosing false information to their managers (29%).

Researchers have recently been interested in researching the reasons behind unethical practices during the COVID-19 pandemic and understanding the relationship with job loss and perceived job insecurity. For example, guided by appraisal theories of emotion, Hillebrandt and Barclay [4] argued that COVID-19 provokes anxiety and can drive employees to prioritize their self-interest and promote cheating behavior in workplace. Elshaer and Azazz [3] surveyed 650 employees working in the Egyptian tourism industry to explore the psychological process that would drive unethical organizational behaviors by employees who contend with job insecurity. They found that perceived job insecurity reduces job embeddedness, strengthens turnover intentions, and encourages unethical behavior.

In addition, previous studies asserted that employees who suffer from stresses due to workplace threats (e.g., job insecurity) may conduct UOB as a way to protect their gains and job assets [12,13]. Employees conducting unethical organization behavior (UOB) can also be driven by self-serving interest to acquire personal gains [14] or benefiting their organization or group [15] while benefiting themselves accordingly [16]. Based on behavioral ethics research, people can generally fail to make an objective assessment of the ethics of their behavior in the workplace [17], since their cognitive biases cause them to underestimate or ignore their unethical behavior. Elshaer et al. [18] added that often, employees do not make an explicit decision to act unethically but rather seek to convince themselves that there is nothing wrong with their behavior. In general, UOB can lead to devastating effects, such as significant financial losses, legal prosecutions, and corporate closures [19,20]. While even simple unethical behaviors in organizations can lead to significant hidden costs, tarnishing employee morale and damaging a company's reputation [21].

Despite the thrive of behavioral ethics research, negative behavior displayed within organizations has such a wide scope that it is virtually not possible to explore within the scope of a few research projects [22], and various studied contexts are needed to unpack the drivers of UOB for mitigating resulting risks. Most previous research on unethical behavior in the workplace focus on unethical pro-organizational behavior (in the name of the company) [9] with little attention to unethical practices in the name of self-interest [22–24] or the family [2,25]. The prevalent unethical behaviors during the COVID-19 pandemic [3] and their possible relations with job insecurity [2] have raised significant questions about the different forms of unethical organizational behavior (UOB) during crises, the possible psychological process that drive such practices, and how it can be mitigated. Therefore, to address this gap of research and based on theories of conservation of resources, social cognitive and behavioral ethics (i.e., the self-maintenance and bounded ethicality theories), the current study aims to further investigate the effect of job insecurity on unethical organizational behavior among employees amid the COVID-19 pandemic, using family financial pressure and family motivation as mediating variables. The results of this study, thus, extend prior research results on conditions that shape unethical practices in the workplace and better explain the widespread UOB during the COVID-19 pandemic. It also provides insights into how organizations can address ethical challenges.

2. Theoretical Background and Hypotheses Development
2.1. Job Insecurity and Unethical Workplace Behavior

Job insecurity has long been a subject of study in a wide variety of research papers [2,4,26,27]. Numerous studies have been conducted in the hotel and tourism industries, notably on job insecurity and its effect on human behavior [2,28]. Job insecurity is a "perceptual phenomenon" that focuses on a person's current job stability threats [29]. Hellgren et al. [30] proposes two categories of job insecurity: quantitative "threats to the job as a whole" and qualitative "threats to desired job characteristics". Quantitative job insecurity focuses on the expected job loss triggered by intentional or unintentional administrative signals or appraisal reports by employees' supervisors, while qualitative job insecurity illustrates how an individual perceives their future job loss in light of a perceived threat [30].

Given the devastating effects of the COVID-19 pandemic on the economy, downsizing has become a common strategy in recent years. Downsizing is a method of reducing labor costs, streamlining operations, and increasing organizational competitiveness [31]. According to [32,33], organizational restructuring and the downsizing process have proved to threaten workers and their careers, resulting in exacerbating perceived job insecurity [34]. The resulting stresses of perceived job instability may motivate employees to engage in unethical actions that they believe might protect them against the threat of job loss or even keep some important features of their job [23,35–39]. Unethical workplace behavior may include actions that benefit the organization, group or employee self-interest, such as diminishing colleagues' efforts to improve personal relationships, reputations, and professional success [40]. Employees' activities and behaviors that are in direct conflict with the organization's norms and values may create significant financial losses [41] and jeopardize organizational image [42]. Accordingly, as shown in Figure 1, the below hypothesis is suggested:

Hypothesis 1 (H1). *Job insecurity has a positive impact on workplace unethical behavior.*

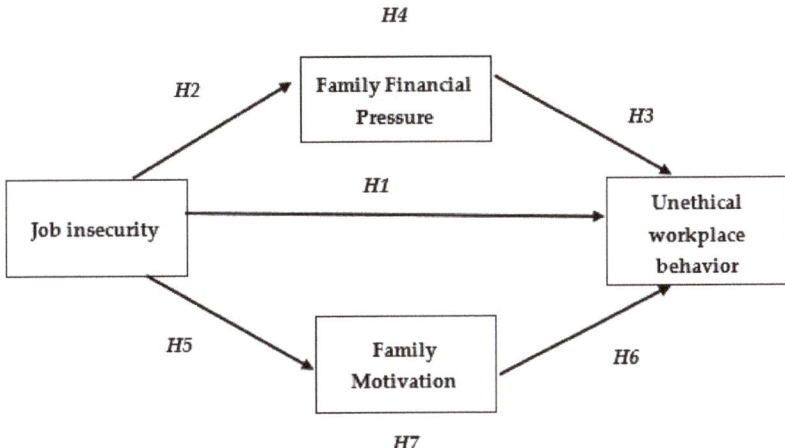

Figure 1. Research framework.

2.2. Job Insecurity, Family Financial Pressure, and Unethical Workplace Behavior

Employees as well as their families face financial difficulties as a result of the high percentage of job insecurity [43]. Despite remarkable advances in our understanding of the impact of job insecurity on well-being, stress, and health over the last several years [30,44], it is difficult to infer causality. Financial stress on the family (i.e., related to satisfying basic needs, family education cost, utilities payments, or family healthcare expenses) is likely to exacerbate job insecurity, which in turn leads to financial pressure [45,46]. A few research studies have explored the relationship between job insecurity and employees' financial well-being and pressure and provide contradicting results between significant [47] and insignificant [45] effects. Therefore, the relationship between job insecurity and family financial pressure requires further investigation.

Families' financial difficulties are not just felt by the impoverished; they are also felt by rich people who want to maintain pace with their friends. When confronted with strong financial difficulties from family members, an employee's principal purpose is to relieve those pressures. The more pressing the need, the more significant this goal will become. Generally, supporting one's family monetarily is a key worth in human culture [48]. Liu et al. [25] elaborated that social expectations are framed, and laws are laid out to uphold the satisfaction of familial monetary obligations. When stressed to assist their families, employees are bound to consider it to be their responsibility to make any strides important to help their family, subsequently obscuring their moral obligation regarding their actions.

Based on the theory of conservation of resources developed by Hobfoll [12], when people face a concern of losing their valuable resources, they become pressured to protect those resources by, for example, acquiring recuperation assets. Accordingly, when employees encounter substantial financial difficulties in their families, they are more likely to concentrate their efforts on obtaining financial compensation from their employer [46]. As a result, self-justification of immoral actions in the workplace can then thrive [49]. Unethical workplace activities may help alleviate the stress and aggravation felt by employees while simultaneously improving the financial well-being of the employees' families. Many sorts of unethical behavior in the name of the family are directly linked to financial advantages that might relieve financial stress, such as bringing organization possessions home for use or accompanying relatives to the workplace to gain benefit from the organization's resources.

According to the social cognitive theory proposed by Bandura [50] and the self-concept maintenance theory developed by Mazar et al. [51], the readiness of self-justifications encourages unethical behavior through an expanded moral disengagement. Self-justifications can make the UB looks less immoral; costs of the dishonest action are limited, disregarded, or confounded; or casualties of the wrongdoing are undervalued or accused. In summary, when family financial pressures are increased because of perceived job insecurity, employees may become more likely to participate in unethical workplace behavior to benefit their family and decrease these related stresses. Thus, the following hypotheses were proposed:

Hypothesis 2 (H2). *Job insecurity has a significant impact on family financial pressure.*

Hypothesis 3 (H3). *Family financial pressure has a significant impact on unethical workplace behavior.*

Hypothesis 4 (H4). *Family financial pressure mediates the impact of job insecurity and unethical workplace behavior.*

2.3. Job Insecurity, Family Motivation, and Unethical Workplace Behavior

Supporting one's family is a significant justification for why many people work, yet surprisingly few researchers have investigated the effects of family motivation [47], particularly in relation to perceived pressures and job insecurity. Moreover, Liu et al. [25] noted that no previous study has thoroughly examined the role of the family as a motivating factor for unethical behavior in organizations. Menges et al. ([47], p. 700) defines family motivation as *"the desire to expend effort to benefit one's family"*. Prior research suggested that workers with a high family motive are more likely to prioritize family concerns and perceive the family's best interests as a main consideration [25,46,48]. This would likely drive employees who place a high value on their families to justify immoral behavior in the workplace since it benefits them personally and socially as well as their own families [52,53].

Relatedly, previous studies [53–55] explained that employees ted to perceive their desire protect to benefit another party's or beneficiaries' interest (family members in this study) as a moral (ease-to-use) justification for unethical behavior. Based on the concept of bounded ethicality, an employee may often behave unethically as he/she either consciously or unconsciously was able to disregard and justify his/her own misconduct [30].

Accordingly, this study suggests that when job insecurity increases, workers with high family motivation may engage in unethical practices to benefit their family interests and will demonstrate less attention to organizational moral standards. In other words, whether individuals choose to be engaged in unethical organizational behavior (UOB) that violates the moral code and interests of the firm can be determined by their familial motives. Employees thus become more prone to justify their unethical workplace behavior in order to alleviate their job insecurity:

Hypothesis 5 (H5). *Job insecurity has a significant impact on family motives.*

Hypothesis 6 (H6). *Family motivation has a significant impact on unethical workplace behavior.*

Hypothesis 7 (H7). *Family motivation mediates the impact of job insecurity on unethical workplace behavior.*

3. Methodological Approach

3.1. Development of Study Measures and Instrument

The formulation of the scales in this study was based on an extensive survey of previously employed theoretical items in the literature. This survey creates four factors, each with their own set of items, which are then revised to fit the context of the hospitality industry (Hotels and travel agents). The operationalization of the study variables is depicted in Table 1.

We use the fundamental processes proposed by Maddox [56] and Churchill [57] to create 21 variables (questions) on a standard five-point Likert scale, where strongly disagree is 1 and strongly agree is 5. The items measuring job insecurity were created with a multi-item scale developed by Hellgren et al. [30] and employed by Elshaer and Azazz [3] in the tourism industry. Family financial pressures were operationalized by three variables based on the work of Conger et al. [58] and employed by Elshaer and Azazz [3] in the hotel industry. We adopted the five items of family motivation of Menges et al. [47]; a sample item is "It is important for me to do good for my family". Finally, unethical workplace behavior in the name of the family was measured by seven items derived from Liu et al. [25]; a sample item is "I took advantage of my position in the company to make things more convenient for my family".

The questionnaire was formerly in English; then, the back-translation approach was adopted [59]. Three qualified academics (obtained Ph.D. degrees from UK) translated the research questionnaire from its original language (English) to respondents' language (Arabic). Furthermore, another three academics conducted the back translation from respondents' language (Arabic) to English. The resulted revealed that the two versions were the same and consistent with no differences. Using extensive pre-testing and piloting stages, the research instrument was internally validated with input from six academics and fifteen employees in the field of the hospitality industry. The pilot participants indicated the measures' high consistency and face and content validity. The final instrument was administered to 1000 employees working in five-star hotels and travel agents in greater Cairo, Egypt.

3.2. Process of Collecting Data

The study data were gathered in a three-waves process from 30 five-star hotels and 35 travel agents classified as category A in greater Cairo, Egypt. It was decided to use the three-wave approach, with at least a one-month period between each wave, in order to reduce the probability of common method variance (CMV) [60]. Participants in the first wave (W1) provided information about their demographics as well as their perceptions of job insecurity. After one month (W2), participants who had completed the first wave were surveyed regarding unethical workplace behavior in the name of the family. After one more month (W3), those who completed both the W1 and W2 surveys answered questions about family financial stress and family motivation. To ensure that the data collected in all three waves came from the same respondents, a coding system was used. The participants were chosen with the help of the hotels/travel agencies mangers who agreed to let us use their staff lists for scientific purpose. A total of 1000 non-managerial employees were randomly chosen to participate in the three waves (W1, W2, and W3) of the survey process; replies were obtained from 890, 800, and 770 people, respectively, demonstrating response rates of 89%, 80%, and 77%, respectively.

Table 1. Descriptive statistics.

Abbreviation	Items	M	S.D	Skewness	Kurtosis	VIF
Job insecurity—Job_Inst—Hellgren et al. [30]						
Job_Inst_1	"I am worried that I will have to leave my job before I would like to."	3.51	1.1496	−0.412	−0.578	1.110
Job_Inst_2	"I worry about being able to keep my job."	3.51	1.163	−0.399	−0.634	3.542
Job_Inst_3	"I am afraid I may lose my job shortly."	3.54	1.125	−0.399	−0.561	3.529
Job_Inst_4	"I worry about getting less stimulating work tasks in the future."	3.46	1.180	−0.424	−0.502	2.979
Job_Inst_5	"I worry about my future wage development."	3.47	1.176	−0.427	−0.487	2.133
Job_Inst_6	"I feel worried about my career development in the organization."	3.46	1.198	−0.471	−0.456	2.891
Family financial pressure—Fin_Pres—Conger et al. [58]						
Fin_Pres_1	"My family can hardly make ends meet."	4.11	0.661	−1.288	1.601	1.589
Fin_Pres_2	"My family has difficulty paying its monthly bills."	4.13	0.671	−1.306	1.404	1.137
Fin_Pres_3	"My family has little money left at the end of the month."	4.10	0.649	−1.283	1.922	1.464
Family Motivation—Fam_Motiv—Menges et al. [47]						
Fam_Motiv_1	"I care about supporting my family."	3.58	1.239	−0.412	−0.966	2.101
Fam_Motiv_2	"I want to help my family."	3.53	1.188	−0.339	−0.940	3.065
Fam_Motiv_3	"I want to have a positive impact on my family."	3.61	1.168	−0.341	−0.977	1.290
Fam_Motiv_4	"It is important for me to do good for my family."	3.48	1.208	−0.338	−0.959	2.141
Fam_Motiv_5	"My family benefits from my job."	3.51	1.202	−0.359	−0.927	3.842
Unethical workplace behavior in the name of the family—Unethic—Liu et al. [25]						
Unethic_1	"To help my family, I took company assets/supplies home for family use."	3.82	1.248	−1.023	0.062	3.196
Unethic_2	"To help my family, I submitted my family's household receipts (e.g., gas) to my company for reimbursement."	3.74	1.263	−0.937	−0.158	3.250
Unethic_3	"I took my family members to work to enjoy company resources and benefits that were intended for employees."	3.78	1.241	−0.987	0.033	3.556

Table 1. Cont.

Abbreviation	Items	M	S.D	Skewness	Kurtosis	VIF
Unethic_4	"I took advantage of my position in the company to make things more convenient for my family."	3.77	1.252	−0.997	0.004	3.740
Unethic_5	"I helped my family member get a job in my organization, even though I knew the family member was not qualified."	3.73	1.270	−0.923	−0.160	3.477
Unethic_6	"I disclosed confidential company information to my family members so that they can have advantages/benefits."	3.72	1.293	−0.934	−0.203	2.471
Unethic_7	"To help my family, I spent work resources to deal with family-related issues when at work."	3.70	1.293	−0.892	−0.290	3.166

4. Results

4.1. Descriptive Statistics

Of the 770 who completed the questionnaires in the final third wave, 70% were male. Ten percent of those who responded in the final wave were between the ages of 18 and 23, 15% were 24–29 years old, 25% were 30–35 years old, 30% were 36–41 years old, and 20% were above 42 years old. In terms of education, 50% of the participants achieved high school level, 30% obtained a college degree, and 20% had a bachelor's level or above. Regarding work experience, 30% of participants had experience for one year or less, 40% had work experience of two to three years, while participants who had work experience for more than five years accounted for 15% of the total targeted participants.

The variables mean ranged from 3.46 to 4.13, while the items' standard deviation (S.D.) scores were from 0.649 to 1.293, suggesting that the study data are more distributed and less gathered around its mean value [61]. The skewness and kurtosis scores are not exceeding -2 or $+2$, suggesting that the study data have satisfactory normal distribution [62]. Furthermore, as depicted in Table 1, variance inflation factors (VIF) scores for all items were below 0.4, which confirm that multicollinearity is not an issue in our study [63].

4.2. Measurement Model Assessment

For construct reliability and validity, we used confirmatory factor analysis (CFA) to combine all dependent and independent unobserved latent variables into a single CFA model that showed a satisfactory model fit: model fit: χ^2 (183, n = 770) = 489.891, $p < 0.001$, normed χ^2 = 2.677, RMSEA = 0.031, CFI = 0.977, TLI = 0.978, NFI = 0.977), as depicted in Table 2 [61,64]. We examined the composite reliability and discriminant validity of our constructs using the estimates from this model [65]. Measuring the construct validity was completed by examining convergent and discriminant validity for each construct. To test the convergent validity of the factors, Table 2 shows that all factor loadings for our constructs' items are statistically significant at the 0.001 level and exceed the minimum criterion of 0.5. Second, the average variance extracted (AVE) for all research constructs is greater than 0.5. Finally, the construct reliability (CR) scores for all the employed four factors—job insecurity (0.959), family financial pressure (0.939), family motivation (0.979), and unethical workplace behavior in the name of the family (0.977)—exceeded the recommended 0.70 cut-off point. Thus, as Anderson and Gerbing [64] and Hair et al. [62] recommend, our CFA output results revealed that all research constructs have a high satisfactory level of convergent validity.

Table 2. CFA Discriminant and Convergent Validity.

Factors and Items	Loading	CR	AVE	MSV	1	2	3	4
1—Job Insecurity (a = 0.905)		0.959	0.799	0.33	**0.894**			
Job_Inst_1	0.948							
Job_Inst_2	0.976							
Job_Inst_3	0.979							
Job_Inst_4	0.823							
Job_Inst_5	0.817							
Job_Inst_6	0.800							
2—Family Financial Pressure (a = 0.917)		0.939	0.837	0.33	0.182	**0.915**		
Fin_Pres1	0.914							
Fin_Pres2	0.935							
Fin_Pres3	0.895							

Table 2. Cont.

Factors and Items	Loading	CR	AVE	MSV	1	2	3	4
3—Family Motivation (a = 0.902)		0.979	0.904	0.13	0.47	0.053	**0.951**	
Fam_Motiv_1	0.939							
Fam_Motiv_2	0.977							
Fam_Motiv_3	0.931							
Fam_Motiv_4	0.937							
Fam_Motiv_5	0.970							
4—Unethical Workplace Behavior (a = 0.918)		0.977	0.857	0.16	0.125	0.11	0.43	**0.926**
Unethic_1	0.913							
Unethic_2	0.884							
Unethic_3	0.940							
Unethic_4	0.923							
Unethic_5	0.976							
Unethic_6	0.971							
Unethic_7	0.868							

Model fit: (χ^2 (183, n = 770) = 489.891, p < 0.001, normed χ^2 = 2.677, RMSEA = 0.031, SRMR = 0.039, CFI = 0.977, TLI = 0.978, NFI = 0.977, PCFI = 0.809 and PNFI = 0.810). CR: composite reliability; AVE: average variance extracted; MSV: maximum shared value. Diagonal values: the square root of AVE for each dimension. Below diagonal values: intercorrelation between dimensions.

The discriminant validity of constructs was assessed using Cronbach alpha values, correlation matrixes, and the square root of AVEs, as recommended by Fornell and Larcker [65]. Table 2 showed the correlation matrix, composite Cronbach alphas, and AVE values of the research four factors. As displayed in Table 2, bold diagonal values (the square root of AVEs) are larger than off-diagonal values (the correlations between those factors), which support a satisfactory discriminant validity for research factors as advocated by Fornell and Larcker [65]. Finally, the AVE values for all the four factors surpass the maximum shared values (MSV), further supporting a satisfactory level of discriminant validity. Overall, our measurement model demonstrates satisfactory levels of composite reliability and discriminant validity, according to the previous findings.

4.3. Structural Model Assessment

Following the establishing of confidence in the adequacy of the employed measures, we conducted structural equation modeling (SEM) to test the impact of job insecurity on unethical workplace behavior in the name of the family via family financial pressure and family motivation. The evaluation of the hypothesized model is confirmed through two main criteria: (1) the overall model goodness of fit (GoF) using the recommended indices such as x^2/df, TLI, CFI, RMR and RMSEA and the statistical significance level for the models' hypotheses. As shown in Table 3, the GoF measures for the structural model yielded satisfactory results. Additionally, the results of the anticipated model are illustrated in Figure 2 and Table 3.

The interrelationship in the suggested model contains seven justified hypotheses that investigate interactions among the research latent variables. The SEM analysis revealed that all seven hypotheses are significant at a statistical p-value less than 0.05. Hypothesis 1 (H1) investigated the direct effect of job insecurity on unethical workplace behavior in the name of the family, which was supported (T-value = 3.759, p < 0.01) with a path coefficient of 0.21, demonstrating that the two variables have a positive direct relationship. Likewise, the SEM analysis revealed that the job insecurity significantly and positively affects family financial pressure (H2) (T-value = 12.479, p < 0.001) with a path coefficient of 0.39, thus supporting hypothesis number 2 (H2). Additionally, in line with our proposition, the effect of family financial pressure on unethical workplace behavior in the name of the family was found to be significant and positive (T-value = 13.018, $p < 0.001$) with a correlation coefficient of 0.45, therefore supporting hypothesis number 3 (H3). Furthermore, as proposed, hypothesis number five tested the impact of job insecurity on family motivation, and the analysis gave signals of a positive and significant (T-value = 10.444, $p < 0.001$) association between the two factors with a correlation coefficient of 0.37, thus supporting hypothesis number 5 (H5). Finally, as proposed in hypothesis number 6 (H6), the impact of family motivation on unethical workplace behavior in the name of the family was found to be significant and positive (T-value = 15.702, $p < 0.001$, coefficient = 0.49); thus, hypothesis number 6 (H6) was confirmed.

Table 3. Result of structural model.

	Hypotheses			Beta (β)	C-R (T-Value)	R^2	Hypotheses Results
H1	Job insecurity	→	Unethical workplace behavior	0.21 **	3.759		Supported
H2	Job insecurity	→	Family financial pressure	0.39 ***	12.479		Supported
H3	Family financial pressure	→	Unethical workplace behavior	0.45 ***	13.018		Supported
H4	Job insecurity → Family financial pressure → Unethical workplace behavior			Path 1: β = 0.39 ***; t-value = 12.479 Path 2: β = 0.45 ***; t-value = 13.018			Supported
H5	Job insecurity	→	Family motivation	0.37 ***	10.444		Supported
H6	Family motivation	→	Unethical workplace behavior	0.49 ***	15.702		Supported
H7	Job insecurity → Family motivation → Unethical workplace behavior			Path 1: β = 0.37 ***; t-value = 10.444 Path 2: β = 0.49 ***; t-value = 15.702			Supported
Unethical workplace behavior						0.52	

Model fit: (χ^2 (184, $n = 770$) = 677.488, $p < 0.001$, normed χ^2 = 3.682, RMSEA = 0.043, SRMR = 0.049, CFI = 0.974, TLI = 0.975, NFI = 0.967, PCFI = 0.709 and PNFI = 0.710). *** $p < 0.001$, ** $p < 0.01$.

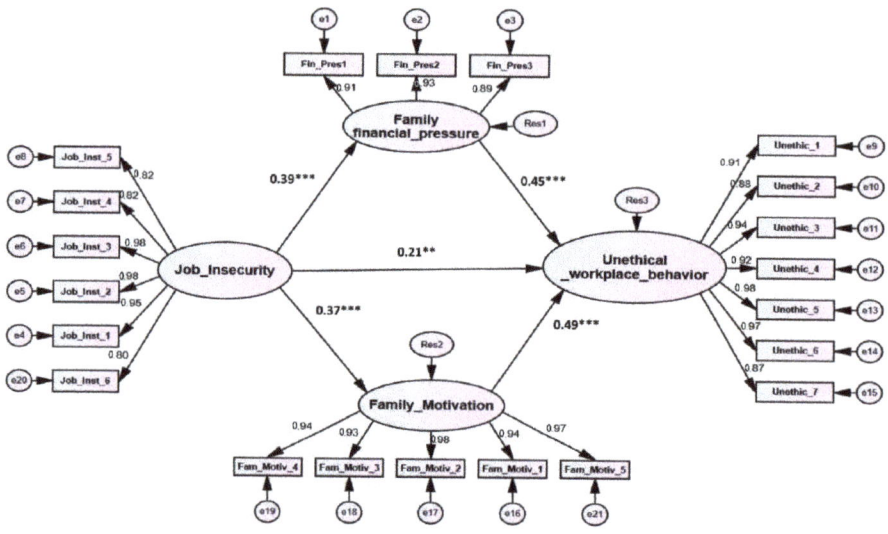

Figure 2. The structural model. ***: significant level below 0.001, **: significant level below 0.01.

To test hypotheses 4 and 7, suggestions introduced by [62,66] were adopted to evaluate the mediation impact of family financial pressure and family motivation in the relationship between job insecurity and unethical workplace behavior in the name of the family. Specifically, Zhao et al. [66] declared that for "direct-only nonmedication effects", only direct path coefficients should be observed, and that only direct path coefficients should be observed with a significant p-value, while all indirect relationships should not be statistically significant. For "complementary mediation", all direct and indirect correlations should be significant p-value with the same sign. Finally, "competitive mediation" is supported when all relationships (direct and indirect) are significant but with opposing signs. As pictured in Figure 2, all the tested paths are significant with the same positive sign, as depicted in Table 4. Specifically, the direct relationship between job insecurity and unethical workplace behavior in the name of the family is significant and positive (β = 0.21, t-value = 3.759, p < 0.001), and job insecurity directly, positively, and significantly, affects family financial pressure (β = 0.39, t-value = 12.479, p < 0.001) and family motivation (β = 0.37, t-value = 10.444, p < 0.001). In the same vein, family financial pressure was found to have a direct, positive, and significant relationship with unethical workplace behavior in the name of the family (β = 0.45, t-value = 13.018, p < 0.001). Similarly, family motivation was found to have a direct, positive, and significant relationship with unethical workplace behavior in the name of the family (β = 0.49, t-value = 15.702, p < 0.001). These results supported the complementary mediation of family financial pressure and family motivation in the relationship between job insecurity and unethical workplace behavior in the name of the family, therefore supporting hypotheses 4 and 7. Furthermore, specific indirect estimates from job insecurity to unethical workplace behavior through family financial pressure was calculated from the SEM Amos output (as shown in Table 4) to detect mediation, in which the lower (0.210) and the upper value (0.393) generated a significant (p > 001) standardized indirect estimates of 0.303. Similarly, the specific indirect estimate from job insecurity to unethical workplace behavior through family motivation was lower (0.216), and the upper value (0.389) created a significant (p > 001) standardized indirect estimate of 0.326. The previous results further support H4 and H7.

Table 4. Calculating mediation effects from Amos output.

Indirect Path	Unstandardized Estimate	Lower	Upper	p-Value	Standardized Estimate
Job Insecurity → Family financial pressure → Unethical workplace behavior	0.341	0.210	0.393	0.001	0.303 ***
Job Insecurity → Family Motivation → Unethical workplace behavior	0.334	0.216	0.389	0.001	0.326 ***

*** p < 0.001.

Finally, the standardized indirect path coefficient and total effects may also be reviewed in the SEM output to detect mediation impacts [62]. The standardized indirect path coefficients from the job insecurity to unethical workplace behavior in the name of the family via the mediating role of family financial pressure and family motivation increase the direct impact from 0.21 (β = 0.21, p < 0.01) to a total impact of 0.65 (β = 0.65, p < 0.001). This suggests that unethical workplace behavior in the name of the family increased by 44% via the mediating role of family financial pressure and family motivation. Furthermore, the proposed structural model showed a high level of explanatory power (R^2), explaining 52% of the variation in unethical workplace behavior in the name of the family (Table 3).

5. Discussion and Implications

The outbreak of COVID-19 has created an opportunity to better understand the relationship between unethical behavior and perceived risk of job insecurity in tourism organizations. Drawing to theories of conservation of resources, social cognitive and behavioral ethics (i.e., the self-maintenance and bounded ethicality theories), this study examined family motivation and financial pressure as mediators of the relationship between job insecurity and unethical organizational behaviors. The results provide insights into the reasons behind the increased UOB during the COVID-19 pandemic [2,3,8,9], and they would add to researchers and practitioners understanding of how to address ethical challenges in their organizations.

A survey was created and distributed to 770 employees of five-star hotels and Category A travel agencies. To evaluate the proposed structural model as well as the measurement model, two main data analysis methods were used. SEM was used to evaluate the proposed structural model, and CFA was used to evaluate the measurement model's convergent and discriminant validity, respectively. The findings revealed that the measurement model exhibited good convergence and discriminant validity, and that the proposed structural model accurately represented the data. A total of seven hypotheses were proposed and evaluated. The results revealed that job insecurity has a direct impact on unethical workplace behavior in the name of family as well as an indirect impact through financial pressure and motivation imposed by the extended family. The indirect effect increases the total effect of job insecurity on unethical organization behavior in the name of the family by 44%, providing evidence that both family financial pressure and family motivation play a role in mediating the relationship between job insecurity and unethical organization behavior in the name of the family. All endogenous variables combined account for 52% of the variance in unethical organizational behavior to benefit family, according to the findings.

These results extend the prior results of Lawrence and Kacmar [38], who found emotional exhaustion as a mediator in the relationship between job insecurity and unethical behavior. This is by highlighting the role of emotional exhaustion that derived from family financial pressures and motivation. Complementing prior research, family financial pressures [25,46] and motivations [9,55] were found to reduce self-regulatory resources and motivate unethical behaviors in the name of the family. The results indicated that participants who suffered high job instability in their workplace experienced higher levels of family pressures and were more prone to practice UOB to benefit their relatives. In support, Zhang et al. [46] articulated that when employees encounter substantial financial difficulties in their families, they are more likely to focus on obtaining financial benefits from their employer. In addition, this study provides empirical support for the argument of Hillebrandt and Barclay [4] that anxiety elicited by COVID-19 may focus employees' attention on their self-related interest and encourage cheating and other unethical behaviors.

5.1. Implications to Theory

The result of this study has a three-fold contribution to theory. First, it extends the discussion of previous studies on conditions that shape unethical practices in workplaces. Most previous studies have identified that perceived job insecurity results in UOB that are either for benefiting the organization or self-serving. While this study adds empirical evidence on the important effect of family-related pressures, financial or motivational, on UOB, with particular attention of the influence of these factors when accompanied with job insecurity. Second, this study tries to answer the calls of prior researchers [3,4,22,25,66] to further examine the influence of environmental factors (e.g., COVID-19 outbreak) on UOB. The results add to explaining the reasons of the widespread unethical behaviors in organizations encountered during the COVID-19 pandemic. In particular, the current study adds to the understanding of the psychological process that employees may go through in making unethical decisions when faced by job insecurity. It is also the first study to discuss the mediating role of family motivation and financial pressure in the relationship between perceived job insecurity and UOB.

Third, this study answers calls to examine the employee's family as a source of motivation to possible UOB [25,46]. Despite previous warnings of its possible strong influence on unethical workplace behavior [46], family motivation has received little empirical and theoretical attention. Instead, most studies have regarded family motivation as a driver of work effectiveness (e.g., [47]). Therefore, by demonstrating the role of family motivation in triggering unethical workplace behavior, this study extends research knowledge about possible psychological aspects that fuel UOB. At the same time, it gives insights to the possible dual role of family motivation as a source of desirable (work effectiveness, for more information see [47]) and undesirable organizational actions (UOB).

5.2. Implications to Practice

The tourism industry was the most affected during the COVID-19 pandemic. The large seen shutdowns and layoffs during the pandemic and their effect on employee's psychology and behavior would have a long-lasting difficult influence on tourism workplaces and hospitality industry if not well understood and dealt with by decision-makers. Although the influence of COVID-19 on job loss and job insecurity has received much attention in recent tourism and hospitality research, a more comprehensive picture of the detrimental effect of job stress and anxiety on employee's behavior still needs to be explored to better inform tourism decision-makers [9,23]. In this regard, this study contributes to the understanding of why the COVID-19 pandemic has induced UOB in the tourism industry and highlights the role of job insecurity and family pressures and motivation in increasing UOB in the name of the family. This would inform tourism decision-makers and managers toward preventing unethical behavior and the possible damaging consequences on financial performance and reputation. Decision-makers should strive to advocate social messages and enact policies that reduce employees' perceived job insecurity, since this is a gateway to UOB.

In addition, based on the concept of bounded ethicality, the current study asserted that ambiguous circumstances (e.g., job insecurity) may veil the ethical aspects of employee's decisions, as people lean to self-justification of their immoral actions in the workplace [17,18,67]. Therefore, pressures of job loss may drive even honest employees to engage in minor dishonesty and simultaneously stay ignorant (ethically blind) of the ethical repercussions of their acts [18,68]. Thus, with this in mind, organizational managers need to carefully observe the actions of all employees and regularly provide moral reminders, which can be a useful tool to reduce or prevent UOB. Organizations also should assess the ethical development of employees, promote moral actions and punish for unethical behavior.

6. Conclusions, Limitations, and Further Research

The prevalent and costly unethical practices in workplaces and their different types have attracted recent research attention, especially during the COVID-19 crises. This study investigated a neglected yet important form of UOB: unethical organizational practices in the name of the family. It proposed a model that may assist academics and practitioners in better understanding of how perceived job insecurity influences UOB through the mediating effect of family financial pressure and family motivation. The results revealed that perceived risk of job insecurity predicts employees' engagement in UOB, while intentions of unethical behaviors increase by high family motivation and financial pressures.

However, this study has some limitations that offers opportunities for future research papers. The current results of the analyzed data showed that family motivation and financial pressure partially mediated the impact of job insecurity and unethical workplace behavior. To further our understanding on the relationship between job insecurity and UOB, future research papers can investigate more mediating variables (e.g., work intensification, trust in management, feeling of guilt, and job embeddedness) that can affect the relationship between job insecurity and unethical workplace behavior in the name of the family. Moreover, future studies should investigate possible boundary conditions such as moral identities and religious commitment, since previous studies, for example, revealed that moral identity undermines the strong influence of the self-control depletion on dishonesty and unethical practices [69].

Although this study ensured the confidentiality and anonymity of the questionnaire for the participants, the self-reported survey used in this study may encourage participants to biases their answers, since questions were about unethical actions to benefit the family. Thus, future studies can allow peer evaluation through colleagues or supervisors for more objectivity. In addition, future research can address the practices of decision makers to diminish UOB for family benefit and suggest methods that can be followed to control unethical practices. Furthermore, the collected data were cross-sectional; therefore, causal association between latent variables cannot be completely confirmed, and it is recommended for future investigations to collect longitudinal objective data or a different data source to validate the study model. Finally, a multigroup analysis approach can be conducted in future studies to validate and compare the results of the current study with data collected from different context (industry/country) [70]. Finally, it is important to highlight that the current study explores the relationship between family pressure and unethical workplace behavior under job insecurity. Accordingly, the UOB examined is not general but rather related to the benefit of the family. Future research would need to study general and other specific unethical behaviors that prevail in times of crisis (e.g., under job insecurity) and apply them to different contexts to understand how prevalent UOB is and how to mitigate its undesired consequences.

Author Contributions: Conceptualization, I.A.E. and M.G.; methodology, I.A.E., M.G. and A.M.S.A.; software, I.A.E. and M.G.; validation, I.A.E., A.M.S.A. and M.G.; formal analysis, I.A.E. and A.M.S.A.; investigation, I.A.E., M.G. and A.M.S.A.; resources, I.A.E.; data curation, I.A.E.; writing—original draft preparation, M.G., I.A.E. and A.M.S.A.; writing—review and editing, I.A.E. and M.G; visualization, I.A.E.; supervision, I.A.E.; project administration, I.A.E., M.G. and A.M.S.A.; funding acquisition, I.A.E. and A.M.S.A. All authors have read and agreed to the published version of the manuscript.

Funding: This work was supported through the Annual Funding track by the Deanship of Scientific Research, Vice Presidency for Graduate Studies and Scientific Research, King Faisal University, Saudi Arabia [GRANT466].

Institutional Review Board Statement: The study was conducted according to the guidelines of the Declaration of Helsinki and approved by the deanship of scientific research ethical committee, King Faisal University (project number: GRANT466, date of approval: 11 January 2022).

Informed Consent Statement: Informed consent was obtained from all subjects involved in the study.

Data Availability Statement: Data are available upon request from researchers who meet the eligibility criteria. Kindly contact the first author privately through e-mail.

Conflicts of Interest: The authors declare no conflict of interest.

References

1. WTTC (World Travel and Tourism Council). Latest Research from WTTC Shows a 50% Increase in Jobs at Risk in Travel Tourism. 2020. Available online: https://wttc.org/News-Article/Latest-research-from-WTTC-shows-a-50-percentage-increase-in-jobs-at-risk-in-Travel-and-Tourism (accessed on 20 February 2022).
2. Richter, F. COVID-19 Has Caused a Huge Amount of Lost Working Hours, World Economic Forum. 2021. Available online: https://www.weforum.org/agenda/2021/02/covid-employment-global-job-loss/ (accessed on 30 March 2022).
3. Elshaer, I.A.; Azazz, A.M. Amid the COVID-19 Pandemic, Unethical Behavior in the Name of the Company: The Role of Job Insecurity, Job Embeddedness, and Turnover Intention. *Int. J. Environ. Res. Public Health* **2021**, *19*, 247. [CrossRef] [PubMed]
4. Hillebrandt, A.; Barclay, L.J. How COVID-19 Can Promote Workplace Cheating Behavior via Employee Anxiety and Self-Interest: And How Prosocial Messages May Overcome This Effect. *J. Organ. Behav.* **2022**. [CrossRef] [PubMed]
5. Saad, S.K.; Elshaer, I.A. Justice and Trust's Role in Employees' Resilience and Business' Continuity: Evidence from Egypt. *Tour. Manag. Perspect.* **2020**, *35*, 100712. [CrossRef]
6. Jung, H.S.; Jung, Y.S.; Yoon, H.H. COVID-19: The Effects of Job Insecurity on the Job Engagement and Turnover Intent of Deluxe Hotel Employees and the Moderating Role of Generational Characteristics. *Int. J. Hosp. Manag.* **2021**, *92*, 102703. [CrossRef]
7. Shin, Y.; Hur, W.-M. When Do Service Employees Suffer More from Job Insecurity? The Moderating Role of Coworker and Customer Incivility. *Int. J. Environ. Res. Public Health* **2019**, *16*, 1298. [CrossRef]
8. Sheetal, A.; Feng, Z.; Savani, K. Using Machine Learning to Generate Novel Hypotheses: Increasing Optimism about COVID-19 Makes People Less Willing to Justify Unethical Behaviors. *Psychol. Sci.* **2020**, *31*, 1222–1235. [CrossRef]
9. Chen, C.-C.; Zou, S.S.; Chen, M.-H. The Fear of Being Infected and Fired: Examining the Dual Job Stressors of Hospitality Employees during COVID-19. *Int. J. Hosp. Manag.* **2022**, *102*, 103131. [CrossRef]
10. EY Global Integrity Report. 2020. Available online: https://www.ey.com/en_gl/global-integrity-report (accessed on 18 April 2022).

11. Covid-19 Crisis Increases Risk of Unethical Conduct in Corporate India: EY Survey-The Economic Times. Available online: https://economictimes.indiatimes.com/news/company/corporate-trends/covid-19-crisis-increases-risk-of-unethical-conduct-in-corporate-india-ey-survey/articleshow/76623451.cms?from=mdr (accessed on 18 April 2022).
12. Hobfoll, S.E. The influence of culture, community, and the nested-self in the stress process: Advancing conservation of resources theory. *Appl. Psychol.* **2001**, *50*, 337–421. [CrossRef]
13. Myung, E. Progress in Hospitality Ethics Research: A Review and Implications for Future Research. *Int. J. Hosp. Tour. Adm.* **2018**, *19*, 26–51. [CrossRef]
14. Elçi, M.; Alpkan, L. The Impact of Perceived Organizational Ethical Climate on Work Satisfaction. *J. Bus. Ethics* **2009**, *84*, 297–311. [CrossRef]
15. Umphress, E.E.; Bingham, J.B.; Mitchell, M.S. Unethical Behavior in the Name of the Company: The Moderating Effect of Organizational Identification and Positive Reciprocity Beliefs on Unethical pro-Organizational Behavior. *J. Appl. Psychol.* **2010**, *95*, 769. [CrossRef] [PubMed]
16. Thau, S.; Derfler-Rozin, R.; Pitesa, M.; Mitchell, M.S.; Pillutla, M.M. Unethical for the Sake of the Group: Risk of Social Exclusion and pro-Group Unethical Behavior. *J. Appl. Psychol.* **2015**, *100*, 98. [CrossRef] [PubMed]
17. Feldman, Y. *The Law of Good People*; Cambridge University Press: Cambridge, UK, 2018.
18. Elshaer, I.A.; Azazz, A.; Saad, S.K. Unethical Organization Behavior: Antecedents and Consequences in the Tourism Industry. *Int. J. Environ. Res. Public Health* **2022**, *19*, 4972. [CrossRef] [PubMed]
19. Treviño, L.K.; Nelson, A.K. *Managing Business Ethics: Straight Talk about How to Do It Right*; Wiley: Hoboken, NJ, USA, 2011.
20. Cialdini, R.B.; Petrova, P.K.; Goldstein, N.J. The hidden costs of organizational dishonesty. *Sloan Manag. Rev.* **2004**, *45*, 67–73.
21. Gürlek, M. How Does Work Overload Affect Unethical Behaviors? The Mediating Role of Pay Dissatisfaction. *Turk. J. Bus. Ethics* **2020**, *13*, 68–78. [CrossRef]
22. Gürlek, M. Shedding Light on the Relationships between Machiavellianism, Career Ambition, and Unethical Behavior Intention. *Ethics Behav.* **2021**, *31*, 38–59. [CrossRef]
23. Mitchell, M.S.; Baer, M.D.; Ambrose, M.L.; Folger, R.; Palmer, N.F. Cheating under Pressure: A Self-Protection Model of Workplace Cheating Behavior. *J. Appl. Psychol.* **2018**, *103*, 54. [CrossRef]
24. Liu, Z.; Liao, H.; Liu, Y. For the Sake of My Family: Understanding Unethical pro-Family Behavior in the Workplace. *J. Organ. Behav.* **2020**, *41*, 638–662. [CrossRef]
25. Law, R. The Perceived Impact of Risks on Travel Decisions. *Int. J. Tour. Res.* **2006**, *8*, 289–300. [CrossRef]
26. Reisel, W.D.; Probst, T.M.; Chia, S.-L.; Maloles, C.M.; König, C.J. The Effects of Job Insecurity on Job Satisfaction, Organizational Citizenship Behavior, Deviant Behavior, and Negative Emotions of Employees. *Int. Stud. Manag. Organ.* **2010**, *40*, 74–91. [CrossRef]
27. Simpson, P.M.; Siguaw, J.A. Perceived Travel Risks: The Traveller Perspective and Manageability. *Int. J. Tour. Res.* **2008**, *10*, 315–327. [CrossRef]
28. Greenhalgh, L.; Rosenblatt, Z. Evolution of Research on Job Insecurity. *Int. Stud. Manag. Organ.* **2010**, *40*, 6–19. [CrossRef]
29. Hellgren, J.; Sverke, M.; Isaksson, K. A Two-Dimensional Approach to Job Insecurity: Consequences for Employee Attitudes and Well-Being. *Eur. J. Work. Organ. Psychol.* **1999**, *8*, 179–195. [CrossRef]
30. Martin, K.D.; Cullen, J.B. Continuities and Extensions of Ethical Climate Theory: A Meta-Analytic Review. *J. Bus. Ethics* **2006**, *69*, 175–194. [CrossRef]
31. Frone, M.R. What Happened to the Employed during the Great Recession? A US Population Study of Net Change in Employee Insecurity, Health, and Organizational Commitment. *J. Vocat. Behav.* **2018**, *107*, 246–260. [CrossRef]
32. Meyer, J.P.; Allen, N.J. Testing the "Side-Bet Theory" of Organizational Commitment: Some Methodological Considerations. *J. Appl. Psychol.* **1984**, *69*, 372. [CrossRef]
33. Niesen, W.; Van Hootegem, A.; Handaja, Y.; Batistelli, A.; De Witte, H. Quantitative and Qualitative Job Insecurity and Idea Generation: The Mediating Role of Psychological Contract Breach. *Scand. J. Work. Organ. Psychol.* **2018**, *3*, 1–14. [CrossRef]
34. Vohs, K.D.; Schmeichel, B.J. Self-Regulation and Extended Now: Controlling the Self Alters the Subjective Experience of Time. *J. Personal. Soc. Psychol.* **2003**, *85*, 217. [CrossRef]
35. Baumeister, R.F. Esteem Threat, Self-Regulatory Breakdown, and Emotional Distress as Factors in Self-Defeating Behavior. *Rev. Gen. Psychol.* **1997**, *1*, 145–174. [CrossRef]
36. Baumeister, R.F.; Vohs, K.D. Self-Regulation, Ego Depletion, and Motivation. *Soc. Personal. Psychol. Compass* **2007**, *1*, 115–128. [CrossRef]
37. Lawrence, E.R.; Kacmar, K.M. Exploring the Impact of Job Insecurity on Employees? Unethical Behavior. *Bus. Ethics Q.* **2017**, *27*, 39–70. [CrossRef]
38. Duffy, M.K.; Ganster, D.C.; Pagon, M. Social Undermining in the Workplace. *Acad. Manag. J.* **2002**, *45*, 331–351.
39. Robinson, S.L.; Bennett, R.J. A Typology of Deviant Workplace Behaviors: A Multidimensional Scaling Study. *Acad. Manag. J.* **1995**, *38*, 555–572. [CrossRef]
40. Ghanem, M.; Elshaer, I.; Shaker, A. The successful adoption of is in the tourism public sector: The mediating effect of employees' trust. *Sustainability* **2020**, *12*, 3877. [CrossRef]
41. Selenko, E.; Mäkikangas, A.; Stride, C.B. Does Job Insecurity Threaten Who You Are? Introducing a Social Identity Perspective to Explain Well-Being and Performance Consequences of Job Insecurity. *J. Organ. Behav.* **2017**, *38*, 856–875. [CrossRef]

42. De Witte, H.; Pienaar, J.; De Cuyper, N. Review of 30 Years of Longitudinal Studies on the Association between Job Insecurity and Health and Well-Being: Is There Causal Evidence? *Aust. Psychol.* **2016**, *51*, 18–31. [CrossRef]
43. Gaunt, R.; Benjamin, O. Job Insecurity, Stress and Gender: The Moderating Role of Gender Ideology. *Community Work. Fam.* **2007**, *10*, 341–355. [CrossRef]
44. Turner, J.B.; Kessler, R.C.; House, J.S. Factors Facilitating Adjustment to Unemployment: Implications for Intervention. *Am. J. Community Psychol.* **1991**, *19*, 521–542. [CrossRef]
45. Zhang, X.; Liao, H.; Li, N.; Colbert, A.E. Playing It Safe for My Family: Exploring the Dual Effects of Family Motivation on Employee Productivity and Creativity. *Acad. Manag. J.* **2020**, *63*, 1923–1950. [CrossRef]
46. Menges, J.I.; Tussing, D.V.; Wihler, A.; Grant, A.M. When Job Performance Is All Relative: How Family Motivation Energizes Effort and Compensates for Intrinsic Motivation? *Acad. Manag. J.* **2017**, *60*, 695–719. [CrossRef]
47. Schwartz, S.H.; Cieciuch, J.; Vecchione, M.; Davidov, E.; Fischer, R.; Beierlein, C.; Dirilen-Gumus, O. Refining the theory of basic individual values. *J. Personal. Soc. Psychol.* **2012**, *103*, 663–688. [CrossRef] [PubMed]
48. Newman, A.; Le, H.; North-Samardzic, A.; Cohen, M. Moral disengagement at work: A review and research agenda. *J. Bus. Ethics* **2020**, *167*, 535–570. [CrossRef]
49. Bandura, A. Moral Disengagement in the Perpetration of Inhumanities. *Personal. Soc. Psychol. Rev.* **1999**, *3*, 193–209. [CrossRef] [PubMed]
50. Mazar, N.; Amir, O.; Ariely, D. The Dishonesty of Honest People: A Theory of Self-Concept Maintenance. *J. Mark. Res.* **2008**, *45*, 633–644. [CrossRef]
51. Lau, S. Utilitarianistic Familism: The Basis of Political Stability. In *Social Life and Development in Hong Kong*; The Chinese University Press: Hong Kong, China, 1981; pp. 195–216.
52. Chen, M.; Chen, C.C.; Sheldon, O.J. Relaxing Moral Reasoning to Win: How Organizational Identification Relates to Unethical pro-Organizational Behavior. *J. Appl. Psychol.* **2016**, *101*, 1082. [CrossRef]
53. Wiltermuth, S.S. Cheating more when the spoils are split. *Organ. Behav. Hum. Decis. Processes* **2011**, *115*, 157–168. [CrossRef]
54. Detert, J.R.; Treviño, L.K.; Sweitzer, V.L. Moral Disengagement in Ethical Decision Making: A Study of Antecedents and Outcomes. *J. Appl. Psychol.* **2008**, *93*, 374. [CrossRef]
55. Maddox, R.N. Measuring Satisfiaction with Tourism. *J. Travel Res.* **1985**, *23*, 2–5. [CrossRef]
56. Churchill, G.A., Jr. A Paradigm for Developing Better Measures of Marketing Constructs. *J. Mark. Res.* **1979**, *16*, 64–73. [CrossRef]
57. Conger, R.D.; Rueter, M.A.; Elder, G.H., Jr. Couple Resilience to Economic Pressure. *J. Personal. Soc. Psychol.* **1999**, *76*, 54–71. [CrossRef]
58. Douglas, S.P.; Craig, C.S. Collaborative and Iterative Translation: An Alternative Approach to Back Translation. *J. Int. Mark.* **2007**, *15*, 30–43. [CrossRef]
59. Podsakoff, P.M.; MacKenzie, S.B.; Lee, J.-Y.; Podsakoff, N.P. Common Method Biases in Behavioral Research: A Critical Review of the Literature and Recommended Remedies. *J. Appl. Psychol.* **2003**, *88*, 879. [CrossRef] [PubMed]
60. Kline, R.B. *Principles and Practice of Structural Equation Modeling*; Guilford Publications: New York, NY, USA, 2015.
61. Hair, J.F.; Matthews, L.M.; Matthews, R.L.; Sarstedt, M. PLS-SEM or CB-SEM: Updated Guidelines on Which Method to Use. *Int. J. Multivar. Data Anal.* **2017**, *1*, 107–123. [CrossRef]
62. Bryman, A.; Cramer, D. *Quantitative Data Analysis with IBM SPSS 17, 18 19: A Guide for Social Scientists*; Routledge: London, UK, 2011; ISBN 978-0-203-18099-0.
63. Anderson, J.C.; Gerbing, D.W. Structural Equation Modeling in Practice: A Review and Recommended Two-Step Approach. *Psychol. Bull.* **1988**, *103*, 411–423. [CrossRef]
64. Fornell, C.; Larcker, D.F. Structural Equation Models with Unobservable Variables and Measurement Error: Algebra and Statistics. *J. Mark. Res.* **1981**, *18*, 382–388. [CrossRef]
65. Zhao, X.; Lynch, J.G., Jr.; Chen, Q. Reconsidering Baron and Kenny: Myths and Truths about Mediation Analysis. *J. Consum. Res.* **2010**, *37*, 197–206. [CrossRef]
66. Lu, J.G.; Lee, J.J.; Gino, F.; Galinsky, A.D. Air pollution, state anxiety, and unethical behavior: A meta-analytic review. *Psychol. Sci.* **2020**, *31*, 748–755. [CrossRef]
67. Keem, S.; Shalley, C.E.; Kim, E.; Jeong, I. Are creative individuals bad apples? A dual pathway model of unethical behavior. *J. Appl. Psychol.* **2018**, *103*, 416–431. [CrossRef]
68. Lois, G.; Wessa, M. Honest mistake or perhaps not: The role of descriptive and injunctive norms on the magnitude of dishonesty. *J. Behav. Decis. Mak.* **2021**, *34*, 20–34. [CrossRef]
69. Gino, F.; Schweitzer, M.E.; Mead, N.L.; Ariely, D. Unable to Resist Temptation: How Self-Control Depletion Promotes Unethical Behavior. *Organ. Behav. Hum. Decis. Processes* **2011**, *115*, 191–203. [CrossRef]
70. Elshaer, I.A.; Augustyn, M.M. Testing the Dimensionality of the Quality Management Construct. *Total Qual. Manag. Bus. Excell.* **2016**, *27*, 353–367. [CrossRef]

MDPI
St. Alban-Anlage 66
4052 Basel
Switzerland
Tel. +41 61 683 77 34
Fax +41 61 302 89 18
www.mdpi.com

International Journal of Environmental Research and Public Health Editorial Office
E-mail: ijerph@mdpi.com
www.mdpi.com/journal/ijerph

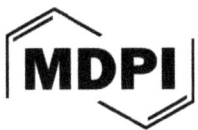